THE HEART &
ESSENCE OF
DAN-XI'S METHODS
OF TREATMENT

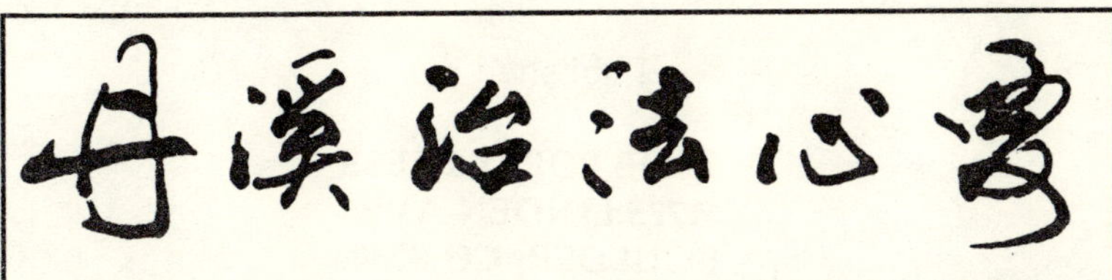

The Heart & Essence Of Dan-xi's Methods of Treatment

A Translation of the *Dan Xi Zhi Fa Xin Yao*

by Yang Shou-zhong

Blue Poppy Press

Published by:

**BLUE POPPY PRESS
1775 LINDEN AVE.
BOULDER, CO 80304**

First Edition, October, 1993

**ISBN 0-936185-50-3
LC 93-72799**

COPYRIGHT 1993   ©   BLUE POPPY PRESS

The information in this book is given in good faith. However, the translators and the publisher cannot be held responsible for any error or omission. Nor can they be held in any way responsible for treatment given on the basis of information contained in this book. The publisher make this information available to English language readers for scholarly and research purposes only.

The publishers do not advocate nor endorse self-medication by laypersons. Chinese medicine is a professional medicine. Laypersons interested in availing themselves of the treatments described in this book should seek out a qualified professional practitioner of Chinese medicine.

Printed at Westview Press, Boulder, CO on acid free, recycled paper.
Cover Printed at C&M Press, Thornton, CO.

10 9 8 7 6 5 4 3 2 1

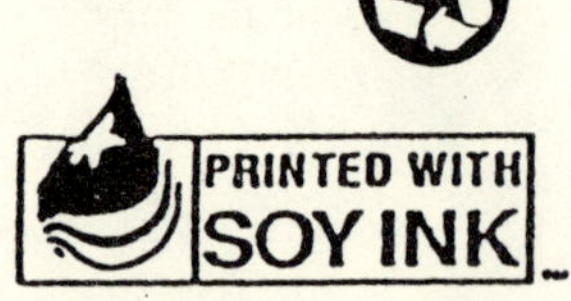

Translator's Preface

Zhu Dan-xi was one of the founders of the four great schools (*si da jia*) of medicine of the Jin-Yuan Dynasties. This book is a translation of the *Dan Xi Zhi Fa Xin Yao (The Heart & Essentials of Dan-xi's Treatment Methods)*. This is primarily a book of treatment methods, formulas, and case histories. This translation is based on the People's Health & Hygiene Press' edition published in Beijing in 1983.

The following somewhat loosely translated account of Zhu Dan-xi's life is based on a biography written by Dai Liang (1317-1384 CE), a famous Chinese historian. It is taken from his *Dan Xi Weng Zhuang (Biography of the Reverend Dan-xi)*. Because Dai Liang lived so close to the time of Zhu, this account is felt to be authoritative.

The Reverend Dan-xi (1281-1358 CE) was born in Dan Xi, Yi Wu, a county in Fujian Province. His surname was Zhu, his (scholarly) name was Zhen-heng, and his infant name, which was taboo, was Yan-xiu.[1] All his students respectfully called him the Reverend Dan-xi to avoid the impropriety of directly calling him Zhu Zhen-heng.

The reverend master was diligent in his pursuit of learning from his early childhood and was able to learn by heart a thousand

---

[1] In old China, it was inappropriate for a person of lower rank to use the same name as a person of higher rank. Thus commoners were not allowed to use any of the characters of the current sovereign's name in their own. The avoidance of such characters was referred to as name taboo. As a child, Zhu was given the name Yan-xiu by his family. This family-bestowed name is referred to as one's *ming* name in Chinese. When he became a Confucian scholar, he was given the name Zhen-heng. This is called one's *zi* name. However, because his infant name contained a taboo character, his students called him by his place of birth, *Dan Xi*, Cinnabar Creek. Thus Reverend Dan-xi might also be rendered the Reverend or Master of Cinnabar Creek.

characters each day. When he was a little older, he began to study the Confucian classics under a master in the neighborhood as preparation for entering the Confucian bureaucracy through the government examinations. Later, he heard of the master Xu Wen-yi[2], who, being the fourth direct descendant of the Zhu Zi School[3], was teaching the doctrines of the founder of Neoconfucianism in the Ba Hua Mountains. Zhu went to this master as a pupil and studied Confucian philosophy concerning human ethics and world view. He soon became proficient in these doctrines and determined to devote his entire life to them.

One day, Master Xu Wen-yi sighed, saying, "I have been stricken with disease for such a long time. Unless I meet a really illustrious doctor, I have no hope of recovery." The master went on, "You are exceptionally intelligent. Couldn't you condescend to train in medicine?"[4] These words reminded the Reverend Dan-xi of his heartbreaking bereavement: the loss of several members of his family in succession, the death of his wife at no more than 20 years of age, and, not long since, the demise of his dear father. This question would change the course of his whole life. He answered

---

[2]   A.k.a. Xu Qian, an outstanding Neoconfucian scholar. He devoted his whole life to the propagation of the doctrines without any aspiration for fame and wealth.

[3]   Zhu Zi (1130-1200CE), whose real name was Zhu Xi. Zi a form of address given to the most respected of great masters, such as Lao Zi, Chuang Zi, Kong Zi, and Meng Zi. Zhu Zi was a standard-bearer and one of the founders of Neoconfucianism in the Song Dynasty. He was generally acclaimed in later generations as an authority in explaining Confucianism.

[4]   In old China, many strict Confucianists believed that it was degrading for a Confucian scholar to study and practice a technical vocation such as medicine. Study of the Confucian classics and philosophy along with the social and moral self-cultivation this entailed was considered a big *dao* or path. Technical knowledge and practice were considered a little *dao*. Therefore, Zhu's Confucian teacher asked him to *condescend* and study such a little *dao*. As the exchange goes on to show, Zhu felt that medicine in the service of others does not have to be a little *dao*.

emotionally, "If a student can be proficient in an art and make full use of it to be of any good to humankind, then he may achieve greatness though not an official in power."

After that, Zhu cared not a jot about the official examinations. He gave up his preparations for them altogether and set about the study of medicine. He wholly devoted himself to the cause of rescuing patients instead of pursuing his studies of how to assist the monarch in ruling the people. At that time, the 297 formulas designed by Chen Shi-wen and Pei Zhong-yuan[5] were the most influential and widely circulated among medical practitioners. Nearly all medical students of that time believed that the memorization and rote application of these formulas was the shortest and most effective way of becoming a good doctor. Zhu followed suit and, with admirable industry and unstinting perseverance, applied himself to the memorization of these formulas more vigorously than anyone else. Quickly he had all these formulas at the tips of his fingers. However, later a doubt somehow crept into his mind. Was it really valid to merely stick to the old, dead, limited formulas for the treatment of all sorts of patients in contemporary times? After all, were not the time honored theories and instructions of such classics as the *Su Wen (Simple Questions)* and *Nan Jing (Classic of Difficult [Issues])* the best criteria for truth in the study and practice of medicine? Thinking like this, Zhu made up his mind to delve into the immortal classics.

---

[5]   Chen and Pei were famous physicians in the Song Dynasty. On the basis of their collated and corrected former government published pharmacopoeia, in 1107-1110 CE they composed a new official pharmacopoeia consisting of 297 formulas. This was titled the *Jiao Zheng Tai Ping Hui Min Ju Fang (Corrected & Collected Formulas of the Great Harmony Imperial Grace Pharmacy)*. This formulary was in wide use throughout the country for a long period and was considered the most authoritative work in formulary. Although this work contributed to the preservation of many ancient proven formulas, at the same time it encouraged a harmful tendency to abandon the soul of TCM, *i.e.*, *bian zheng lun zhi*, the basing of treatment on pattern discrimination, and the mechanical employment ancient, "dead" formulas.

However, of the many doctors in the neighborhood, not one had an adequate knowledge of these classics. Therefore Zhu had no one from whom to learn. Thus he made some necessary preparations and set off in search of a learned doctor. He crossed the River Ze, travelled through Wu County (now Wuxi City, Jiangsu Province), passed Wan Ling, visited Nan Xu Prefecture, and arrived in Jian Ye (now Nanjing), the then political, economic, and cultural center of south China. Zhu walked on foot all this way, but in vain. Yet he did not give up hope.

Then he travelled further, and while staying in Wu Ling (now Hangzhou, the capital of Zhejiang Province), he heard of a doctor named Luo Zhi-di. This master was respectfully called Master Great Void. He was the inheritor of the teachings of the great master Liu Wan-su.[6] In addition, he was erudite in the theories of Zhang Cong-zheng[7] and Li Gao[8] and was celebrated for his specialization in many areas of medicine. However, Luo Zhi-di was a person of an eccentric character, haughty, cold to visitors, and difficult to please. At first our reverend master was denied a reception.

---

[6]   Liu Wan-su, a.k.a Liu Shou-zhen (circa 1120-1200 CE). A native of He Jian, Hebei Province, Liu was the originator of the *Han Liang Pai*, the School of Cold & Cool (Medicine). He believed that disease is primarily caused by evil heat in the body and that therefore one should use most cold and cool natured medicinals to clear that heat. Liu was one of the four great masters of the Jin-Yuan.

[7]   Zhang Cong-zheng, a.k.a. Zhang Zi-he (circa 1156-1228 CE). A native of Kao Cheng in Henan Province, Zhang was the originator of the *Gong Xia Pai*, the School of Attack & Precipitation or Purgation. Zhang believed that disease is primarily caused by the presence of evil qi which should be rid from the body. Therefore, he emphasized diaphoresis, ejection (emesis), and precipitation (purgation) as the main methods of treatment. Zhang was another of the four great masters.

[8]   Li Gao, a.k.a. Li Dong-yuan (1180-1252 CE). A native of Zheng Ding, Hebei Province, Li was the originator of the *Bu Tu Pai*, the School of Supplementing Earth. Li emphasized the pivotal role of the spleen and stomach in the creation of evil heat and thus also emphasized the regulation of digestion as a primary treatment method. Li was yet another of the four great masters.

Undaunted, he continued to go and call upon Luo again and again. But it was no use. Then Zhu went to him more and more frequently until he was finally admitted a reception.

"Are you that Zhu Yan-xiu?" asked the old man, who, moved by the persistence of our Reverend Dan-xi, had learned a lot about him and particularly about his bright intelligence and proficient medical skills. At this, the Reverend Dan-xi knelt down immediately, kowtowing to the north. This is a special form of etiquette paid to a superior, for instance, one's father. When Zhu saw acquiescence in the face of the old man, he began to kowtow once again to pay a pupil's respect.

Soon after taking him as a pupil, Luo became more than ever delighted and gratified. This new pupil was found to be a real genius, bright and assiduous, and Luo tried to impart all he had learned in his life, cultivating without any reserve the doctrines of each school, enlightening Zhu on the pith and essence of the *Nei Jing (Inner Classic)* and other such medical classics. He even made Zhu a present of his precious collection of books by Liu Wan-su, Zhang Cong-zheng, and Li Gao. Before long, our Reverend Dan-xi had familiarized himself with all these teachings. He then parted with his strict yet enthusiastic teacher.

When the physicians in his home country heard that he had betrayed their worshipped Chen Shi-wen and Pei Zhong-yuan, they became surprised. Everyone of them laughed at and mocked him as wayward. The only one who was delighted by Zhu's new knowledge was his old Confucian teacher, Xu Wen-yi, who remarked, "I have been diseased of the limbs for more than ten years and no one has been able to offer me a cure." He declared with joy and confidence, "Now I have hope of recovery at last!" Happily, our Reverend Dan-xi did not fail his former master's expectation and accomplished a successful treatment. This gave a good lesson to those who had shown contempt towards Zhu, and they soon changed their attitude, admiring his astonishing progress and unconventional approach to medicine. In a few years, he became known to the whole country.

Nonetheless, the Reverend Dan-xi did not rest content with what he had learned and achieved. He took in the theory of damp heat and ministerial fire from Zhang Cong-zheng, Li Gao, and Liu Wan-su. However, these three revolutionary medical men had evolved their innovative theories based on patients and disorders seen in the north where wind and cold prevail, while the Reverend Dan-xi lived and worked in the south where damp heat is overwhelming and people are subject to fire. Zhu realized that just as it was wrong to blindly follow ancient predecessors, it was also not productive to passively accept the teachings of modern masters without original thinking on one's own. He respected the ancient sages but he did not allow his medical practice to be confined to their views, formulas, and theories of pathogenesis. He learned from the past and enriched upon that past, making a beautiful combination of the experience of the past great masters with his own practice and new findings.

Owing to his marvelous medical skills, attractive personality, and the fact that he cherished the same warm heart in treating rich or poor, young or old alike, attending each case with a moving sense of responsibility, patients from far and near came to him like a stream, and respectful physicians and scholars followed him everywhere like shadows. Yet the Reverend Dan-xi was always seen indefatigably elucidating issues patiently and in great detail.

Besides what Dai Liang has pointed out above, it is also important to note that, although Zhu Zhen-heng is hailed as a great medical innovator, he nonetheless vigorously trained in and faithfully inherited the legacy left in the ancient medical classics, such as the *Nei Jing (Inner Classic)*, the *Ling Shu (Spiritual Pivot)*, and the *Nan Jing (Classic of Difficult [Issues])*. These constituted the core of his doctrines even though he practiced them in a unique and creative way. As to contemporary doctrines, most of which he had a good command, the one which had the most profound impact on the formation of Zhu's distinctive medical system was the theory of damp heat expounded by Liu Wan-su and Li Gao. Both Liu and Li considered damp heat to be the main cause of disease and taught that clearing damp heat is the overwhelming priority in treatment. With that as a starting point, Zhu Zhen-heng went further and advanced the well-known aphorism, "Yang is constantly in superabundance, while yin tends to be insufficient." This statement became the germ and cornerstone of the later *Wen Bing Xue* or Warm Disease School.

This theory of Zhu's concerning the tendency to yin insufficiency deserves our particular attention. It is based on Zhu's explanation of the important concept of ministerial fire. Zhu held that any movement, whether internal and external, is the display of yang. This includes labor, thought, and desire for sex, wealth, and fame. Zhu observed,

> Heaven governs living things and, for that reason, it never stands still. Human beings are bestowed life (by heaven) and, therefore, (also) never stand still. That which makes things constantly move is none other than the work of ministerial fire.

He explained this concept further, saying,

> Fire is associated with yin in the interior and yang in the exterior. It governs movement, and conversely, any movement is ascribed to fire.

Zhu continued, saying that fire is called sovereign fire when it is generated by the interaction between form and qi and, as such, is listed as one of the five phases. Ministerial fire, on the other hand, is a fire that is generated out of vacuity and emptiness caused by the necessity to maintain life, and it becomes observable in movement. Any movement beyond a certain limit, which is commonly overstepped, may stir this ministerial fire, and stirring of ministerial fire never fails to do harm to the balance between yin and yang. Therefore, it follows that supplementation of yin is a necessary component of almost every treatment.

Many TCM scholars have rightly pointed out that this theory has virtually provided the basis for the TCM practice of preventive medicine. This assessment is borne out by the fact that most proven formulas that either help people recuperate or maintain fitness with no specific remedial indications are primarily composed of yin-supplementing medicinals.

Nevertheless, Zhu Dan-xi did not go to the extreme of only employing supplementation and enrichment of yin. He incorporated all the useful elements from the theories expounded by his predecessors, and especially the other three great masters of the Jin-Yuan. He did not at all object to the use of drainage or attacking in general, Zhang Zi-he's emphasis, although he repeatedly warned against recklessly introducing hot, dry medicinals to treat frenetically stirring ministerial fire. He is even known for the invention of the so-called *Dan Xi San Fa* or Dan-xi's Three Methods. These were diaphoresis, ejection (or emesis), and precipitation (or purgation) and these directly parallel and allude to Zhang Zi-He's, founder of the School of Attack & Purgation, Three Methods. However, it does not need a thorough examination to see that Zhu's understanding and use of these three methods were different from Zhang Zi-he's and are peculiar to Zhu's theory of nurturing yin. For instance, to promote perspiration, he did not merely use medicinals to effuse evils through the exterior but also those that supplement yin. These were for the purpose of enriching the source of water and boosting the root of the body to achieve the combined effect of attacking evil and protecting the righteous simultaneously. He also said that to eject (or cause vomiting), not only emetics but any kind of medicinals as well can be used at the same time. Based on this, Zhu designed many formulas which were supplementing in nature but were administered for the clinical purpose of provoking emission.

Thus, it is important to reiterate that, although Zhu Dan-xi is hailed as the founder of one of the four great schools of the Jin-Yuan, his theory and practice in no way repudiated or was mutually exclusive to that of the other three great schools. Readers familiar with Li Dong-yuan's *Pi Wei Lun (Treatise on the Spleen & Stomach)* will see that Zhu accepted and used many of the theories, favorite medicinals, and formulas of Li, such as *Bu Zhong Yi Qi Tang* (Supplement the Center & boost the Qi Decoction), *Zhi Zhu Wan* (Aurantium & Atractylodis Pills), and *Ju Pi Zhi Zhu Wan* (Citrus,

Aurantium, & Atractylodis Pills). Even though Zhu is remembered today primarily for his emphasis on enriching yin, like Li, Zhu also advocated that damp heat can be cleared by warm medicinals, such as Radix Panacis Ginseng (*Ren Shen*), Rhizoma Atractylodis Macrocephalae (*Bai Zhu*), and the like. In addition, Li's theories concerning counterflow inversion were extremely important to Zhu who accepted Li's method of using qi medicinals to treat this but also advanced the method of using blood medicinals for this as well depending upon the circumstances. Thus, Zhu Dan-xi can be seen not just as one of four co-equal great masters of the Jin-Yuan but the fruition and amalgamation of Jin-Yuan medicine. Students of the *Pi Wei Lun* in particular will find this book a continuation and deepening of the theories and methods contained in that book.

Zhu has also long been regarded as the past master of treating the so-called miscellaneous diseases or *za bing*. These are the traditionally named and enumerated diseases commonly appearing in Chinese *nei ke* or internal medicine clinical manuals. They are miscellaneous in that they are a mixed collection of diseases not grouped by any other over-riding principle. For instance, the recent *Zhong Yi Nei Ke Lin Chuang Shou Ce (Clinical Handbook of TCM Internal Medicine)* published in 1990 by the Shanghai Science & Technology Press, still uses this term as the heading for its list of diseases covered. As a treatment manual, Books 1-6 of the *Dan Xi Zhi Fa Xin Yao* cover an assortment of both internal and external diseases or *nei ke* and *wai ke*. Book 7 is devoted to *fu ke* or gynecology. And Book 8 deals with *er ke* or pediatrics as well as miscellaneous formulas and case histories.

In the treatment of disease, Zhu applied in a masterly way the principle of basing treatment on pattern identification (*bian zheng lun zhi*) and came up with new, enlightening approaches to a variety of diseases. These have since been recognized as these diseases' classic treatment by later generations. Readers of this book familiar with modern TCM clinical manuals with their descriptions of disease causes and mechanisms, pattern discrimination, methods of treatment, and standard guiding formulas will find that many of these are based on Zhu's insights recorded herein.

xiii

In addition, Zhu advanced the notion of qi, blood, phlegm, and depression as the four key points in analyzing disease patterns and focused on the genesis of the six environmental excesses as the guideline in designing particular formulas. Based on this idea, he used four basic formulas as his foundation in clinical practice: *Si Jun Zi Tang* (Four Gentlemen Decoction) for qi disease, *Si Wu Tang* (Four Materials Decoction) for blood disease, *Er Chen Tang* (Two Aged Decoction) for phlegm disease, and *Yue Ju Wan* (Outthrust Tribulation Pills) for depression disease. Zhu then modified these prescriptions in accordance with the conditions of the six environmental excesses. This is a very simple methodology and is easy to follow by modern practitioners. It goes along with the saying that new practitioners know 20 formulas to treat one disease, but old practitioners can treat 20 disease with but one formula. Though Zhu's prescriptive methodology for the treatment of a large variety of diseases is simple and easy to remember, it has been proven, nonetheless, by generations of practitioners as being exceptionally efficacious.

In treating disease, Zhu also took geographical location into full account. Different living environments, different customs, and different historical backgrounds all contribute to differences in the contraction and progression of disease. This is easy to see. Obesity may be a problem in developed countries, while under-nourishment is killing many people in the developing world. People living in damp coastal lowlands may suffer from different maladies than others living in dry, arid, upland deserts. Zhu Dan-xi did not originate these ideas which come from such classics as the *Nei Jing*, but not everyone is able to implement a synthesized analysis of all these factors, reach a cogent, scientific diagnosis of a particular case, and thereby devise an effective treatment plan. This is the work of a master, and Zhu Zhen-heng has set us a brilliant example in this regard.

As a practitioner of long-standing and rich experience, Zhu was a prolific designer of a great number of effective therapies and, in particular, of herbal formulas. This present work contains numerous examples of these. Other of his achievements include his written legacy. This includes the *Dan Xi Xin Fa (Dan Xi's Heart Methods [of Treatment])* or *Xin Fa* for short, completed in 1347 in 5 volumes. This book deals with the treatment of a great variety of diseases and is one of the most dearly treasured of TCM classics. The *Jin Gui Gou Xuan (Probing into the Subtleties of the Golden Cabinet)* in 3 volumes is a work treating various miscellaneous diseases. The *Yi Xue Fa Ming (The Study of Medicine Made Clear)* is a collection of his reading notes. The *Ju Fang Fa Hui (Criticisms & Revelation of the Corrected Collection of Formulas)* was written in the form of questions and answers. It is a discussion of medical theories. The *Ju Fang (Collected Formulas)* is the abbreviated name of the *Tai Ping Hui Min Ju Fang (Corrected Collection of Formulas of the Great Harmony Imperial Grace Pharmacy)* compiled the Chen and Pei mentioned above. Dan-xi's *Yi Yao (Essentials of Medicine)* unfortunately has long been lost.

Any one of these works is worthy of transmission. It is a well known fact that the four great masters of the Jin-Yuan Dynasties raised Chinese medicine to new heights in terms of both theory and practice, and of these four — Liu Wan-su, Zhang Cong-zheng, Li Gao, and Zhu Dan-xi — Li Gao and Zhu Dan-xi are generally considered the greatest. Li Gao's *magnum opus*, the *Pi Wei Lun (Treatise on the Spleen & Stomach)*, has already been published as part of Blue Poppy Press' Great Masters Series. However, till now, no book by Zhu Dan-xi has existed in English. Therefore, it is fitting that a title by Zhu Dan-xi take its place in this Great Masters Series.

After serious consideration, we selected the *Dan Xi Zhi Fa Xin Yao (The Heart & Essentials of Dan-xi's [Treatment Methods] Methods)* for our first Zhu Dan-xi translation. Some of the reasons for our selection are covered in the following Ming and Qing Dynasty prefaces by Gao Bin and Xiao Shu-lin. However, the quote below from the People's Health & Hygiene Press Chinese edition of 1983 also clarifies why we have chosen this book above Zhu's other writings to transmit first to English readers:

> Master Zhu left behind him the *Dan Xi Xin Fa*, the *Yi Yao*, the
> *Dan Xi Zhi Fa Xin Yao*, and other works. But the *Dan Xi Xin Fa*
> has undergone such repeated adulteration and garbling by later
> generations that it has lost its original look, while the *Yi Yao* has

been long lost, incapable of being restored. The only work that survives largely intact is the *Dan Xi Zhi Fa Xin Yao* which covers the contents of both the *Dan Xi Xin Fa* and the *Yi Yao*. Besides, because it was completed during his advanced years, it is comparatively very rich, reliable, and comprehensive, and is worthy of being regarded as a representative work of the school led by Zhu Dan-xi.

This work is composed largely of formulas, case histories, and treatment methods. It is extremely valuable to clinical practitioners of TCM. However, to do the great theoretician justice, the publication of this translation will be followed by the translation of Zhu's *Ge Zhi Yu Lun (Extra Treatises Based on Investigation & Inquiry)*. Compiled in 1347, that is a one volume work made up of a collection of Zhu's essays specifically on his medical theories. Here the reader will be able to find out more about Zhu's theoretical concepts than we have introduced in this volume. Once both volumes are available, we feel we will have presented English-speaking readers with the best of Zhu Dan-xi's theory and practice.

Although I have based my translation of the *Xin Yao* on the above mentioned People's Health & Hygiene Press edition, observant readers of both will discover a number of places where I have disagreed with the reading of that Chinese editor. As is well known, classical Chinese is devoid of punctuation. Therefore, how one groups the words affects the meaning conveyed. Like so many modern Chinese editions of premodern books, the Chinese editor of the 1983 edition has inserted modern punctuation to make the book more easily readable. However, in doing so, I believe he has made many errors in reading, and my understanding of the text is different in quite a number of places. In the process of translation, I often found and had to put right wrong punctuations which revealed the carelessness or lack of TCM knowledge on the part of that editor. My policy in translation was to be as faithful to Zhu Zhen-heng as possible, based on my own knowledge of classical Chinese and my understanding of Chinese medicine, rather than to that modern Chinese editor.

My translational terminology and methodology have been based on Nigel Wiseman and Ken Boss' *Glossary of Chinese Medical Terms and Acupuncture Points* published by Paradigm Publications, Brookline, MA. Formulas are identified first by their Pinyin names followed by their English translation in parentheses. Ingredients in these formulas are identified first in Latin pharmacological nomenclature followed by Pinyin in parentheses. The main sources for the identifications of medicinal ingredients used in preparing this book have been Bensky & Gamble's *Chinese Herbal Medicine: Materia Medica*; Hong-yen Hsu's *Oriental Materia Medica; A Concise Guide*; Stuart & Read's *Chinese Materia Medica*; and the Shanghai Science & Technology Press' *Zhong Yao Da Ci Dian (A Dictionary of Chinese Herbs)*. Acupuncture points mentioned in the text are identified first by their Pinyin name followed by their numerical notation in parentheses. In comparison to the World Health Organization's International Acupuncture Nomenclature, we have separated the syllables of the Pinyin and use the following abbreviations which are different from that system: Lu for Lung, Per for Pericardium, TH for Triple Heater, and Liv for Liver.

As mentioned above, classical Chinese has no punctuation. Nor does it use the Western concept of paragraphs. Therefore, the reader will see that frequently the author jumps from one topic to another more abruptly than is common in English expository writing. I have tried to make meaningful paragraph breaks without unduly wasting paper. As the reader will also see, some of these are rather arbitrary. In addition, the reader will notice that, due to differences in premodern and modern standards of scholarship, the text of this book bears the trace of authors other than Zhu Dan-xi. This underscores that the primary intent and importance of books such as this are the conveyance of practical, clinically useful information. Thus this text exemplifies the fact that, in the premodern Chinese medical literary tradition, books were living things which grew and changed over generations.

Yang Shou-zhong
North China Coal Mines Medical College
Tangshan, Hebei, PRC

Preface to the
Dan Xi Zhi Fa Xin Yao
from the Gao[1] Edition

Dan-xi is to medicine what Zhu Zi is to our Confucianism. Zhu Zi is profound in the Confucianist doctrines, and has [3 characters missing[2]] his marvelous true and unique attainments. His speeches and writings [1 character missing] suffice as a summary of the past and blaze a new path to the future. He has established himself as a paragon for a hundred succeeding generations to emulate and no one has ever been sacrilegious against [1 character missing].

Dan-xi [5 characters missing] as a physician, there are many in the south. Moreover, during the reign of Cheng Hua[3] the *Xin Fa (Heart Methods)* was brought out, and during the reign of Hong Zhi[4] the *Yi Yao (Essentials of Medicine)* came out as well. Besides these, there was the work, the *Xin Yao (The Heart & Essentials)*[5], which was in my family's collection and had never been published. It was not till quite recently a published edition (of this) has been in circulation. But it is

---

[1] Gao Bin, a.k.a Gao Shu-zong, Ming Dynasty. He supposedly wrote the *Bian Chan Xu Zhi (Compulsory Knowledge About Smooth Delivery)*. However, the authorship of this work is questionable.

[2] Owing to long circulation, a few parts of this text are missing or illegible. When such is the case, the number of characters which are either missing or illegible is given in parentheses.

[3] 1465-1487 CE, the reign of Emperor Xian Zong, Ming Dynasty

[4] 1488-1505 CE, the reign of Emperor Xiao Zong, Ming Dynasty

[5] The abbreviated title of the *Dan Xi Zhi Fa Xin Yao*

full of all sorts of misprinted characters; there are an extraordinary many typographical errors in it.

My nephew has long been deep in (the study of) medicine, day and night contemplating the heart of Dan-xi's doctrines, and for that purpose he has found this work particularly significant. I did not have the heart to sit and do nothing but just look on while the many mistakes in (the already published edition) were misleading the whole world, and therefore I embarked upon the collation and republication of this work in the hope that, together with my colleagues, I might lend my assistance to the people in the area of enhancing their moral strength and prolonging their life span. Extremely laborious and expensive as the project was, I would not withdraw from it, because (I thought) it a sublime deed.

In a comparison of the above three works, I found that the *Xin Fa* comprises the *xin* (heart) without the *yao* (essentials) in the title, and the *Yi Yao* comprises the *yao* without the *xin* in the title, while this present work comprises both the *xin* and the *yao* or the heart and the essentials. The teachings that one and the same person comes up with may be different (in different) works (composed at different times), but compared with the other two books, this work is most obviously particularly choice and comprehensive. For it truly embraces all that is subtle and fine of the art acquired by Dan-xi through his spirit and heart and is a product gushing from the depth of his heart. This is just what the title of *Xin Yao* is intended to suggest. If later generations are to track the heart of Dan-xi, what other book can lead them to success other than this one?

There is, however, another saying. Senior physicians explain that one should take their time, and, when they get a light hand (in the medical art), their heart will be in command of it. That which can be called perfection is unaccessible to my son through my explanation, neither is it accessible to me through my son's explanation. It must need the heart to build it up and cannot be passed on through words. What is preserved in books is but the traces of wonderful application, and it is wrong to take them as the heart *per se*. To track down the heart of Dan-xi, the key lies in that our hearts must try to accommodate the heart of Dan-xi first. Only later on, can one make a wonderful application of Dan-xi's (teachings), extremely profound and of broad reading, with a sharp idea of the fine, a clear understanding of the dim and obscure, and a penetrating insight into anything in touch. This is the heart of Dan-xi. The derivation of wonderful application definitely always comes after learning.

People must grind elaborately, deliberate intently, and pursue the learning devotedly. Then, one day, it is not difficult for them to have in their possession the heart of Dan-xi. Suppose, to obtain the heart, one did not strive after the heart but only after the traces. (In that case,) I am afraid that this book would only be a lump of waste paper. It is this fear that leads me to go out of my way to give this piece of advice to readers of this work.

Written by Gao Bin, Master Silkworm in the Woods,
Jiang Yin; 1st, 11th month, the year of Gui Mou[6],
the reign of Jia Qing[7]

---

[6]   1542 CE

[7]   1522-1566 CE, the reign of Emperor Shi Zong, Ming Dynasty

Preface to the Republication of the
Dan Xi Zhi Fa Xin Yao

This work is the pristine edition by Gao Shu-zong of the Ming Dynasty, but it has been hardly seen in circulation in the country. In the summer of Wu Xu[1], Shu(-lin)[2] came across it in an old trunk. After having gone over it several times, poring over and reviewing it with interest, he acquired a rough knowledge of it. Then he sometimes meted out treatments according to the methods (it instructs) and very often he achieved unexpected results. A small number of literati and officials presented compliments to him for his medical knowledge, but actually, credit should largely be given to this book.

Nowadays available in the book stores, the only work (by Dan-xi) is the *Xin Fa*. The *Yi Yao* is rarely, if at all, seen. In his later years, the master collected what he felt was not satisfactorily dealt with in those two books and, after careful deliberation, made some additions and subtractions to them to compile this his final work. Although teachings that one and the same person comes up with may be different in their old and new works, this work is pithy and choice, excelling those other two beyond comparison.

It is a popular comment that Dan-xi is to medicine what Zhu Zi of Kao Ting[3] was to our Confucianism. (Zhu Zi) spent scores of years in

---

[1]   1898 CE

[2]   The author of this preface. Little is known about him except that he helped publish the Qing edition we have based our translation on.

[3]   Kao Ting is located in the southwest of Jian Yang county, Fujian Province, a historical spot from the days of the Tang Dynasty. In his late years, Zhu Xi, *i.e.*, Zhu Zi, lived there and set up a school named *Zhu Lin Jing She* (Bamboo Forest Mansion of the Elite). Emperor Li Zong of the Song Dynasty issued a decree that the school be named *Kao Lin Shu Yuan* (Kaolin Academy) as a special favor

compiling works, but he did not conclude his most profound thinking in one tome until the evening of his life. From this it is seen that the ancient took great scruple and prudence, without the least bit of perfunctoriness, in establishing a teaching that would have a bearing on the future.

Having been lying for long years, buried and pressed (under of pile of other books), the original (copy of this) book was badly worm-eaten at the margins and corners (of its pages). Fortunately, however, the characters were clear and unobscured. On opening it, a bright beam of light and the odor of treasure issued forth from the paper. But for the protection of god and spirit, it would not have been so preserved. It happened that some influential officials of Jiangsu Province were establishing a medical research institute in the south of the city, and there gathered all the distinguished physicians from every corner of the province. Xiao Shu-lin was among those present. By chance, he happened to mention this work in quoting something, and all the people around expressed their pity for having never read it. What is more, because they feared that it might be buried in oblivion forever in the distant future, they raised funds and put it to press for a new edition in order that they may enjoy the pleasure of sharing it with the colleagues and that the scholars teaching Dan-xi might learn something from it.

Respectfully written by Xiao Shu-lin, inferior student of Qian Tang[4], 1st month of summer, Ji You[5], 1st year of Xuan Tong[6]

---

shown to Zhu Xi in recognition of his great contribution to Chinese culture and education.

[4]   Now Hangzhou, Zhejiang Province

[5]   1909 CE

[6]   Reign name of the last emperor of China

Table of Contents

Book 3

Book 4

Book 5

Book 6

Book 7 Women's Disorders

Book 8 Children's Disorders

Appendix: Collection of Missing Case Studies, 443

BOOK ONE

Collated & Corrected
by Gao Shu-zong
Inferior student, Jiang Yin

Re-collated by Xiao Shu-lin,
Inferior student, Qian Tang

Chapter One

Wind Stroke

Largely, (this disease) is governed by blood vacuity and the existence of phlegm. (Therefore,) the treatment of phlegm should take precedence, and blood should be nurtured and moved afterwards. It may (also) be produced by blood vacuity embracing fire and dampness, and the great method is to eliminate phlegm as the ruling (therapy). (In that case,) for simultaneous supplementation (of the blood), Succus Zingiberis (*Jiang Zhi*) is indispensable. The *Nei Jing (Inner Classic)* says, "Wherever evils converge, there the qi must become vacuous." Liu He-jian[1] considered (wind stroke) an internal damage heat disease. Zhang Zhong-jing[2] considered it an external contraction of evils.

When wind hurts people, in most cases it lodges in the lungs. Hemiplegia is usually accompanied by copious phlegm [For details, see the *Yi Yao (Essentials of Medicine)*[3] {later editor}]. Congestion and exuberance of phlegm, deviated mouth and eyes, and inability to speak justify ejection (*i.e.*, emesis). A moderate or a conscious

---

[1]   Liu He-jian, a.k.a. Liu Wan-su (circa 1120-1200CE), founder of one of the four great schools of the Jin-Yuan Dynasties, was the pioneer of the Cold & Cool Doctrine. His main contribution to TCM is his research in the *Nei Jing* and his exposition that fire heat is the principal cause of disease.

[2]   Zhang Zhong-jing (circa 150-219 CE), one of the greatest of all TCM scholars whose *Shang Han Lun (Treatise on Cold Damage)* is regarded as the first systematic book treating medication in China.

[3]   Another work by Zhu Dan-xi which is long lost

case (require) *Gua Di San* (Melon Pedicle Powder)[4] and *Xi Xian San* (Dilute Drool Powder).[5] Another (way to induce vomiting is) to boil one half *jin* of shrimp together with fermented soybean jam[6], Chinese green onion, and Chinese prickly ash, first eating the prawns and next drinking the soup. (Then) perform mechanical emesis to lead out the wind and phlegm. However, in case of vacuity, it is not all right to cause vomiting.

Temporary collapse justifies ejection. Sudden collapse with qi vacuity should be treated by supplementation with Radix Panacis Ginseng (*Ren Shen*) and Radix Astragali Membranacei (*Huang Qi*). (Collapse with) enuresis is ascribed to qi vacuity and requires supplementation with Radix Panacis Ginseng (*Ren Shen*) and Radix Astragali Membranacei (*Huang Qi*). In case of qi vacuity with the existence of phlegm, boil a thick decoction of Radix Panacis Ginseng with Succus Bambusae (*Zhu Li*) and Succus Zingiberis (*Jiang Zhi*). Blood vacuity makes it necessary to supplement with *Si Wu Tang* (Four Materials Decoction)[7], stir-frying (the ingredients) with Succus Zingiberis (*Jiang Zhi*), and, for fear that phlegm should become stagnant, adding Succus Bambusae (*Zhu Li*) and Succus Zingiberis (*Jiang Zhi*). This (also) treats (blood vacuity) with phlegm embraced within it.

---

4 This formula is composed of Pediculus Melonis (*Gua Di*), stir-fried to yellow, and Semen Phaseoli Calcarati (*Chi Xiao Dou*), in equal amounts.

5 There are several kinds of *Xi Xian San* (Dilute Drool Powder). Here it may refer to *Jiu Ji Xi Xian San* which is composed of Fructus Gleditschiae Sinensis (*Zao Jiao*), stripped of its black skin, and Alumen (*Bai Fan*).

6 This is made from soybean, flour, etc. The sauce is then extracted from these ingredients.

7 This is composed of equal amounts of Radix Angelicae Sinensis (*Dang Gui*), Rhizoma Ligustici Wallichii (*Chuan Xiong*), Radix Albus Paeoniae Lactiflorae (*Ba Shao*), and prepared Radix Rehmanniae (*Da Shu Di*).

To treat phlegm with qi repletion and ability to eat, use Succus Viticis Negundae (*Jing Li*). (But) in case of qi vacuity with low food intake, use Succus Bambusae (*Zhu Li*). These two ingredients eliminate phlegm, open the connecting vessels, and move blood and qi, but, when they are introduced into *Si Wu Tang* and the like, they need to be assisted by a small amount of Succus Zingiberis (*Jiang Zhi*). In persons with wind stroke, pain in the sinews arising whenever they move is due to absence of blood to nourish the sinews. This is called sinew desiccation and is absolutely incurable.

Fat, white (*i.e.*, pale) persons usually have phlegm dampness. (For them,) use Radix Praeparatus Aconiti Carmichaeli (*Fu Zi*) and Radix Aconiti (*Wu Tou*) to move the channels. At the beginning of (wind) stroke collapse, keep on pinching *Ren Zhong* (GV 26) till (the patient) comes to. Then administer a phlegm-removing formula like *Er Chen* (Two Aged [Decoction])[8], *Si Jun Zi* (Four Gentlemen [Decoction])[9], and *Si Wu Tang* (Four Materials Decoction). Additions and subtractions to these should be made before using them.

Thin persons (usually suffer from) yin vacuity and fire heat. (For them, use) *Si Wu Tang* plus Radix Achyranthis Bidentatae (*Niu Xi*), Succus Bambusae (*Zhu Li*), Radix Scutellariae Baicalensis (*Huang Qin*), and Cortex Phellodendri (*Huang Bai*). In case of existence of phlegm, add phlegm(-removing) medicinals.

A fat person who was struck by wind with a deviated mouth and numb and insensitive hands and feet, was treated as a phlegm case at both sides (with the following prescription:) Bulbus Fritillariae (*Bei Mu*), Fructus Trichosanthis Kirlowii (*Gua Lou*), Rhizoma Arisaematis (*Nan Xing*), Rhizoma Pinelliae Ternatae (*Ban Xia*),

---

[8] This refers to *Er Chen Tang* which is composed of Rhizoma Pinelliae Ternatae (*Ban Xia*), Pericarpium Citri Rubri (*Ju Hong*), Sclerotium Poriae Cocoris (*Fu Ling*) and mix-fried Radix Glycyrrhizae (*Zhi Cao*).

[9] This is composed of equal amounts of Radix Panacis Ginseng (*Ren Shen*), mix-fried Radix Glycyrrhizae (*Zhi Cao*), Sclerotium Poriae Cocoris (*Fu Ling*), and Rhizoma Atractylodis Macrocephalae (*Bai Zhu*).

Pericarpium Citri Reticulatae (*Chen Pi*), Rhizoma Atractylodis Macrocephalae (*Bai Zhu*), Radix Scutellariae Baicalensis (*Huang Qin*), Rhizoma Coptidis Chinensis (*Huang Lian*), Cortex Phellodendri (*Huang Bai*), Radix Et Rhizoma Notopterygii (*Qiang Huo*), Radix Ledebouriellae Sesloidis (*Fang Feng*), Herba Seu Flos Schizonepetae Tenuifoliae (*Jing Jie*), Rhizoma Clematidis Chinensis (*Wei Ling Xian*), Herba Menthae (*Bo [He]*), Ramulus Cinnamomi (*Gui [Zhi]*), Radix Glycyrrhizae (*Gan Cao*) and Radix Trichosanthis Kirlowii (*Tian Hua Fen*). (He was told to) eat much wheat flour food. Radix Aconiti Coreani (*Bai Fu Zi*), Succus Bambusae (*Zhu Li*), Succus Zingiberis (*Jiang Zhi*), and a spoonful of wine were added to move the channels.

A woman more than 60 years of age (suffered from) hemiplegia of the left hand and foot with loss of voice but good appetite (literally, strong in eating. Her formula consisted of) Radix Ledebouriellae Sesloidis (*Fang Feng*), Herba Seu Flos Schizonepetae Tenuifoliae (*Jing Jie*), Radix Et Rhizoma Notopterygii (*Qiang Huo*), Rhizoma Arisaematis (*Nan Xing*), Myrrha (*Mo Yao*), Gummum Olibani (*Ru Xiang*), Caulis Akebiae Mutong (*Mu Tong*), Sclerotium Poriae Cocoris (*Fu Ling*), Cortex Magnoliae Officinalis (*Hou Po*), Radix Platycodi Grandiflori (*Jie Geng*), Radix Glycyrrhizae (*Gan Cao*), Herba Ephedrae (*Ma Huang*), dried Buthus Martensi (*Quan Xie*), and Flos Carthami Tinctorii (*Hong Hua*). All the above were powdered and taken with warmed wine and effect followed.

It was spring. Her pulse was hidden and faint. (Therefore she was) administered thin (*i.e.*, not very strong), salty pickle, one bowl each morning, to provoke vomiting. From the fifth day on, Rhizoma Atractylodis Macrocephalae (*Bai Zhu*), Pericarpium Citri Reticulatae (*Chen Pi*), Sclerotium Poriae Cocoris (*Fu Ling*), Radix Glycyrrhizae (*Gan Cao*), Cortex Magnoliae Officinalis (*Hou Po*), and Rhizoma Acori Graminei (*Chang Pu*) were administered, 2 doses daily. Later Rhizoma Ligustici Wallichii (*Chuan Xiong*), Fructus Gardeniae Jasminoidis (*Shan Zhi*), Semen Praeparatus Sojae (*Dou Chi*), Pediculus Melonis (*Gua Di*), powdered Semen Phaseoli Radiati (*Lu Dou Fen*), and salty pickle were administered. Massive vomiting was induced. As inability to take in food arose, *Si Jun Zi Tang* was administered, and then succeeded by Radix Angelicae Sinensis (*Dang Gui*), wine-processed Radix Scutellariae Baicalensis (*Huang Qin*), Flos Carthami Tinctorii (*Hong Hua*), Caulis Akebiae Mutong (*Mu Tong*), Cortex Magnoliae Officinalis (*Hou Po*), Semen Arctii Lappae (*Shu Nian Zi*), Rhizoma Atractylodis (*Cang Zhu*), ginger-processed Rhizoma Arisaematis (*Nan Xing*), Radix Achyranthis Bidentatae (*Niu Xi*), and Sclerotium Poriae Cocoris (*Fu Ling*) which were made into pills the size of Chinese parasol tree seeds with wine paste. At night after 10 days' administration, (the patient) sweat moderately and regained the ability to move her limbs and to speak.

A person suffered from wind stroke. (They were given) Bulbus Fritillariae (*Bei Mu*), Fructus Trichosanthis Kirlowii (*Gua Lou*), Rhizoma Arisaematis (*Nan Xing*), Rhizoma Pinelliae Ternatae (*Ban Xia*), wine-processed Rhizoma Coptidis Chinensis (*Huang Lian*), wine-processed Radix Scutellariae Baicalensis (*Huang Qin*), wine-processed Cortex Phellodendri (*Huang Bai*), Radix Ledebouriellae Sesloidis (*Fang Feng*), Herba Seu Flos Schizonepetae Tenuifoliae (*Jing Jie*), Radix Et Rhizoma Notopterygii (*Qiang Huo*), Herba Menthae (*Bo [He]*), Ramulus Cinnamomi (*Gui [Zhi]*), and Rhizoma Clematidis Chinensis (*Wei Ling Xian*).

A fat person who suffered from wind stroke was first treated with ejection and then administered Rhizoma Atractylodis (*Cang Zhu*), (two characters missing), wine-processed Radix Scutellariae Baicalensis (*Huang Qin*), wine-processed Cortex Phellodendri (*Huang Bai*), Caulis Akebiae Mutong (*Mu Tong*), Sclerotium Poriae Cocoris (*Fu Ling*), Radix Achyranthis Bidentatae (*Niu Xi*), Flos Carthami Tinctorii (*Hong Hua*), Rhizoma Cimicifugae (*Sheng Ma*), Cortex Magnoliae Officinalis (*Hou Po*), and Radix Glycyrrhizae (*Gan Cao*).

A fat person suffered from a deviated mouth and paralysis of the hands with a strong pulse. (They were given) Rhizoma Arisaematis (*Nan Xing*), Rhizoma Pinelliae Ternatae (*Ban Xia*), Herba Menthae (*Bo [He]*), Ramulus Cinnamomi (*Gui [Zhi]*), Rhizoma Clematidis Chinensis (*Wei Ling Xian*), wine-processed Radix Scutellariae Baicalensis (*Huang Qin*), wine-processed Cortex Phellodendri

(*Huang Bai*), Radix Trichosanthis Kirlowii (*Tian Hua Fen*), Bulbus Fritillariae (*Bei Mu*), Herba Seu Flos Schizonepetae Tenuifoliae (*Jing Jie*), Fructus Trichosanthis Kirlowii (*Gua Lou*), Rhizoma Atractylodis Macrocephalae (*Bai Zhu*), Pericarpium Citri Reticulatae (*Chen Pi*), fresh Rhizoma Zingiberis (*Sheng Jiang*), Radix Glycyrrhizae (*Gan Cao*), Radix Ledebouriellae Sesloidis (*Fang Feng*), Radix Et Rhizoma Notopterygii (*Qiang Huo*), and Succus Bambusae (*Zhu Li*).

A person with hemiplegia of the right side (was prescribed) wine-processed Rhizoma Coptidis Chinensis (*Huang Lian*), wine-processed Cortex Phellodendri (*Huang Bai*), and Radix Ledebouriellae Sesloidis (*Fang Feng*), one half *liang* for each of the above, Rhizoma Pinelliae Ternatae (*Ban Xia*), 1 *qian*, Radix Et Rhizoma Notopterygii (*Qiang Huo*), 5 *qian*, wine-processed Radix Scutellariae Baicalensis (*Huang Qin*), Radix Panacis Ginseng (*Ren Shen*), Rhizoma Atractylodis (*Cang Zhu*), 1 *liang* for each of the above, Rhizoma Ligustici Wallichii (*Chuan Xiong*), Radix Angelicae Sinensis (*Dang Gui*), each 5 *qian*, Herba Ephedrae (*Ma Huang*), 3 *qian*; Radix Glycyrrhizae (*Gan Cao*), 1 *qian*, Rhizoma Arisaematis (*Nan Xing*), 1 *liang*, and Radix Praeparatus Aconiti Carmichaeli (*Fu Zi*), 3 slices. The above were made into pills the size of pellets, dissolved in wine, and taken.

A fat person with qi depression due to worry and thought (suffered from) paralysis of the right hand (two characters missing). (They were given) *Bu Zhong Yi Qi Tang* (Supplement the Center and Boost the Qi Decoction).[10] Because of the existence of phlegm, Rhizoma Pinelliae Ternatae (*Ban Xia*) and Succus Bambusae (*Zhu Li*) (two characters missing) were added.

The wind stroke patterns of deviated mouth and eyes, abnormality in speech, and drooling, generalized paralysis, or hemiplegia can all be treated (with the formula below). All this is due to vacuity

---

[10] This is composed of Radix Astragali Membranacei (*Huang Qi*), mix-fried Radix Glycyrrhizae (*Zhi Gan Cao*), Radix Panacis Ginseng (*Ren Shen*), Rhizoma Atractylodis Macrocephalae (*Bai Zhu*), Radix Angelicae Sinensis (*Dang Gui*), Pericarpium Citri Reticulatae (*Chen Pi*), Rhizoma Cimicifugae (*Sheng Ma*), and Radix Bupleuri (*Chai Hu*).

weakness of the original qi in the past and subjection to external evils (in the present) plus overindulgence in wine and sex. (For this,) use Radix Panacis Ginseng (*Ren Shen*), Radix Ledebouriellae Sesloidis (*Fang Feng*), Radix Ephedrae Chinensis (*Ma Huang*), Radix Et Rhizoma Notopterygii (*Qiang Huo*), Rhizoma Cimicifugae (*Sheng Ma*), Radix Platycodi Grandiflori (*Jie Geng*), Gypsum (*Shi Gao*), Radix Scutellariae Baicalensis (*Huang Qin*), Herba Seu Flos Schizonepetae Tenuifoliae (*Jing Jie*), Rhizoma Gastrodiae Elatae (*Tian Ma*), Rhizoma Arisaematis (*Nan Xing*), Herba Menthae (*Bo [He]*), Ramulus Cinnamomi (*Gu [Zhi]*), Radix Puerariae Lobatae (*Ge Gen*), Radix Rubrus Paeoniae Lactiflorae (*Chi Shao Yao*), Semen Pruni Armeniacae (*Xing Ren*), Radix Angelicae Sinensis (*Dang Gui*), Rhizoma Ligustici Wallichii (*Chuan Xiong*), Rhizoma Atractylodis Macrocephalae (*Bai Zhu*), Herba Cum Radice Asari Sieboldi (*Xi Xin*) and Fructus Gleditschiae Sinensis (*Zhu Ya Zao Jiao*), all in equal amounts. Boil together with Rhizoma Zingiberis (*Jiang*) and Bulbus Allii Fistulosi (*Cong*) and take. In addition, (one) should drink it with half a cup of Succus Bambusae (*Zhu Li*). One should also receive moxibustion. Recovery will follow a moderate sweat.

A person approximately 60 years of age was used to fat meat and fine grain. He (also) used to suffer from chronic constipation in the middle of summer and had committed the offence of chamber taxation[11] in addition. One day in the latrine, all of a sudden his hands became floppy and his eyes became wide open and lusterless. Urine came out unconsciously, sweat exuded like rain, a rale was heard in his throat like sawing, his respiration was extremely faint, and his pulse was large, irregular, and terribly arrhythmic. This was yin depletion followed by sudden expiry of yang. While (I) immediately ordered the boiling of some Radix Panacis Ginseng (*Ren Shen*) to a paste[12], I moxaed *Qi Hai* (CV 6) with the moxa cones as big as the small finger. When the eighteenth cone was burned up, his right hand was able to move.

---

[11] *I.e.*, sexual intercourse

[12] A *gao* is a thick paste made by boiling a decoction down until it becomes something like a jelly.

Another 3 cones and his lips began to move a little. By that time, the ginseng paste was ready and 1 cupful was administered. By midnight, 3 cupfuls were taken, and his eyes became able to move. It was not until 2 *jin* (of ginseng) had been taken that his ability to speak was restored and he began to ask for gruel. After taking 5 *jin*, his urinary incontinence was checked. After taking 10 *jin*, safety was secured.

Postpartum wind stroke in women should not be treated as wind but by (administration of) *Xiao Xu Ming Tang* (Minor Reinforce Life Decoction).[13] The only choice is to greatly supplement qi and blood and after that to treat phlegm. Such treatment should be carried out in accordance with the (relative) quantities of qi and blood determined by the pulses at both hands.

A fundamental method for the treatment of wind stroke is to drain heart fire. Lung metal is consequently cleared and, since liver wood is no longer replete, the spleen will be free from injury.[14] (In addition), supplement kidney water and heart fire is consequently downborne. Therefore the lungs are no longer subjected to heat. With the spleen and lungs calmed down, the *yang ming* becomes replete (*i.e.*, in this case, solid, better). With the *yang ming* replete, the gathering sinews are moistened and enabled to bind the bones and disinhibit the joints.

---

[13] This is composed of Herba Ephedrae (*Ma Huang*), Radix Stephaniae Tetrandrae (*Fang Ji*), Radix Panacis Ginseng (*Ren Shen*), Radix Scutellariae Baicalensis (*Huang Qin*), Cortex Cinnamomi (*Gui Xin*), Radix Glycyrrhizae (*Gan Cao*), Radix Paeoniae Lactiflorae (*Shao Yao*), Rhizoma Ligustici Wallichii (*Chuan Xiong*), Semen Pruni Armeniacae (*Xing Ren*), processed Radix Praeparatus Aconiti Carmichaeli (*Zhi Fu Zi*), Radix Ledebouriellae Sesloidis (*Fang Feng*), and fresh Rhizoma Zingiberis (*Sheng Jiang*).

[14] The logic underlying this is that heart fire restrains the lung metal, while lung metal in turn restrains liver wood. When heart fire is drained, lung metal is freed from torment and, consequently, liver wood is no longer subject to harm done by the injured lungs.

Du Qing Bi Tong Shen San (Du Qing-bi's[15] Free the Spirit Powder, consists of) Bombyx Batryticatus (*Bai Jiang Can*), 7 pieces, baked dry, ground to powder. Take brewed with half a cup of fresh Succus Zingiberis (*Sheng Jiang Zhi*) and wind phlegm will immediately be vomited. A little later, another 7 pieces of Bombyx Batryticatus should be taken in the same way to eject (the wind phlegm) completely. Then take Radix Et Rhizoma Rhei (*Da Huang*), the size of two fingers, wrap in paper, and roast well. Soak with saliva and swallow this down. About the time (it takes to eat) a meal later, administer still more Radix Et Rhizoma Rhei. If (the patient's) mouth is tightly shut, boil this with Bombyx Batryticatus and pour through a bamboo pipe down one of the nostrils, the left for males and the right for females.

Since the *Nei Jing*, wind stroke disease has been regarded as an external strike by wind evils. However, the country is divided into the south and the north, and (therefore, this disease) cannot be treated in one and the same way. (We) should follow (Liu) He-jian, who is unquestionably right in ascribing (this disease) to inappropriate nursing and (inadequate) rest with water unable to restrain fire. According to (the cases) available (to me) so far, (although) there is indeed external wind stroke, it is only extremely rarely seen. Therefore, neither is it right to ascribe all cases to inappropriate nursing and (inadequate) rest and exclude external stroke.

Master Xu has spoken of a qi stroke variety and there is also this kind as well.[16] This is a damage by the seven affects[17] (as manifest-

---

[15] A.k.a. Du Ben (1276-1350 CE), a versatile scholar studied in history, literature, and medicine and founder of tongue diagnosis in Chinese medicine. His main contribution to TCM is his augmentation of the *Jin Jing Lu (Golden Mirror Records)* by Ao Ji-wong.

[16] Xu Shu-wei (1079-circa 1154 CE), who was distinguished for his profound research into the *Shang Han Lun* by Zhang Zhong-jing. He is addressed as a master because he was titled Master in the then royal academy.

[17] A.k.a. the seven affects. These are joy, anger, anxiety, thought, sorrow, fear, and fright.

ed by) a large, floating pulse; a floating, tight pulse; or a moderate, slow pulse. These are all wind pulses. Slow and floating pulses indicate that a cure is possible, while a large, rapid, urgent pulse (foretells) death.

In the case of true external stroke, (Li) Dong-yuan's[18] logic (of categorizing) stroke of the blood vessels, stroke of the bowels, and stroke of the viscera is a beautiful approach. In some cases, inability to lift the limbs looks like atony, and these should be distinguished carefully. In the *Ju Fang (Collected Formulas)*[19], wind stroke and atony are treated in the same way. This is fundamentally erroneous. The *Fa Hui (Criticisms & Revelations)*[20] deals with this at length. Zhang Zi-he's[21] three methods[22] are applicable to sudden stroke of evil qi with exuberant phlegm and repletion heat, but they are inapplicable otherwise.

---

[18]   Li Dong-yuan (1180-1251 CE), founder of one of the four great schools of the Jin-Yuan Dynasties, whose main works were the *Pi Wei Lun (Treatise on the Spleen & Stomach)* and the *Lan Shi Mi Cang (Secret Collection of the Exquisite Orchid Library)*. His doctrine can be best summarized as the belief that any contraction of evil qi, including even external evils, is ultimately due to internal injury in turn due to vacuity of the spleen and stomach. Therefore, he based his treatment of whatever disease on supplementation of the stomach qi.

[19]   *Tai Ping Hui Min He Ji Ju Fang* in full, a work compiled by Chen Shi-wen *et al.* in 1151 CE. This was a collection of formulas mainly used by the then official pharmacy. For further information on this book, see the Translator's Preface.

[20]   *Ju Fang Fa Hui (Criticism & Revelation of the Ju Fang)* in full by Zhu Dan-xi, a work devoted to criticism and identification of errors in the *Tai Ping Hui Min He Ji Ju Fang*.

[21]   A.k.a. Zhang Cong-zheng (circa 1156-1228 CE), the first of all four great schools of the Jin-Yuan Dynasties who argued that all diseases should be attacked.

[22]   *I.e.*, diaphoresis, ejection, and precipitation

Chapter Two

Lai Wind

The great wind disease[1] is an affliction by the killing qi between heaven and earth [{a discussion of} which is found in the *Yi Yao (Essentials of Medicine)* {later editor}]. The treatment methods are (to use) *Zui Xian San* (Drunken Immortal Powder[2], if the evil is) in the upper or *Tong Tian Zai Zao San* (Free Heaven Re-creation Powder, if it is) in the lower, formulas in the *San Yin Fang (Three Causes Formulas)*[3], and afterwards *Tong Shen San* (Free the Spirit Powder)[4], *i.e.*, *Fang Feng Tong Shen San* (Ledebouriella Communicate with the Divinity Powder). At the same time, prick *Wei Zhong* (Bl 40) to let out blood with a three-edged needle. Those who do not keep an abstemious diet

---

[1] *Lai* or great wind is defined in some publications as leprosy, but, in fact, it covers a much wider range of cutaneous disorders. These are usually stubborn with pathological changes in skin color, etc.

[2] This is composed of Semen Sesami Indicae (*Hu Ma Zi*), Fructus Arctii Lappae (*Niu Bang Zi*), Fructus Lycii Chinensis (*Gou Qi Zi*), Semen Viticis (*Man Jing Zi*), Fructus Tribuli Terrestris (*Bai Ji Li*), Radix Sophorae Flavescentis (*Ku Shen*), Radix Ledebouriellae Sesloidis (*Fang Feng*), Fructus Trichosanthis Kirlowii (*Gua Lou*), and Calomelas (*Qing Fen*. It is so named because the taker may become as if intoxicated.

[3] A.k.a. the *San Yin Ji Yi Bing Zheng Fang Lun (Treatise on Diseases, Signs, and Formulas According to the Unified Theory of the Three Causes)* by Chen Wu-ze (1131-1189 CE)

[4] This is composed of Radix Ledebouriellae Sesloidis (*Fang Feng*), Rhizoma Ligustici Wallichii (*Chuan Xiong*), Radix Angelicae Sinensis (*Dang Gui*), Radix Paeoniae Lactiflorae (*Shao Yao*), Radix Et Rhizoma Rhei (*Da Huang*), Mirabilitum (*Mang Xiao*), Fructus Forsythiae Suspensae (*Lian Qiao*), Herba Menthae (*Bo He*), Herba Ephedrae (*Ma Huang*), Gypsum (*Shi Gao*), Radix Platycodi Grandiflori (*Jie Geng*), Radix Scutellariae Baicalensis (*Huang Qin*), Rhizoma Atractylodis Macrocephalae (*Bai Zhu*), Fructus Gardeniae Jasminoidis (*Shan Zhi Zi*), Herba Seu Flos Schizonepetae Tenuifoliae (*Jing Jie Sui*), Talcum (*Hua Shi*), and dry Rhizoma Zingiberis (*Gan Jiang*).

or refrain from chamber taxation are incurable. (The amounts of the ingredients in) *Zui Xian San* [which can be found in the *Yi Yao* {later editor}] should vary quantitatively in accordance with the age as well as (the state of) vacuity and repletion (of the patient). For those with severe and acute signs, *Zai Zao San* should be administered first to precipitate (the evil). This formula should not be administered till supplementation and nurturing has affected rehabilitation. In the course of taking this formula, (one) should not eat salt, fermented soybean jam, vinegar, various fish, meats, spices, fruits, and roasted and fried foods. (They should) eat only bland gruel or cooked vegetables which should also be taken bland. Eggplants are forbidden but Zaocys Dhumnades (*Wu Shao She*) and Coluber Spinalis (*Cai Hua She*) can be taken bland (*i.e.*, without salt) after being cooked in wine to assist the strength of the medicinals.

A (variant) version says: Although *Zui Xian San* has a singular effect, it must have silver dust (*Yin Fen*) as its envoy. Because it is an important ingredient for penetrating the diaphragm to free the large intestine, silver dust is employed to drive the various ingredients into the (hand) *yang ming* channel to open the depression of wind heat and diaphragmatic glomus. As a result, the toxins of the malign qi and foul filth are eliminated, and the worms generated by them are killed. (Silver dust) can ascend along the channel to the teeth, the tender and thin parts, to eliminate the foul and toxic drool. If the teeth are injured by taking this drug, (one can) rub (the teeth) with powdered Rhizoma Coptidis Chinensis (*Huang Lian*) or solidify water[5] in advance to resolve (*i.e.*, anticipate) the toxins of silver dust.

Tong Tian Zai Zao San is composed of good quality, blast-fried Radix Et Rhizoma Rhei (*Da Huang*), 1 *liang*, and blast-fried, solitarily growing Spina Gleditschiae Sinensis (*Zao Jiao Ci*), 1.5 *liang*. These should preferably be the large black ones of the previous year. Powder the above finely (and take) 2 *qian* per dose, brewed with cold wine in the evening. Prepare a night stool to wait for the worms to be discharged. Those with black mouths are years old worms. Those with red mouths are young ones. Several days later, another dose should be taken. (The

---

[5] Silver is greatly cold and is able to enter the kidneys. To counteract its undesirable effects, one can fortify water, *i.e.*, fortify the kidneys with water-boosting medicinals.

disease) cannot be exterminated till these worms are all removed. A variant version says: According to our master, *Tong Tian Zai Zao San* includes, in addition, Tuber Curcumae (*Yu Jin*), one half *liang*, used raw, and Semen Pharbitidis (*Bai Qian Niu*), 6 *qian*, used half raw and half stir-fried.

One formula to treat numbness wind (consists of) *Si Wu Tang* (Four Materials Decoction) plus Radix Et Rhizoma Notopterygii (*Qiang Huo*), Radix Ledebouriellae Sesloidis (*Fang Feng*), Pericarpium Citri Reticulatae (*Chen Pi*), and Radix Glycyrrhizae (*Gan Cao*). Another formula (consists of) Radix Et Rhizoma Rhei (*Da Huang*), Radix Scutellariae Baicalensis (*Huang Qin*), and Realgar (*Xiong Huang*), three ingredients altogether. Powder the above. Then boil Folium Cinnamomi Camphorae (*Zhang Shu Ye*) to a thick decoction and put in the preceding medicinals for steaming and washing. To treat numbness wind with a large and vacuous pulse, (use) Fructus Xanthii Sibirici (*Cang Er*), Fructus Arctii Lappae (*Niu Bang*), steamed with wine, each 3 *qian*, Rhizoma Polygonati (*Huang Jing*) and Herba Spirodelae Polyrrhizae (*Fu Ping*), 1 *liang* each, and Radix Sophorae Flavescentis (*Ku Shen*), 7.5 *qian*. Powder the above. Boil in wine Zaocys Dhumnades (*Wu She*) or, if not available, snakeheaded fish instead, with this make (the above medicinals) into pills and take. After the pulse is found replete, also use *Tong Tian Zao San* to remove worms.

A formula to treat pestilential wind (consists of) equal amounts of Fructus Xanthii Sibirici (*Cang Er*), Folium Spirodelae Polyrrhizae (*Ye Fu Ping*), and Fructus Arctii Lappae (*Shu Nian Zi*), stir-fried with sprayed on bean wine.[6] Powder the above and take with sprayed on bean wine. In a (variant) formula, there is snake meat (in addition). *Huang Jing Wan* (Polygonatum Pills, consist of) equal amounts of stir-fried Fructus Xanthii Sibirici (*Cang Er*), Folium Spirodelae Polyrrhizae (*Ye Fu Ping*), and Fructus Arctii Lappae (*Shu Nian Zi*, plus) half as much snake meat, stripped of skin and bone after being soaked in wine. Weigh out twice as much of Rhizoma Polygonati (*Huang Jing*) as the preceding 3 medicinals. Pound these without anything added but the Herba Xanthii Sibirici (etc.) and bake dry. Powder and make into pills with flour.

---

[6] The processing method is as follows: Obtain a certain amount of black soybeans, boil, stir-fry till no smoke is seen any more, collect in a ceramic pot, quench with wine, soak overnight, and remove the beans. The remaining wine is left for use.

Vacuity itching of the upper body is the result of blood failing to nurture the muscle interstices. Administer *Si Wu Tang* plus Radix Scutellariae Baicalensis (*Huang Qin*) brewed with powdered Folium Spirodelae Polyrrhizae (*Fu Ping*). To treat itching all over the body, powder 1 *qian* of Flos Campsis Grandiflorae (*Ling Xiao Hua*), brew with wine (and take). A (variant) version gives an instruction on the administration of *Tong Tian Zai Zao San*: Towards sunrise, (one) should face east, taking it with limeless wine[7], as much as one can. (Thus) a moderate condition will be checked when there is diarrhea of foul and filthy substance like fish intestines. Keep away from toxins for half a month, taking merely thin gruel and soft food. Then eyebrows, hair, and skin will gradually grow (back) to normal. Even a severe case does not need administration more than 2-3 times, but care should be taken about nursing and rectifying (*i.e.*, reposing). Do not toil and tax (on oneself) unwisely and do not take the meat of calf, horse, ass, and mule for (the rest of one's) life. Those who violate (these prohibitions) will die without a remedy.

Chapter Three

Cold Damage

Warming and dissipation are the ruling (methods for the treatment of this disease). There may be sudden stroke by cold qi between heaven and earth and damage by cold and raw foods through the mouth. For external contraction with no internal damage, use the methods of (Zhang) Zhong-jing. If internal damage is embraced within (vacuity, use) *Bu Zhong Yi Qi Tang* (Supplement the Center & Boost the Qi Decoction) plus (wind cold) effusing medicinals. It is necessary to first

---

[7]   In the past, during the final stage of wine-production, some lime was put in to make the wine clearer. The wine thus made was called limed wine, while wine made without lime was called limeless wine.

to prop up the righteous qi with Radix Panacis Ginseng (*Ren Shen*) and Radix Astragali Membranacei (*Huang Qi*).

Cold in the center with great vacuity of stomach qi justifies warming and dissipating with *Li Zhong Tang* (Rectify the Center Decoction).[1] For serious cases, add Radix Praeparatus Aconiti Carmichaeli (*Fu Zi*). With center cold, sudden (external) contraction may start a disease immediately and violently. This is because, in persons with a cold center, if (external evils) take advantage of loose and wide open interstices, all parts of the body are subject to evils. It is difficult to identify which channel or connecting vessel is involved, and there is no heat to dissipate. Warming and supplementation can effect resolution naturally. Because this is great vacuity of the stomach qi, unless it is treated without delay, death is quite close. Dai[2] comments: This is spoken of as a disease arising out of the body being subjected to astringing and killing qi and eating cold substances, like iced water, melons, and fruits. The pulse must be deep and thin with cold hands and feet, faint breathing, bodily fatigue, absence of thirst despite fever, and disinclination to speak. If this method is applied by mistake to a heat disease, a moderate case is exacerbated and a serious case dies. A rapid pulse, (excessive) drinking of water, or vexed agitation and restlessness indicate a heat disease in any case.

The two patterns, cold and heat, are like water and fire, and the contraction of them cannot be treated in the same way. Inappropriate treatment may kill a patient. Students must be very cautious! It may be questioned why supplementation is recommended since subjection

---

[1] This is composed of Radix Panacis Ginseng (*Ren Shen*), dry Rhizoma Zingiberis (*Gan Jiang*), mix-fried Radix Glycyrrhizae (*Zhi Gan Cao*), and Rhizoma Atractylodis Macrocephalae (*Bai Zhu*).

[2] Dai Si-gong (circa 1324-1405CE), styled Yuan-li, faithful pupil of Zhu Zhen-heng. He was director of the imperial medical board of his time and helped to bring out and propagate the doctrines of his master. As a matter of fact, the present work is believed to be written by Dai Yuan-li rather than Zhu Zhen-heng in person. From the many comments inserted in the texts, it is obvious that Dai at least helped collect the materials and participated in the compilation of this work.

to evils means a disease of superabundance. The *Nei Jing (Inner Classic)* says: Wherever evils converge, the qi invariably becomes vacuous there. (Therefore,) internal damage is extremely common, while external contraction is but occasionally met. Moderate patterns, such as colds and flu, should not rashly be considered cold damage and treated as such.

A disease wrought by cold damage presupposes the body (already) offended by cold qi and eating inappropriately cold substances and must necessarily be (treated) with a version of *Bu Zhong Yi Qi Tang* with additions and subtractions and with effusing medicinals added. Cold damage embracing internal damage [{a discussion of which} is found in the *Yi Yao (Essentials of Medicine)* {later editor}], irrespective of the conditions of external contraction, first requires Radix Panacis Ginseng (*Ren Shen*) and Radix Astragali Membranacei (*Huang Qi*) to prop up the righteous qi. (Only) afterwards should one introduce effusing medicinals. Moderate illnesses, like the patterns of colds and flu, must not be considered cold damage and treated rashly as such. The west and the north are regions of extreme cold with astringing and killing (qi). Therefore, external damage is extremely common there. The east and the south are warm and temperate regions where external damage is extremely rarely seen, only one or two out of a hundred or even thousand cases.

Some miscellaneous diseases may look like diseases of the six channels[3], and for that reason, lay and vulgar persons are often confused and find it difficult to distinguish these. If a pattern displays much similarity to cold damage (only in its signs), it is always (determined as) a miscellaneous pattern. Detailed discussions of it are all derived from the "Treatise On Heat Disease (*Re Lun*)" in the *Nei Jing (Inner Classic)*.[4] Since Chang Sha[5], many a scholar has carried out research,

---

[3] According to Zhang Zhong-jing, cold damage is transmitted in order of the six channels. Therefore, cold damage is implied here.

[4] *I.e., Su Wen (Simple Questions)*, Ch. 31

but over the past thousand years, that which has tapped the pith and essence (of the issue) is none other than the teachings of (Li) Dong-yuan. He says that internal damage is extremely common, while external damage is but occasionally seen. This (statement) reveals a truth that no predecessors have ever shed light on before. (Li) Dong-yuan has given a comprehensive description on how to identify the pulses of internal and external damage. People after him have followed a vulgar point of view. Unable to see the truth and confused before the similarities, they commit the diabolical mistake of taking (internal) for external damage. They may have occasionally implemented a cure, (but) that is because they did not act too recklessly and they used many harmonizing and resolving or moderating and pacifying medicinals to effect dissipation. A reckless person will be a murderer. Be cautious by all means!

Chapter Four

Internal Damage

This (disease) is especially governed by what is discussed at great length by (Li) Dong-yuan concerning the differentiation between internal and external damage. The majority of people in the world contract this kind of disease. However, it may contain within it phlegm or external evils or be started by depression internally. In all such cases, supplementation of the original qi is the ruling (modality), and other medicinals should be introduced depending upon what is contained within (this vacuity).

---

[5] Zhang Ji, better known as Zhang Zhong-jing. Sometimes he is named Zhang Chang-sha because he once held the office of governor of Changsha Prefecture, present Changsha City, Hunan.

In case of contained phlegm (use) *Bu Zhong Yi Qi Tang* (Supplement the Center & Boost the Qi Decoction) with large amounts of Rhizoma Pinelliae Ternatae (*Ban Xia*) and Succus Zingiberis (*Jiang Zhi*) to transport and convey (phlegm).

Chapter Five

Summerheat

For summerheat qi or sudden turmoil (*i.e.*, acute gastroenteritis with vomiting and diarrhea, use) *Huang Lian Xiang Ru Yin* (Coptis & Elsholtzia Drink).[1] In case of embraced phlegm, add Rhizoma Pinelliae Ternatae (*Ban Xia*). If (evil qi) has taken advantage of qi vacuity, add Radix Panacis Ginseng (*Ren Shen*) and Radix Astragali Membranacei (*Huang Qi*).

For summerheat illness with internal damage (use) *Qing Shu Yi Qi Tang* (Clear Summer Heat & Boost the Qi Decoction).[2] If there is thirst, add Radix Rehmanniae (*Sheng Di Huang*), Tuber Ophiopogonis Japonicae (*Mai Men Dong*), Radix Cyathulae (*Chuan Niu Xi*), stir-fried Cortex Phellodendri (*Huang Bai*), Rhizoma Anemarrhenae (*Zhi Mu*), Radix Puerariae Lobatae (*Ge Gen*), and Radix Glycyrrhizae (*Sheng Gan Cao*).

To treat all kinds of summerheat, (use) *Yu Long Wan* (Jade Dragon Pills): Semen Lepidis Apetali (*Chi Ting*), Sulphur (*Wo Liu Huang*), Nitre (*Xiao Shi*),

---

[1] This is composed of stir-fried Semen Dolichoris Lablabis (*Bian Dou*), Cortex Magnoliae Officinalis (*Hou Po*), and Herba Elsholtziae Splendensis (*Xiang Ru*).

[2] This is composed of Radix Panacis Quinquefolii (*Xi Yang Shen*), Herba Dendrobii (*Shi Hu*), Tuber Ophiopogonis Japonicae (*Mai Men Dong*), Rhizoma Coptidis Chinensis (*Huang Lian*), Folium Bambusae (*Zhu Ye*), Ramus Nelumbinis Nuciferae (*He Geng*), Rhizoma Anemarrhenae (*Zhi Mu*), Radix Glycyrrhizae (*Gan Cao*), Semen Oryzae Sativae (*Jing Mi*), and Pericarpium Citrulli Vulgaris (*Xi Gua Cui Yi*).

Talcum (*Hua Shi*), and Alum (*Ming Fan*), 1 *liang* (each). Powder and make into pills with 6 *liang* of fine (wheat) flour and rain water.

For qi vacuity with low food intake, body heat, spontaneous sweating, and fatigue, (use) *Qing Shu Yi Qi Tang*. (But) for qi vacuity with low food intake, spontaneous heat, spontaneous sweating, and a thin, weak or large, surging pulse, (use) *Bu Zhong Yi Qi Tang* plus Tuber Ophiopogonis Japonicae (*Mai Men Dong*), Fructus Schizandrae Chinensis (*Wu Wei Zi*), and Rhizoma Anemarrhenae (*Zhi Mu*).

For summerheat qi with vexing thirst and a vacuous pulse, (use) *Zhu Ye Shi Gao Tang* (Bamboo Leaf & Gypsum Decoction).[3] (But) a summerheat illness with vexation and agitation day and night and incessantly drinking water which comes to an end at daybreak, generalized swelling, dripping of the bladder, absence of thirst, and requesting a fan at night should be treated by *Leng Xiang Yin Zi* (Cool Fragrance Drink).[4]

In the sixth month, a person more than 50 years of age had an attack of fever with massive sweating, aversion to cold, uncheckable shivering, and vexing thirst. This was summer heat illness. All his pulses were vacuous, faint, thin, and weak as well as rapid. This person was an addicted gambler, and hence caused himself taxation which led to vacuity. Then (he) was administered a decoction of Radix Panacis Ginseng (*Ren Shen*) brewed with *Ren Shen Si Ling San* (Added Ginseng Four *Ling* Powder).[5] Eight doses and he was quiet (*i.e.*, recuperated).

---

[3] This is composed of Folium Bambusae (*Zhu Ye*), Gypsum (*Shi Gao*), Tuber Ophiopogonis Japonicae (*Mai Men Dong*), Rhizoma Pinelliae Ternatae (*Ban Xia*), Radix Panacis Ginseng (*Ren Shen*), mix-fried Radix Glycyrrhizae (*Zhi Gan Cao*), and Semen Oryzae Sativae (*Jing Mi*).

[4] This is composed of mix-fried Radix Glycyrrhizae (*Zhi Gan Cao*), Radix Praeparatus Aconiti Carmichaeli (*Fu Zi*), Fructus Amomi Tsao-ko (*Cao Guo Ren*), Pericarpium Citri Rubri (*Ju Hong*), and fresh Rhizoma Zingiberis (*Sheng Jiang*).

[5] This is composed of Radix Panacis Ginseng (*Ren Shen*), Sclerotium Poriae Cocoris (*Fu Ling*), Sclerotium Polypori Umbellati (*Zhu Ling*), Rhizoma Alismatis (*Ze Xie*), and Rhizoma Atractylodis Macrocephalae (*Bai Zhu*).

Dai comments: Summerheat is the raging heat in the summer months, and the qi of this exuberant heat is liable to catch people (during those months. Due to that qi,) there may be affliction, damage, and stroke, which are different in terms of severity and distinguishable in terms of vacuity and repletion. The two (disorders) of abdominal pain with water diarrhea, (*i.e.,*) sufferings of the stomach and the large intestine, and nausea which is (due to) phlegm and rheum in the stomach opening are (both) afflictions by summer heat. (For them,) *Huang Lian Xiang Ru Yin* can be used. Rhizoma Coptidis Chinensis (*Huang Lian*) can abate summer heat and Herba Elsholtziae Splendensis (*Xiang Ru*) is able to disperse accumulated water.

Body heat with headache, agitation and restlessness, or pricking pain all over the body, this is heat damaging the flesh partings. It requires the toxin-resolving *Bai Hu Tang* (White Tiger Decoction)[6] plus Radix Bupleuri (*Chai Hu*). In case of qi vacuity, add Radix Panacis Ginseng (*Ren Shen*). Coughing, alternating cold and heat, and thief sweating (*i.e.*, night sweating) with a constantly rapid pulse is heat fixing to the lung channel. This requires *Qing Fei Tang* (Clear the Lungs Decoction)[7], *Chai Hu Tian Shui San* (Bupleurum Heavenly Water Powder)[8], and the like. If treated in a timely (manner) it will be alright, but any delay will lead to inability to cure. (In this case,) exuberant fire is overwhelming metal. This is summerheat stroke.

To treat any disease, it is vital to have a clear identification and not to mete out a treatment without discrimination. (Summer heat illness) can also be found occasionally in spring or autumn. (Therefore, one) should not adhere to a one-sided view. The wise policy is to design

---

[6] This is composed of Rhizoma Anemarrhenae (*Zhi Mu*), Gypsum (*Shi Gao*), mix-fried Radix Glycyrrhizae (*Zhi Gan Cao*), and Semen Oryzae Sativae (*Jing Mi*).

[7] This is composed of Semen Coicis Lachryma-jobi (*Yi Yi Ren*), Radix Stephaniae Tetrandrae (*Fang Ji*), Semen Pruni Armeniacae (*Xing Ren*), and Semen Benincasae Hispidae (*Dong Gua Ren*).

[8] This is composed of Radix Bupleuri (*Chai Hu*), Talcum (*Hua Shi*), and mix-fried Radix Glycyrrhizae (*Zhi Gan Cao*).

formulas in accordance with diseases (in this case meaning patterns). One formula (is to) boil Herba Elsholtziae Splendensis (*Xiang Ru*, first down) to a thick decoction, then down to a paste, and then make into pills. These remove summerheat and disinhibit minor water.[9]

Summerheat is classified into a yang and a yin pattern and both require *Huang Lian Xiang Ru Yin, Qing Shu Yi Qi Tang, Wu Ling San* (Five *Ling* Powder)[10], and the like. There may be cases of embraced phlegm or where vacuity is taken advantage of (by evils). In case of embraced phlegm, add Rhizoma Pinelliae Ternatae (*Ban Xia*). If (evil qi) is taking advantage of vacuity, add such (medicinals) as Radix Panacis Ginseng (*Ren Shen*) and Radix Astragali Membranacei (*Huang Qi*). Pulse method: when one palpates, one acquires a pulse image which is faint and weak, is feeble when pressure is applied, comes on hidden and deeplying, or is vacuous.

Chapter Six

Summer Sickness[1]

This (condition) is ascribed to yin vacuity, (*i.e.,*) original qi insufficiency. Dai comments: It is (an illness contracted) between late summer and early autumn (consisting) of headache, weak legs, low food intake,

---

[9] *I.e.*, urination

[10] This is composed of Sclerotium Polypori Umbellati (*Zhu Ling*), Rhizoma Atractylodis Macrocephalae (*Bai Zhu*), Sclerotium Poriae Cocoris (*Fu Ling*), Rhizoma Alismatis (*Ze Xie*), and Ramulus Cinnamomi (*Gui Zhi*).

[1] A.k.a summer atony (*xia wei*). This is due to the weakness of the spleen and stomach and retention of rheum and damp heat with manifestations as described in the text.

bodily fatigue, and generalized fever. The pulse is large and wiry. Subtract Radix Bupleuri (*Chai Hu*) and Rhizoma Cimicifugae (*Sheng Ma*) from *Bu Zhong Yi Qi Tang* (Supplement the Center & Boost the Qi Decoction) and add stir-fried Cortex Phellodendri (*Huang Bai*). *Sheng Mai San* (Generate the Pulse Powder) is (also) appropriate: Tuber Ophiopogonis Japonicae (*Mai Men Dong*), Fructus Schizandrae Chinensis (*Wu Wei Zi*), and Radix Panacis Ginseng (*Ren Shen*). (It) comes from the *Qian Jin Fang (Prescriptions [Worth] A Thousand [Pieces of] Gold)*.[2] One may also subtract Radix Bupleuri (*Chai Hu*) and Rhizoma Cimicifugae (*Sheng Ma*) from *Bu Zhong Yi Qi Tang* and add stir-fried Cortex Phellodendri (*Huang Bai*) and Radix Paeoniae Lactiflorae (*Shao Yao*). In case of embraced phlegm, add Rhizoma Pinelliae Ternatae (*Ban Xia*), Rhizoma Arisaematis (*Nan Xing*), Pericarpium Citri Reticulatae (*Chen Pi*), and the like.

Chapter Seven

Summerheat Wind[1]

Summerheat wind, if it is (an illness of) phlegm, requires ejection. If fire and phlegm are embraced, one can use the ejection method for those with repletion. Those cases of summer heat wind that can be treated by ejection are actually summer heat stroke. Such patients must (already) have had fire heat and phlegm repletion internally. When they try to escape from summer heat and enjoy coolness in the shade,

---

[2] The medical *magnum opus* by Sun Si-miao of the Tang Dynasty

[1] As the author explains, this is a type of summerheat stroke, but usually accompanied by symptoms such as clenched jaw, spasm, or even loss of consciousness and arched back rigidity. In other words, this is a combination of summerheat stroke with wind symptoms.

the eight winds[2] assault them. (Thus internal fire) is depressed and develops into generalized fever with possible cloudedness and dizziness. (In that case,) along with ejection one should (also use) diaphoresis. Depressed fire is resolved once helped by diaphoresis. Wind is dissipated once helped by diaphoresis. (And) phlegm is discharged once helped by gushing sweat. (Hence) one effort accomplishes three results. This is an expedient treatment for those with phlegm repletion contained within, rather than a general treatment modality for summer heat wind. For summer heat wind without anything contained within, it is appropriate to apply diaphoresis (alone) to dissipate (wind).

Chapter Eight

Stomach Wind

The pulse of stomach wind is wiry, moderate, and floating in the right *guan* section.[1] This is caused by enjoying cool breezes immediately after taking food or drink. Its signs are inability to take in food and drink, emaciation, an enlarged belly, aversion to wind, copious sweating on the head, and an obstructed diaphragm. *Wei Feng Tang* (Stomach Wind Decoction)[2] is the very (formula) to treat this. (However,) it should be modified in accordance with any pattern contained within.

---

[2] *I.e.*, winds from eight points of the compass

[1] *I.e.*, the middle section of the radial artery pulse at the wrist

[2] This is composed of Rhizoma Atractylodis Macrocephalae (*Bai Zhu*), Rhizoma Ligustici Wallichii (*Chuan Xiong*), Radix Panacis Ginseng (*Ren Shen*), Radix Albus Paeoniae Lactiflorae (*Bai Shao Yao*), Radix Angelicae Sinensis (*Dang Gui*), Cortex Cinnamomi (*Rou Gui*), and Sclerotium Poriae Cocoris (*Fu Ling*).

Chapter Nine

Dampness

In the *Ben Cao (Materia Medica)*[1], Rhizoma Atractylodis (*Cang Zhu,* is prescribed) to treat dampness (and) applicable for (dampness) either in the upper or lower. *Er Chen Tang* (Two Aged Decoction) plus wine-processed Radix Scutellariae Baicalensis (*Huang Qin*), Radix Et Rhizoma Notopterygii (*Qiang Huo*), and Rhizoma Atractylodis (*Cang Zhu*) can dissipate wind and move dampness. In treating dampness, *Er Chen Tang* is able to moisten the stool and make voiding of the urine long if up-raising agents are added. For dampness in the upper, Rhizoma Atractylodis (*Cang Zhu*) is tremendously meritorious, (while) dampness in the lower (requires) upraising. Dampness in the external requires effusing through the exterior, (but) dampness in the internal requires bland percolators. Bland percolators treat dampness in the upper and middle burners. If the dampness is in the upper, moderate diaphoresis is appropriate for resolving it, copious sweating being undesirable. Therefore, medicinals such as Herba Ephedrae (*Ma Huang*) and Radix Puerariae Lobatae (*Ge Gen*) are not used. For treatment methods for various patterns of excessive dampness, one should refer to the pertinent chapters on these.

Dai comments: Medicinals to treat dampness are varied. Each medicinal can be regarded as important depending upon what it treats. (Therefore,) one cannot rightly use the single flavor, Rhizoma Atractylodis (*Cang Zhu*), in all cases. Our master deliberately came up with the above instruction to enlighten people.

Dai comments (further): In the causation of disease, dampness may

---

[1] *Shen Nong Ben Cao (The Divine Husbandman's Materia Medica)* in full, presumably compiled in the Han Dynasty by unknown author(s). This is the first pharmacopeia in Chinese medicine.

intrude from the outside or emerge from within. It is necessary to study pathogenesis in (the light of a particular) geographical region. The east and south are of low lands where rain abounds excessively and the ground is damp. (The dampness) suffered from (in these regions) invariably comes from outside and usually starts from below. Therefore heavy leg foot qi[2] is quite common. To treat this, it is necessary to dissipate (dampness) through diaphoresis. (However,) for chronic cases it is appropriate to course, percolate, and drain. The west and north are high lands where people eat much raw and cold food and sodden wheat food. After (eating these) or drinking wine, if the cold qi (from such food) is depressed, then dampness cannot be evicted. This (then) causes distention and pain in the abdominal skin; if extreme, water drum distention and fullness; or puffy swelling all over the body (as limp) as mud and which remains indented after pressure is relieved. This is (dampness) emerging from within. Depending upon the amount of original qi, (one should) disinhibit urination and defecation (and thus) chase the root cause in the internal. However, internal and external (disease causes) are co-existent in many parts of the country. Only the proportion between these vary (from one part to another). It is necessary to practice a treatment appropriate to the pattern, and (one) should not adhere to one exclusive way.

On getting up one morning in the ninth month, a male aged 35 suddenly (experienced) loss of brightness of his eyes and inability to see. He was very eager for his eyesight (to return), but he did not get (even) a (dim) perception of things and figures till quite a while later. He was unable to identify what he saw. His food intake reduced to half as much as usual and his spirit and thought, (*i.e.*, mind,) were extremely languid. Five days after (contraction of) this disease, his pulse was retarded and large, over four beats (per breath). This was treated as subjection to dampness. Inquiry revealed that he in fact contracted (this condition) after having slept on damp ground for half

---

[2]   This pattern is characterized by insensitivity and swelling of legs and feet and, in extreme cases, cardiac and mental disorders. One should note that in modern Chinese, *jiao qi* (foot qi) in most cases refers to athlete's foot.

a month. With Rhizoma Atractylodis Macrocephalae (*Bai Zhu*) as the sovereign, Radix Astragali Membranacei (*Huang Qi*) and Pericarpium Citri Reticulatae (*Chen Pi*) as the ministers, Radix Praeparatus Aconiti Carmichaeli (*Fu Zi*) as the assistant, a little more than 10 doses achieved recuperation.

For dampness lodging and causing heaviness and pain in the low back and knees with puffy, swollen feet and lower legs, *Chu Shi Dan* (Remove Dampness Elixir, is appropriate), for which see the chapter on foot qi (*i.e.*, Ch. 85, Bk. 5).

Chapter Ten

Fire

Yin vacuity with stirring fire is difficult to treat. Vacuity fire can be treated by supplementation; repletion fire by drainage; a moderate case by downbearing; a severe case by following the propensity (of fire) to upbear.[1] Depressed fire can be treated by effusing but necessarily through the channel involved. Once qi becomes superabundant, there is fire. Extremely excessive fire must be treated by moderating. Radix Glycyrrhizae (*Sheng Gan Cao*) can be used to simultaneously drain and moderate, and Radix Panacis Ginseng (*Ren Shen*) and Rhizoma Atractylodis Macrocephalae (*Bai Zhu*) can also do this. Two conditions allow for effusion: wind cold invading from the external and depressed (fire). There are (also cases) where fire will descend of itself once yin is supplemented. Stir-fried Cortex Phellodendri (*Huang Bai*) and Radix Rehmanniae (*Di Huang*) are among those (medicinals which can accomplish this). In case of exuberant fire, cold and cool medicinals should not be administered rashly. (Rather,) it is imperative to use warm, dissipating ones. (For instance,) *Zuo Jin Wan* (Left Gold Pills) treat liver fire: Rhizoma Coptidis Chinensis (*Huang Lian*), 2 *liang*, and Fructus Evodiae Rutecarpae (*Wu Zhu Yu*), 1 *liang*. Powder the above and make into pills. Take 50 pills per dose with warm boiled water.

The yin vacuity pattern (of fire) is difficult to treat. *Si Wu Tang* (Four Materials Decoction) plus Cortex Phellodendri (*Huang Bai*) is a wonderful formula to downbear fire and supplement yin. Plastrum Testudinis (*Gui Ban*) supplements yin and is consummate yin within yin (in nature). Yin fire can be treated with *Si Wu Tang* plus the lower leg bone of the white horse, which, after being calcined, can be used instead of Radix Scutellariae Baicalensis (*Huang Qin*) and Rhizoma Coptidis Chinensis (*Huang Lian*) to downbear yin fire. Rhizoma Coptidis Chinensis, Radix Scutellariae Baicalensis, Fructus Gardeniae Jasminoidis (*Zhi Zi*), Radix Et Rhizoma Rhei (*Da Huang*), and Cortex Phellodendri can downbear fire, but they should not be used except (to treat) fire within the yin. Fructus Gardeniae Jasminoidis descends in a winding way so as to drain fire within the yin through urination. By nature, it descends and is able to downbear fire. This is little known to people. It also treats the fire inside glomus lumps. Radix Glycyrrhizae (*Sheng Gan Cao*) moderates fire evils. Caulis Akebiae Mutong (*Mu Tong*) descends, draining small intestine fire. Crystallized urine (*Ren Zhong Bai*) drains liver fire and downbears yin fire as well. (It can be used) only after exposure to wind and dew (*i.e.*, the weather) for 2-3 years. *Ren Zhong Huang* (*i.e.*, Radix Glycyrrhizae [*Gan Cao*] contained in a tightly sealed bamboo tube and submerged in a manure pit for at least 2 months, after which it is washed thoroughly) downbears yin fire. It is good for treating years old warm disease. Urine downbears fire extremely speedily.

Qi starting from the left side is liver fire. Qi starting from below the umbilicus is yin fire. Qi starting from the feet (travelling) to the abdomen is (due to) extreme vacuity. Fire starting from the nether septenary spring[1] is a disease that is not (usually) relievable in one (case) out of ten. One method (to treat this) is to apply powdered Radix Praeparatus Aconiti Carmichaeli (*Fu Zi*) on *Yong Quan* (Ki 1)[2] and administer *Si Wu Tang* with fire-downbearing medicinals added. This is wonderful.

A woman with qi repletion was irritable but without bursting (*i.e.*, giving in to outbursts of anger). One day, all of a sudden, she broke into a violent outburst. With a loud scream, she was at the point of inversion. This was because phlegm was obstructed above, while fire started from below, surging up. She was administered powdered Rhizoma Cyperi Rotundi (*Xiang Fu*), 5 qian, Rhizoma Glycyrrhizae (*Sheng Gan Cao*), 3 qian, and Rhizoma Ligustici Wallichii (*Chuan Xiong*), 7 qian. These were boiled in child's urine and Succus Zingiberis (*Jiang Zhi*). Then Pulvis Indigonis (*Qing Dai*), crystallized urine (*Ren Zhong Bai*), and Rhizoma Cyperi Rotundi (*Xiang Fu*) were powdered, added, and made into pills. After recovering to some extent, violent ejection was performed which (then) was followed by recuperation. Later *Dao Tan Tang* (Conduct Phlegm Decoction)[3] plus gingerfried Rhizoma Coptidis Chinensis (*Huang Lian*), Rhizoma Cyperi Rotundi (*Xiang Fu*), and fresh Rhizoma Zingiberis (*Sheng Jiang*) was administered in the form of a decoction taken with *Long Hui Wan* (Gentiana & Aloe Pills).[4]

---

[1] *I.e.*, the kidneys. In Chinese, this term originally meant death or the under or otherworld. Since the kidneys are located below the spleen which is earth and are the water viscera, they acquired this name.

[2] Located in the center of the sole of the foot, this point's name means gushing spring.

[3] This is composed of Rhizoma Pinelliae Ternatae (*Ban Xia*), Rhizoma Arisaematis (*Nan Xing*), Fructus Immaturus Citri Seu Ponciri (*Zhi Shi*), Sclerotium Poriae Cocoris (*Fu Ling*), Pericarpium Citri Rubri (*Ju Hong*), Radix Glycyrrhizae (*Gan Cao*), and fresh Rhizoma Zingiberis (*Sheng Jiang*).

[4] This is composed of Radix Angelicae Sinensis (*Dang Gui*), Radix Gentianae Scabrae (*Long Dan Cao*), Fructus Gardeniae Jasminoidis (*Shan Zhi Zi*), Rhizoma Coptidis Chinensis (*Huang Lian*), Cortex Phellodendri (*Huang Bai*), Radix Scutellariae Baicalensis (*Huang Qin*), Radix Et Rhizoma Rhei (*Da Huang*), dried Succus Alois (*Lu Hui*), Radix Saussureae Seu Vladimiriae (*Mu Xiang*), and Secretio Moschi Moschiferi

A person frequently had a murmuring sound like that of crabs in their lower abdomen. This was treated as yin fire. They were prescribed equal amounts of vanquished (*i.e.*, processed) Plastrum Testudinis (*Bai Gui Ban*), crisp-fried or moxaed[5] with salt and wine, Cacumen Biotae Orientalis (*Ce Bai*), steamed 9 times with wine and baked 9 times, wine-processed Cortex Phellodendri (*Huang Bai*), wine-processed Rhizoma Anemarrhenae (*Zhi Mu*), and wine-processed Rhizoma Ligustici Wallichii (*Chuan Xiong*). These were made into pills with paste; 80 pills per dose, taken with bland salt water.

Chapter Eleven

Depression

(So long as) qi and blood are in equilibrium and harmony, none of the ten thousand diseases can arise. But once depression exists, various diseases will be generated. The ten thousand diseases of the human body are all generated by depression. In general, Rhizoma Atractylodis (*Cang Zhu*) and Rhizoma Ligustici Wallichii (*Fu Xiong*) resolve the various kinds of depression. Other medicinals can be added in accordance with the signs. Depression always takes place in the middle burner. Rhizoma Atractylodis and Rhizoma Ligustici Wallichii can open and up-raise the (depressed) qi so as to up-lift it. If food is (obstructed) over the qi, it will descend of itself when the qi is up-raised. This serves as an example for other (conditions).

For qi depression, use Rhizoma Cyperi Rotundi (*Xiang Fu*). It works its way freely in the chest, but it must undergo soaking in child's urine

---

(*She Xiang*).

[5] The translator suspects that stir-fried should be read for moxaed.

(before use) or its nature can be too dry. Rhizoma Atractylodis (*Cang Zhu*) descends and should be soaked in rice water (before use). For damp depression, use Sclerotium Rubrum Poriae Cocoris (*Chi Fu Ling*), Rhizoma Atractylodis (*Cang Zhu*), Rhizoma Ligustici Wallichii (*Fu Xiong*), and Radix Angelicae (*Bai Zhi*). For phlegm depression, use Pumice (*[Fu] Hai Shi*), Rhizoma Cyperi Rotundi (*Xiang Fu*), Rhizoma Arisaematis (*Nan Xing*), Succus Zingiberis (*Jiang Zhi*), and Fructus Trichosanthis Kirlowii (*Gua Lou*). For heat depression, use Pulvis Indigonis (*Qing Dai*), Rhizoma Cyperi Rotundi (*Xiang Fu*), Rhizoma Atractylodis (*Cang Zhu*), Rhizoma Ligustici Wallichii (*Fu Xiong*), and stir-fried Fructus Gardeniae Jasminoidis (*Zhi Zi*). For blood depression, use skinned Semen Pruni Persicae (*Tao Ren*), Flos Carthami Tinctorii (*Hong Hua*), Pulvis Levis Indigonis (*Qing Dai*), Rhizoma Cyperi Rotundi (*Xiang Fu*), and Rhizoma Ligustici Wallichii (*Fu Xiong*). For food depression, use Rhizoma Atractylodis (*Cang Zhu*), Rhizoma Cyperi Rotundi (*Xiang Fu*), Fructus Crataegi (*Shan Zha*), Massa Medica Fermentata (*Shen Qu*), and iron dust (*Zhen Sha*)[1] which must be quenched in vinegar 7 times and be ground very finely. In spring, add (more) Rhizoma Ligustici Wallichii (*Fu Xiong*). In summer, add Radix Sophorae Flavescentis (*Ku Shen*). In autumn and winter, add Fructus Evodiae Rutecarpae (*Zhu Yu*).

Yue Ju Wan (Outthrust Tribulation Pills) resolve various kinds of depression. (These consist of) equal amounts of Rhizoma Atractylodis (*Cang Zhu*), Rhizoma Cyperi Rotundi (*Xiang Fu*), Rhizoma Ligustici Wallichii (*Fu Xiong*), stir-fried Massa Medica Fermentata (*Shen Qu*), and stir-fried Fructus Gardeniae Jasminoidis (*Zhi Zi*). Powder and make into pills.

One formula that treats qi depression, food accumulation, and phlegm heat (consists of) Rhizoma Cyperi Rotundi (*Xiang Fu*), 1 *liang*, Radix Scutellariae Baicalensis (*Huang Qin*), 1 *liang*, Fructus Trichosanthis Kirlowii (*Gua Lou*), Bulbus Fritillariae (*Bei Mu*), Rhizoma Arisaematis (*Nan Xing*), Massa Medica Fermentata (*Shen Qu*), Fructus Crataegi (*Shan Zha*), 1 *liang*

---

[1]   This refers to iron dust collected in a workshop where needles are made. Before use, it must undergo tempering and calcination with vinegar.

for each of the above, and Sodium Sulphate (*Feng Xiao*), 3 *qian*. Make into pills and take. An(other) formula that treats qi depression (is composed of) Radix Albus Paeoniae Lactiflorae (*Bai Shao Yao*), 1.5 *liang*, Rhizoma Cyperi Rotundi (*Xiang Fu*), 1 *liang*, Radix Glycyrrhizae (*Sheng Gan Cao*), 1.5 *qian*. Powder the above, make into pills with paste, and take with Rhizoma Atractylodis Macrocephalae (*Bai Zhu*) soup. A formula that treats suppressed qi (consists of) Radix Albus Paeoniae Lactiflorae (*Bai Shao Yao*), 1.5 *liang*, Rhizoma Cyperi Rotundi (*Xiang Fu*), 1.5 *liang*, stir-fried Bulbus Fritillariae (*Bei Mu*) and Radix Scutellariae Baicalensis (*Huang Qin*), 5 *qian* each, and Radix Glycyrrhizae (*Sheng Gan Cao*), 3 *qian*. Make the above into pills and take.

A fat woman who suffered from qi depression, numbness of the tongue, dizziness, numbness of the hands and feet, qi obstruction with existence of phlegm, and bound stools (was given) *Liang Ge San* (Cool the Diaphragm Powder)[2] plus Rhizoma Arisaematis (*Nan Xing*), Rhizoma Cyperi Rotundi (*Xiang Fu*), and Rhizoma Ligustici Wallichii (*Tai Xiong*) to open (depressed qi).

(Li) Dong-yuan's *Liu Qi Yin Zi* (Flowing Qi Drink) treats all kinds of asthma in males and females alike, puffy swelling, abdominal distention, and qi attacking and causing migratory pain in the shoulder and hypochondrium. It is composed of Fructus Perillae Frutescentis (*Zi Su*), Pericarpium Viridis Citri Reticulatae (*Qing Pi*), Radix Angelicae Sinensis (*Dang Gui*), Radix Paeoniae Lactiflorae (*Shao Yao*), Radix Linderae Strychnifoliae (*Wu Yao*), Sclerotium Poriae Cocoris (*Fu Ling*), Radix Platycodi Grandiflori (*Jie Geng*), Rhizoma Pinelliae Ternatae (*Ban Xia*), Radix Glycyrrhizae (*Gan Cao*), Radix Astragali Membranacei (*Huang Qi*), Fructus Immaturus Citri Seu Ponciri (*Zhi Shi*), Radix Ledebouriellae Sesloidis (*Fang Feng*), Semen Arecae Catechu (*Bing Lang*), Fructus Citri Seu Ponciri (*Zhi Qiao*), and Pericarpium Arecae (*Da Fu Pi*). Process all the above with Succus Zingiberis (*Jiang Zhi*) and bake dry, each one half *liang*. In case

---

[2] This is composed of Radix Et Rhizoma Rhei (*Da Huang*), slaked lime (*Po Xiao*), Radix Glycyrrhizae (*Gan Cao*), Fructus Gardeniae Jasminoidis (*Shan Zhi Zi*), Herba Menthae (*Bo He*), Radix Scutellariae Baicalensis (*Huang Qin*), and Fructus Forsythiae Suspensae (*Lian Qiao*).

of pain in the heart and the spleen, introduce Rhizoma Acori Graminei (*Chang Pu*). In case of blood vacuity in females, introduce Folium Artemisiae Argyii (*Ai*). In case of the five blocked qi[3], introduce a small amount of Pericarpium Citri Reticulatae (*Chen Pi*).

Dai comments: Depression is bind and gathering which refuses to be effused and evicted. (Thus) that which ought to ascend is not able to ascend. That which ought to descend is not able to descend. That which ought to change and transmit is not able to do so. As a result, conveyance and transformation become abnormal and diseases of the six kinds of depression[4] appear. Depressed qi is (manifest by) pain in the chest and hypochondrium. Damp depression (is manifest by) pain all over the body or pain in the joints which starts with yin cold.[5] Phlegm depression (is manifest by) asthma arising on any movement and a deep, slippery pulse in the *cun* opening.[6] Heat depression (is manifest by) cloudedness with distorted vision, reddish urine, and a deep, rapid pulse. Blood depression (is manifest by) weakness of the limbs and ability to take in food. Food depression (is manifest by) acid eructation, a full stomach with inability to take in food, and a tranquil and normal pulse at the left *cun* while the (right) *cun* pulse is tight and exuberant. *Cang Sha Wan* (Atractylodis Sand Pills) regulate the center and dissipate depression. (They are composed of) Rhizoma Atractylodis (*Cang Zhu*), 4 *liang*, Rhizoma Cyperi Rotundi (*Xiang Fu*), 4 *liang*, and Radix Scutellariae Baicalensis (*Huang Qin*), 1 *liang*. Powder the above and make into pills with cake. Take 30 pills (per dose) with ginger soup after a meal.

---

3   *I.e.*, worry, indignation, qi, cold, and heat blockages. Another classification gives worry, thought, anger, fright, and joy blockages.

4   *I.e.*, qi, blood, dampness, fire, phlegm, and food depressions

5   Yin, as it is here, is often used to describe rainy or wet weather or chilling dampness.

6   This refers to the section of radial artery pulse at the styloid process distal to the styloid process.

Chapter Twelve

Wind Damage

In most cases, (this condition) is ascribed to the lungs. A (variant) version says: It is governed exclusively by the lungs.

A male who was addicted to wine felt fatigued because of (having worn) thin clothing in face of wind cold. For half a month, he had had no desire for food. Then suddenly, he had a fit of high fever just before sleeping with a pain as if being flogged and a moderate aversion to cold. The next morning during examination, his six pulses were all large and floating and felt empty when pressure was applied. This was particularly so on the left (hand). (He) was treated for extreme vacuity and subjection to wind cold and administered Radix Panacis Ginseng (*Ren Shen*) as the sovereign, Rhizoma Atractylodis Macrocephalae (*Bai Zhu*), Radix Astragali Membranacei (*Huang Qi*), and Radix Angelicae Sinensis (*Dang Gui Shen*) as the ministers, and Rhizoma Atractylodis (*Cang Zhu*), Radix Glycyrrhizae (*Gan Cao*), Pericarpium Citri Reticulatae (*Chen Pi*), Medulla Tetrapanacis Papyriferi (*Tong Cao*), and Radix Puerariae Lobatae (*Ge Gen*) as the assistants and envoys. After 5 doses, sweat exited from all over his body like rain, and the quilts had to be changed 3 times. (However,) after a sleep, all his symptoms were eliminated.

Chapter Thirteen

Seasonal Disease

(Seasonal disease) is called warm disease or majority of people disease. That kind whose symptoms are common (to everyone who has it) is separately named heaven-propagating seasonal epidemic. Its treatment is comprised of three methods: appropriate supplementation, appropriate dissipation, and appropriate downbearing. Introduced in the formula (for this disease) are Radix Et Rhizoma Rhei (*Da Huang*), Rhizoma Coptidis Chinensis (*Huang Lian*), Radix Scutellariae Baicalensis (*Huang Qin*), Radix Panacis Ginseng (*Ren Shen*), Radix Platycodi Grandiflori (*Jie Geng*), Radix Ledebouriellae Sesloidis (*Fang Feng*), Rhizoma Atractylodis (*Cang Zhu*), Talcum (*Hua Shi*), Rhizoma Cyperi Rotundi (*Xiang Fu*), and manure-processed Radix Glycyrrhizae (*Ren Zhong Huang*). Powder the above and make into pills with Massa Medica Fermentatae (*Shen Qu*) paste. Take 50-70 pills per dose with one or another decoction depending on (whether the disease involves) the qi, blood, or phlegm. In case of qi vacuity, take with *Si Jun Zi Tang* (Four Gentlemen Decoction). In case of blood vacuity, take with *Si Wu Tang* (Four Materials Decoction). In case of copious phlegm, take with *Er Chen Tang* (Two Aged Decoction. And) in case of severe heat, take with child's urine.

One formula that treats seasonal disease (is composed of) Rhizoma Pinelliae Ternatae (*Ban Xia*), Rhizoma Ligustici Wallichii (*Chuan Xiong*), Sclerotium Poriae Cocoris (*Fu Ling*), one half *qian* for each of the above, Pericarpium Citri Reticulatae (*Chen Pi*), Fructus Crataegi (*Shan Zha*), Rhizoma Atractylodis Macrocephalae (*Bai Zhu*), 1 *qian* for each of the above, Radix Glycyrrhizae (*Gan Cao*), 1 *qian*; Rhizoma Atractylodis (*Cang Zhu*), 1.5 *qian*. Take all the above in one dose. In case of headache, add wine-processed Radix Scutellariae Baicalensis (*Huang Qin*). In case of thirst, add dry Radix Puerariae Lobatae (*Gan Ge*). In case of generalized pain, add Radix Et Rhizoma Notopterygii (*Qiang Huo*), Ramulus Cinnamomi (*Gui Zhi*), Radix Ledebouriellae Sesloidis (*Fang Feng*), and Radix Paeoniae Lactiflorae (*Shao Yao*). A formula that treats warm disease as well as food accumulation and phlegm heat and downbears yin fire (is composed of) manure-processed Radix Glycyrrhizae (*Ren Zhong Huang*) prepared in the shape of pills with cooked rice; 15 pills per dose.

(The treatment of) heaven-propagating seasonal disease requires distinguishing the internal from the external (type). That which intrudes from outside is (characterized by) headache, body pain, aversion to cold when exposed to wind, relief due to warmth, and all the pulses being deep and rapid. If (the evil) is in the upper, massive sweating is invariably required to overcome it. Disregarding the number of days of duration, (one should) use *Liu Shen Tong Jie San* (Six Spirits Overall Resolving Powder): Herba Ephedrae Chinensis (*Ma Huang*), 1.5 *qian*, Rhizoma Atractylodis (*Cang Zhu*), Radix Glycyrrhizae (*Gan Cao*), 1 *qian* each, Radix Scutellariae Baicalensis (*Huang Qin*), Gypsum (*Shi Gao*), and Talcum (*Hua Shi*), 2 *qian* for each of the above. Take all the above as one dose. Boil with fresh Rhizoma Zingiberis (*Sheng Jiang*) and Bulbus Allii Fistulosi (*Cong Tou*) and take while hot.

In case of delirious speech and disquieted spirit and thought (*i.e.*, mind), heat evil exists in the interior, and diaphoresis is not able to completely resolve this. The additional introduction of two ingredients, Radix Panacis Ginseng (*Ren Shen*) and Rhizoma Coptidis Chinensis (*Huang Lian*), will effect quieting. *Liu Shen Tong Jie San* is a formula invented by Zhang Dai-ren.[1] The medicinals introduced in it are light (in quantity), and hence many people are not familiar with it and easily neglect it, failing to see that a divine subtlety resides within it. If a resolving diaphoresis fails to occur, add medicinals such as Folium Perillae Frutescentis (*Zi Su Ye*), dry Radix Puerariae Lobatae (*Gan Ge*), and Radix Angelicae (*Bai Zhi*) to enhance its power. Once perspiration is induced, the disease will disappear as if swept away.

In the course of cold damage, as a result of taxation and toiling and, moreover, due to contraction of excessive cold and dampness, there may arise heat and inability to eat. Several days later, there occur loss of consciousness of human affairs, manic and confused speech, clouded and confounded spirit and thought, a green-blue facial complexion, and exposed teeth. People may assume this is a pattern doomed to death. The pulse is deep and thin. If the administration of *Xiao Chai Hu Tang* (Minor Bupleurum Decoction)[2] and other (formulas)

---

[1]   Zhang Cong-zheng, a.k.a. Zhang Zi-he; see Note 21, Ch. 1, present Bk.

[2]   This is composed of Radix Bupleuri (*Chai Hu*), Radix Scutellariae Baicalensis (*Huang Qin*), Radix Panacis Ginseng (*Ren Shen*), mix-fried Radix Glycyrrhizae (*Zhi Gan Cao*), fresh Rhizoma Zingiberis (*Sheng Jiang*), Rhizoma Pinelliae Ternatae (*Ban Xia*), and

have failed to bring effect, (one should) boil without delay *Si Jun Zi Tang* (Four Gentlemen Decoction) plus several slices of Radix Praeparatus Aconiti Carmichaeli (*Zhi Fu Zi*), after retaining it for a little while in a basin of water to strip it of its hot nature. Then make (the patient) drink this decoction warm. The pulse as well as the spirit and thought will return immediately. Only then can other formulas be used as (further) treatment. This is a yin pattern of cold damage.

Cold damage with unresolvable depression with the three yang merged into the three yin[3], the viscera and bowels bound and dried up, a red face, thirst, palpitations, delirious speech, and more internal than external heat needs resolving (such depression) from within. *San Yi Cheng Qi Tang* (Three To One Support the Qi Decoction)[4] precipitates dry stools. Or (together with it), swallow 2 doses of *Mu Xiang Bing Lang Wan* (Saussurea & Areca Pills).[5] One *qian* of Sodium Sulphate (*Xian Ming Fen*) can be added to this formula as well. Should precipitating and diaphoretic formulas fail to rid the threat of heat, use *Zhi Zi Chi Tang* (Gardenia & Fermented Soybean Decoction)[6] with additions and subtractions. Boil this and take. Or drink *Liang Ge San* (Cool the Diaphragm Powder) with additions and subtractions. If the exterior and interior are not resolved (even then), merely drink *Gua Di*

Fructus Zizyphi Jujubae (*Zao*).

[3] This means that the three yin channels are involved, while the three yang are still subject to evils. In such a case, there must be both yin signs and yang conditions.

[4] This is composed of Radix Et Rhizoma Rhei (*Da Huang*), Mirabilitum (*Mang Xiao*), Cortex Magnoliae Officinalis (*Hou Po*), Fructus Immaturus Citri Seu Ponciri (*Zhi Shi*), and Radix Glycyrrhizae (*Gan Cao*).

[5] This is composed of Radix Saussureae Seu Vladimiriae (*Mu Xiang*), Semen Arecae Catechu (*Bing Lang*), Pericarpium Viridis Citri Reticulatae (*Qing Pi*), Pericarpium Citri Reticulatae (*Chen Pi*), Rhizoma Curcumae Zedoariae (*Peng E Zhu*), Rhizoma Coptidis Chinensis (*Huang Lian*), Cortex Phellodendri (*Huang Bai*), Radix Et Rhizoma Rhei (*Da Huang*), Rhizoma Cyperi Rotundi (*Xiang Fu*), and Semen Pharbitidis (*Qian Niu Zi*).

[6] This is composed of 14 pieces of Fructus Gardeniae Jasminoidis (*Zhi Zi*) and one half *he* (1 *he*=10 *sheng*) of Semen Praeparatus Sojae (*Dou Chi*).

San (Melon Pedicle Powder). Vomiting of phlegm will be followed by perspiration, and the condition and its evils will both be abated.

When cold damage transmits into yin or heat enters the viscera and bowels causing acute dysentery, use center-harmonizing medicinals like Radix Panacis Ginseng (*Ren Shen*), Rhizoma Atractylodis Macrocephalae (*Bai Zhu*), Cortex Magnoliae Officinalis (*Hou Po*), and Pericarpium Citri Reticulatae (*Chen Pi*). If (the dysentery) is (extremely) acute, use roasted Semen Myristicae Fragrantis (*Rou Dou Kou*) and stir-fried Massa Medica Fermentatae (*Shen Qu*) as a stop-gap (measure). After the dysentery is checked, use medicinals to eliminate any remaining heat.

Wherever evils converge, the qi there must become vacuous. In case of internal damage, add Herba Ephedrae Chinensis (*Ma Huang*) and Radix Bupleuri (*Chai Hu*) to *Bu Zhong Yi Qi Tang* (Supplement the Center, Boost the Qi Decoction). In case of severe heat, add Radix Praeparatus Aconiti Carmichaeli (*Fu Zi*).

Cold damage with intense heat, a replete pulse, and mania or withdrawal is a pattern of superabundance. It is necessary to use *Da Cheng Qi Tang* (Major Support the Qi Decoction).[7] A person had originally suffered from internal damage. Diaphoresis resulted in delirious speech. At the beginning, he could recognize people, but 3-5 days later, his speech became more frenetic. This was the spirit failing to keep to its abode. By all means, (one) should avoid attacking and hacking (in such a case). The pulse ought to be conspicuously thin and rapid, with insomnia, cold feet, distressed rapid breathing, a brownish green-blue facial complexion, and dry mouth. Use *Bu Zhong Yi Qi Tang* plus one half *liang* of Radix Panacis Ginseng (*Ren Shen*) and 30 pieces of Folium Lophatheri Gracilis (*Zhu Ye*). Boil and take and effect will follow.

A person who was weak internally suffered as a result of taxation and toiling from great vacuity arising following diaphoresis with a thin and rapid pulse, heat like burning fire, and distressed short and rapid

---

[7]   This is composed of Radix Et Rhizoma Rhei (*Da Huang*), Cortex Magnoliae Officinalis (*Hou Po*), Fructus Immaturus Citri Seu Ponciri (*Zhi Shi*), and Mirabilitum (*Mang Xiao*).

breathing. (Their formula consisted of) Radix Panacis Ginseng (*Ren Shen*), Radix Angelicae Sinensis (*Dang Gui*), Rhizoma Atractylodis Macrocephalae (*Bai Zhu*), Radix Astragali Membranacei (*Huang Qi*), Radix Glycyrrhizae (*Gan Cao*), Fructus Schizandrae Chinensis (*Wu Wei Zi*), Rhizoma Anemarrhenae (*Zhi Mu*), and Folium Lophatheri Gracilis (*Zhu Ye*). (These) were boiled with water and child's urine and taken. Two doses and recuperation ensued.

Vacuity desertion in great disease ought to be attributed to yin vacuity. Perform medicinal moxaing at the cinnabar field[8] to supplement yang. When yang is engendered, yin grows. Do not use Radix Praeparatus Aconiti Carmichaeli (*Fu Zi*) to check (the desertion), but (one) can administer a lot of Radix Panacis Ginseng (*Ren Shen*).

For epidemic disease, the only methods usable are those in the *San Yin Fang (The Three Causes Formulary)*. To resolve various heat diseases, use 5 *liang* of Radix Glycyrrhizae (*Fen Cao, i.e.*, de-barked licorice). Cut very finely, stir-fry for a little while, pound, grind with good quality limeless wine, (the wine's) quantity depending on the patient's capacity for liquor, remove the dregs, and take warm. After a little while, stool will be discharged massively and, with it, the toxin also exits. Even in the presence of great thirst, do not drink water or it will become very difficult to cure.

One formula to treat warm disease (is composed of) manureprocessed Radix Glycyrrhizae (*Ren Zhong Huang*) as the ruler to cure epidemic heat toxin, Rhizoma Atractylodis (*Cang Zhu*) and Rhizoma Cyperi Rotundi (*Xiang Fu*) as ministers to dissipate depression, and Rhizoma Coptidis Chinensis (*Huang Lian*) and Radix Scutellariae Baicalensis (*Huang Qin*) to downbear fire, Radix Panacis Ginseng (*Ren Shen*) to supplement vacuity, and Radix Platycodi Grandiflori (*Jie Geng*) and Radix Ledebouriellae Sesloidis (*Fang Feng*) to disinhibit qi and move the channels, all as assistants. When heat is depressed and bound, the qi and fluids internally and externally become obstructed and dried

---

8   The *dan tian*. This is the area approximately two *cun* or inches under the umbilicus or the lower abdomen in general.

up. Radix Et Rhizoma Rhei (*Da Huang*), bitter and cold, is able to wash and sweep away dry heat. Talcum (*Hua Shi*), slippery in nature and bland in flavor, can disinhibit the portals and resolve bind, freeing the flow of the qi and fluids to moisten dryness. These two, one being yin, the other yang, act as envoys.

Warm disease may be (due to) damage by cold in winter or failure to store essence in winter. (Here one should) be clear about the differentiation between vacuity and repletion (conditions). There may be (cases of) qi depression caused by untimely seasonal qi or (cases) of superimposition of sovereign and ministerial fires.[9] (Here) the host and guest should be identified. There may be (cases) where the five movements and the six qi[10] are just about to veer, when that which is expected

---

[9]   Sovereign fire is the fire of the heart, while ministerial is the fire of the life gate or the kidneys. However, another definition says that the fire of the liver, gallbladder, and triple burner is called the ministerial fire which begins in the life gate.

[10]   According to five movements and six qi theory (*wu yun liu qi xue*), the classical Chinese theory of bioarhythms as they both apply to changes in the weather and human physiology, host movements are the expected prevailing weather in the five seasons, namely, warmth in spring, heat in summer, dampness in long summer, coolness in autumn, and cold in winter. These changes are constant. The guest movements are decided by the so-called great movements which, in turn, are decided by the progression of the heavenly stems. These guest movements are believed to cause abnormal weather changes in the four or five seasons.

The six qi, namely, wind, cold, summer heat, dampness, dryness, and fire, are also classified into host and guest, similar to the five movements. However, their progression is based on the earthly branches which are, in turn, associated with the three yin and three yang. These are the *jue yin*, *shao yin*, and *tai yin* and the *shao yang*, *yang ming*, and *tai yang*. Thus, each qi prevails for a period of one sixth of the year. According to this theory, it is the combination of the host and guest movements and qi that are responsible for the distinctive weather in each season of any particular year.

Moreover, the different relationships between the host and guest movements and qi are reflected in the physiology and pathology of human beings. For instance, take the year *si hai* (S6-B7). In the first half, the *jue yin*, which is wind wood associated with the liver, operates the heaven. Therefore, wind is excessive and it overwhelms spleen earth. Thus, we often see diseases of heart pain, fullness in the hypochondri-

to be overwhelming is thwarted, no longer able to ascend or descend. (In such a case,) it is necessary to determine which qi started (the disease). How can all this be treated by means of treating heat (alone)?

Chapter Fourteen

Maculopapular Eruption

A macule is a product of wind heat containing within it phlegm. It effuses from the interior to the exterior. *Tong Sheng San* (Communicate with the Divinity Powder) dissipates and appeases it in the center. It is necessary to achieve resolution and dissipation by means of promoting moderate perspiration, and it is absolutely not allowed to apply precipitation.

Internal damage macular eruption, (due to) stomach qi vacuity, is started by the fire of all the body ranging over the exterior. It requires supplementation to downbear it. (One) should seek out (the appropriate treatment) in the *Yin Zheng Lue Li (Outlined Discussion & Illustration of Yin Patterns)*.[1] The yin pattern of macular eruption is actually a pattern of internal damage. If this condition becomes more serious after diaphoresis and precipitation, supplement with *Bu Zhong Yi Qi Tang* (Supplement the Center, Boost the Qi Decoction). In case of (desire) to drink iced water, vexation, agitation, clouded spirit, a rapid pulse, and cold feet, add Radix Praeparatus Aconiti Carmichaeli (*Fu*

um, obstruction of the diaphragm, inability to take in food, vomiting, abdominal distention, diarrhea, etc. during this period of time. In that case, we should level the liver with acrid and cool medicinals and pacify the spleen and stomach with sweet medicinals.

[1] This is a work compiled by Wang Hao-gu in 1292 CE. It is a book specially on the yin pattern of cold damage.

Zi). As for failure to effect precipitation or earlier than necessary precipitation in the case of stomach heat and stomach ulceration resulting in macular eruption, there is a detailed discussion (of this) in the *Ba Cui Fang (Collection of Outstanding Works)*.[2] Succus Fructi Curcumae Sativae (*Huang Gua Shui*) brewed with true Terra Flava Usta (*Fu Long Gan*) can eliminate red macules (due to) wind heat.

A person who had macular eruption with a red face, cloudedness and fatuity, delirious speech, and a surging yet vacuous pulse which felt feeble when pressure was applied was prescribed Radix Panacis Ginseng (*Ren Shen*), Radix Rehmanniae (*Sheng Di*), each one half *liang*, Radix Praeparatus Aconiti Carmichaeli (*Fu Zi*), 1 *qian*, and Radix Et Rhizoma Rhei (*Da Huang*), one and a half *qian*. After they were boiled and taken, a bit of diarrhea was induced. This is effective when administered in summer months.

Macular eruption is ascribed to heat and phlegm in the lungs. This requires clearing lung fire and downbearing phlegm or diaphoresis to achieve a resolution. There are (also) cases indicating precipitation with *Tong Sheng San* with additions and subtractions.

Chapter Fifteen

Big Head Heavenly Movement Disease

This is (due to) dampness qi existing in the top. It is a hot swelling starting from the jowls and cheeks and is popularly called cormorant scourge. (Li) Dong-yuan designed a formula (for this composed of)

---

[2] *Ji Sheng Ba Cui (Life-succoring Collection of Outstanding Works)* compiled by Du Si-jing (?-1315 CE) in 1308 CE. This is a series of nineteen important works published in that historical period, mainly the works of Liu Wan-su and his pupils, including Li Gao.

Radix Et Rhizoma Notopterygii (*Qiang Huo*), wine-processed Radix Scutellariae Baicalensis (*Huang Qin*), and wine-steamed Radix Et Rhizoma Rhei (*Da Huang*). This should be modified in accordance with the (particular) disease. Do not use downbearing agents in any case. Fifteen to 16 days (after the contraction), administer *Xiao Chai Hu Tang* (Minor Bupleurum Decoction). In case of no effect, still continue to use effusing and dissipating (medicinals). Fructus Perillae Frutescentis (*Zi Su*) and Pericarpium Citri Reticulatae (*Chen Pi*) offer an efficacious treatment.

(Li) Dong-yuan explains: It is *yang ming* evil heat which is extremely great. This supports and makes replete the ministerial fire of the *shao yang* so as to produce (this disease). One should choose the channel involved depending upon which part is swollen. The treatment should be of a moderate kind. (One) should not use heavy formulas beyond that which is necessary for the disease. The *yang ming* is the chief of the evil and the *shao yang* is the root of it in the case of great swelling in front and behind the ears. Boil wine-processed Radix Scutellariae Baicalensis (*Huang Qin*), wineprocessed Rhizoma Coptidis Chinensis (*Huang Lian*), and mix-fried Radix Glycyrrhizae (*Zhi Gan Cao*) in water and take this little by little continually. Or, after a dose is finished, obtain some Fructus Arctii Lappae (*Shu Nian Zi*), stir-fry on a new clay tile till it emits a fragrance, boil together with Radix Et Rhizoma Rhei (*Da Huang*), remove the dregs, put in Mirabilitum (*Mang Xiao*), all of equal amounts, and take sip by sip at short intervals. Do not eating (immediately) after (taking this). If the bowels are loosened a bit and the evil qi is gone, administer only the former formula. If not, administer (both formulas) as instructed above. Stop (the medication) once the stool is loosened and the evil qi is gone.

In case of *yang ming* (pattern) thirst, add Talcum (*Hua Shi*) and Gypsum (*Shi Gao*). In case of *shao yang* (pattern) thirst, add Radix Trichosanthis Kirlowii (*Gua Lou Gen*). To move the *yang ming* channel[1],

---

[1] This implies that the *yang ming* is affected. In epidemic disease, this is the same as the *yang ming* pattern of cold damage which manifests with generalized fever, aversion to heat rather than cold, spontaneous sweating,

use Rhizoma Cimicifugae (*Sheng Ma*), Radix Paeoniae Lactiflorae (*Shao Yao*), Radix Puerariae Lobatae (*Ge Gen*), and Radix Glycyrrhizae (*Gan Cao*). To move the *tai yang* channel[2], use Radix Et Rhizoma Notopterygii (*Qiang Huo*), Herba Seu Flos Schizonepetae Tenuifoliae (*Jing Jie*), and Radix Ledebouriellae Sesloidis (*Fang Feng*). These medicinals should be used in combination with the above (medicinals).

Chapter Sixteen

Disease Caused by a Warm Winter

When (warm) qi appears (in winter) which is not expected to appear in that season, (disease may be caused). If winter qi, which gentlemen should seal and store, is contrarily drained, (the disease will arise. For it,) use exclusively supplementing formulas aided by exteriorizing and dissipating medicinals, such as *Bu Zhong Yi Qi Tang* (Supplement the Center, Boost the Qi Decoction).

Take a bamboo tube with a joint preserved at each end and cut a hole in the middle. Put in sliced, debarked Radix Glycyrrhizae (*Da Fen Cao*), seal the hole with a wood or bamboo peg and putty. Then put (this) into a big jar of manure on the day of Beginning of Winter. Keep (there) until the eve of Beginning of Spring. Take out and dry at a place in the wind but sheltered from the sun for 21 days (at least), the

------

thirst, and a large, surging pulse. One should note that when the evil has not intruded into the bowel, *i.e.*, the stomach, precipitation should not be administered.

[2] The implication is similar to that in Note 1 above. The *tai yang* channel pattern is characterized by evils still persisting in the exterior, having not yet entered the interior. Its manifestations include aversion to cold, generalized aching, and absence of thirst.

longer, the better. Break (open) the bamboo tube, take out the licorice, and powder finely. This treats yang pattern of epidemic toxins with great effect. A variant version says: This also treats swelling toxin and (can be used) as a dressing after being mixed with water for incised wounds. The pulse (of warm winter disease) is larger at the left *cun* (opening) than at the right, and it is floating, moderate, and exuberant but feels feeble when pressure is applied.

Chapter Seventeen

Malaria

(This condition) is classified into wind, summerheat, food, phlegm, old malaria, and malaria mother. Old malaria is a disease of wind and summerheat entering into the yin viscera. Use blood(-boosting) medicinals to lead (wind summerheat) out into the yang phase, and then dissipate it, (that is to say,) at once supplement and effuse. (For this use) Rhizoma Ligustici Wallichii (*Chuan Xiong*), Flos Carthami Tinctorii (*Hong Hua*), and Radix Angelicae Sinensis (*Dang Gui*) plus Rhizoma Atractylodis (*Cang Zhu*), Rhizoma Atractylodis Macrocephalae (*Bai Zhu*), Radix Angelicae (*Bai Zhi*), Cortex Phellodendri (*Huang Bai*), and Radix Glycyrrhizae (*Gan Cao*). Boil, allow to settle overnight, and then take the next morning.

If there is no sweating, it is essential to cause sweating. Dissipation of evils is being the ruling (method) with supplementation adjunctive. (Whereas,) sweating demands perspiration-checking. In this case, supplementation of the righteous qi is the ruling (modality) with dissipation adjunctive. To dissipate evils through diaphoresis, (use) Fructus Perillae Frutescentis (*Zi Su*), Herba Ephedrae Chinensis (*Ma Huang*), etc. To supplement the righteous qi, (use) Radix Panacis Ginseng (*Ren Shen*), Radix Astragali Membranacei (*Huang Qi*), and the like.

Malaria mother is usually located under the lateral costal region. It causes people profuse sweating and pain in the hypochondrium and should be dispersed and conducted with pills (made from) vinegar-boiled Carapax Amydae (*Bie Jia*) as the sovereign, Rhizoma Sparganii (*San Leng*), Rhizoma Curcumae Zedoariae (*Peng Zhu*), Ovum Notarchi Leachii Freeri (*Hai Fen*), vinegarboiled Rhizoma Cyperi Rotundi (*Xiang Fu*), Pericarpium Viridis Citri Reticulatae (*Qing Pi*), Semen Pruni Persicae (*Tao Ren*), Flos Carthami Tinctorii (*Hong Hua*), Massa Medica Fermentata (*Shen Qu*), and Fructus Germinatus Hordei Vulgaris (*Mai Ya*). Administer (this formula) with additions and subtractions in accordance with the signs. A variant version stipulates that all the ingredients below Rhizoma Cyperi Rotundi be boiled in vinegar (for use).

Thus it is said, if evil qi has lasted long, malaria attacks infrequently because the evil lodges deeply. Conversely, if evil qi has lasted for a short time, malaria attacks frequently. (Therefore, malaria) attacks every three days if (one) has been subjected to the disease for one year. It attacks once every other day if the disease has lasted for half a year. It will attack once a day if the disease has lasted for one month. It will attack two days running and halt for one day if the disease involves both qi and blood. Attacks every other day (should be treated with) supplementing medicinals with exteriorizing ones as aids, and afterwards, (treatment) should end with *Jie Nue Dan* (Terminate Malaria Elixir)[1]; while that (lodging) in the yin phase requires certain medicinals to drive and upraise (the evil) into the yang phase before it can be terminated. Introduced into the formula are Radix Dichroae Febrifugae (*Chuan Chang Shan*), Fructus Amomi Tsao-ko (*Cao Guo*), Rhizoma Anemarrhenae (*Zhi Mu*), Semen Arecae Catechu (*Bing Lang*), Fructus Pruni Mume (*Wu Mei*), stir-fried Squama Manitis (*Chuan Shan Jia*), mix-fried Radix Glycyrrhizae (*Gan Cao Zhi*). Boil in a big bowl of water down to half a bowlful, allow to settle overnight, and take warm

---

[1] This is composed of Mylabris (*Ban Mao*), 2 *qian*, Semen Crotonis (*Ba Dou*), Cinnabar (*Zhu Sha*), each 1 *qian*, Secretio Moschi Moschiferi (*She Xiang*), 2 *fen*, Realgar (*Xiong Huang*), 1.5 *qian*, Secretio Bufonis Bufonis (*Chan Su*), 5 *fen*. Make into pills with Semen Diospyri Loti (*Hei Zao*).

in the morning of the attacking day or two watches before the attacking. In case of vomiting, treat by following the tendency (*i.e.,* apply ejection).

The great method (*i.e.,* fundamental principle) is that summerheat wind always requires diaphoresis. In the summer months, (people) are inclined to repose in windy, cool places and, therefore, their portals are shut up, unable to drain (wind heat). Aversion to food arises invariably from food and drink. (However,) for malaria with vacuity, it is necessary first to administer one or two doses of Radix Panacis Ginseng (*Ren Shen*) and Radix Astragali Membranacei (*Huang Qi*) to prop up the qi to keep it from sinking and, after that, use other medicinals for treatment. If internal damage arises together with external evils, phlegm is invariably produced in the internal, and (this condition) must be resolved through the exterior by means of diaphoresis with the formula *Er Chen Tang* (Two Aged Decoction) plus Fructus Amomi Tsao-ko (*Cao Guo*), Radix Dichroae Febrifugae (*Chang Shan*), Radix Bupleuri (*Chai Hu*), and Radix Scutellariae Baicalensis (*Huang Qin*).

Malaria when severe may display (alternating) cold and heat, splitting headache, thirst and drinking water (excessively), and spontaneous sweating. This can be treated with Radix Panacis Ginseng (*Ren Shen*), Radix Astragali Membranacei (*Huang Qi*), Rhizoma Atractylodis Macrocephalae (*Bai Zhu*), Radix Scutellariae Baicalensis (*Huang Qin*), Rhizoma Coptidis Chinensis (*Huang Lian*), Fructus Gardeniae Jasminoidis (*Zhi Zi*), Rhizoma Ligustici Wallichii (*Chuan Xiong*), Rhizoma Atractylodis (*Cang Zhu*), Rhizoma Pinelliae Ternatae (*Ban Xia*), Radix Trichosanthis Kirlowii (*Tian Hua Fen*), etc.

For chronic malaria, (use) *Er Chen Tang* plus Rhizoma Ligustici Wallichii (*Chuan Xiong*), Rhizoma Atractylodis (*Cang Zhu*), Radix Bupleuri (*Chai Hu*), Rhizoma Atractylodis Macrocephalae (*Bai Zhu*), and dried Radix Puerariae Lobatae (*Gan Ge*). This (formula) is at once supplementing and effusing. (For malaria) attacking towards noon or attacking towards noon with sweating and distressing thirst, (use)

Huang Qi San Bai Tang (Astragalus Three White Decoction)[2] plus Radix Scutellariae Baicalensis (*Huang Qin*) and Rhizoma Coptidis Chinensis (*Huang Lian*). In case of abundant cold, a weak pulse, fatigued body, and low food intake, (use) *Ren Shen Yang Wei Tang* (Ginseng Nurture the Stomach Decoction)[3] from the *Ju Fang (Collected Formulas)*. For malaria resulting from taxation and toiling or from worry and thought with copious sweating, low food intake, extreme fatigue, and disinclination to speak, (use) *Bu Zhong Yi Qi Tang* (Supplement the Center, Boost the Qi Decoction). For stagnated phlegm, chest fullness, more heat than cold, and dry solid stools, (use) *Da Chai Hu Tang* (Major Bupleurum Decoction).[4]

For malarial disease with ability to eat and hidden phlegm, (use) *Xiao Wei Dan* (Minor Stomach Elixir).[5] For malaria with great thirst and great heat to an extreme degree, (use) *Xiao Chai Hu Tang* (Minor Bupleurum Decoction) minus Rhizoma Pinelliae Ternatae (*Ban Xia*) but

---

[2]   This is probably composed of wine-processed Radix Astragali Membranacei (*Huang Qi*), Radix Panacis Ginseng (*Ren Shen*), stir-fried Rhizoma Atractylodis Macrocephalae (*Bai Zhu*), Sclerotium Poriae Cocoris (*Fu Ling*), Radix Glycyrrhizae (*Gan Cao*), Fructus Amomi (*Sha Ren*), Fructus Amomi Tsao-ko (*Cao Guo*), Pericarpium Citri Rubri (*Ju Hong*), Fructus Schizandrae Chinensis (*Wu Wei Zi*), and Fructus Pruni Mume (*Wu Mei*). One should note that the translator is not entirely certain about the composition of this formula.

[3]   This is composed of Rhizoma Pinelliae Ternatae (*Ban Xia*), Cortex Magnoliae Officinalis (*Hou Po*), Rhizoma Atractylodis (*Cang Zhu*), Herba Agastachis Seu Pogostemi (*Huo Xiang*), Semen Amomi Tsao-ko (*Cao Guo Ren*), Sclerotium Poriae Cocoris (*Fu Ling*), Radix Panacis Ginseng (*Ren Shen*), Radix Glycyrrhizae (*Gan Cao*), and Pericarpium Citri Rubri (*Ju Hong*).

[4]   This is composed of Radix Bupleuri (*Chai Hu*), Radix Scutellariae Baicalensis (*Huang Qin*), Radix Paeoniae Lactiflorae (*Shao Yao*), Rhizoma Pinelliae Ternatae (*Ban Xia*), fresh Rhizoma Zingiberis (*Sheng Jiang*), Fructus Immaturus Citri Seu Ponciri (*Zhi Shi*), Radix Et Rhizoma Rhei (*Da Huang*), and Fructus Zizyphi Jujubae (*Zao*).

[5]   This is composed of Flos Daphnis Genkwae (*Yuan Hua*), Rhizoma Euphorbiae Kansui (*Gan Sui*), Radix Euphorbiae Pekinensis (*Da Ji*), Radix Et Rhizoma Rhei (*Da Huang*), and Cortex Phellodendri (*Huang Bai*).

plus Rhizoma Anemarrhenae (*Zhi Mu*), Tuber Ophiopogonis Japonicae (*Mai Men Dong*), and Rhizoma Coptidis Chinensis (*Huang Lian*). Generally speaking, summerheat malaria usually requires *Xiao Chai Hu Tang, Ren Shen Bai Hu Tang* (Ginseng White Tiger Decoction)[6], and the like. (Again) for malaria with thirst, (use) Radix Rehmanniae (*Sheng Di Huang*), Tuber Ophiopogonis Japonicae (*Mai Men Dong*), Radix Trichosanthis Kirlowii (*Tian Hua Fen*), Radix Cyathulae (*Chuan Niu Xi*), Rhizoma Anemarrhenae (*Zhi Mu*), stir-fried Cortex Phellodendri (*Huang Bai*), dry Radix Puerariae Lobatae (*Gan Ge*), and Radix Glycyrrhizae (*Gan Cao*).

For post-malaria (conditions, use) Rhizoma Atractylodis Macrocephalae (*Bai Zhu*), Rhizoma Pinelliae Ternatae (*Ban Xia*), each 1 *liang*, Rhizoma Coptidis Chinensis (*Huang Lian*), 5 *qian*, Radix Albus Paeoniae Lactiflorae (*Bai Shao Yao*), 3 *qian*, and Pericarpium Citri Reticulatae (*Chen Pi*), 5 *qian*. Powder the above and make into pills with gruel. For chronic malaria with sweat refusing to exude, (use) *Er Chen (Tang)* plus Semen Arecae Catechu (*Bing Lang*) and with Rhizoma Atractylodis (*Cang Zhu*) and Rhizoma Atractylodis Macrocephalae (*Bai Zhu*) in double amounts. A person suffered from post-malaria trembling hands. This was phlegm depression barring drool. Ejection ensued in recovery.

Jie Nue Qing Hao Wan (Terminate Malaria Artemisia Apiacea Pills): Herba Artemisiae Apiaceae (*Qing Hao*), 1 *jin*, Folium Benincasae Hispidae (*Dong Gua Ye*), 2 *liang*, Cortex Cinnamomi (*Guan Gui*), 2 *liang*, and Herba Verbenae Officinalis (*Ma Bian Cao*), 2 *liang*. Bake dry the leafy ingredients, powder (all), and make into pills the size of Chinese parasol tree seeds. (Take) 1 *liang* divided into 4 doses. Take one watch before the (expected) attack of malaria.

---

[6] The translator is aware of at least four variant versions of *Ren Shen Bai Hu Tang*. As an example of these, one is composed of Radix Panacis Ginseng (*Ren Shen*), Rhizoma Anemarrhenae (*Zhi Mu*), Gypsum (*Shi Gao*), Radix Trichosanthis Kirlowii (*Tian Hua Fen*), Radix Puerariae Lobatae (*Ge Gen*), Tuber Ophiopogonis Japonicae (*Mai Men Dong*), Folium Lophatheri Gracilis (*Zhu Ye*), and Semen Oryzae Sativae (*Mi*).

Another formula (is composed of) Semen Arecae Catechu (*Bing Lang*), Pericarpium Citri Reticulatae (*Chen Pi*), Rhizoma Atractylodis Macrocephalae (*Bai Zhu*), Radix Dichroae Febrifugae (*Chang Shan*), 2 *qian* for each of the above, Sclerotium Poriae Cocoris (*Fu Ling*), Fructus Pruni Mume (*Wu Mei*), and Cortex Magnoliae Officinalis (*Hou Po*), 1 *qian* for each of the above, all used as two doses. Boil one dose in 1 cup each of wine and water down to half a cupful. Take 1 dose on the eve of the attack and another on the attacking day. A short nap after taking (the decoction) ensures effect.

A malaria-terminating formula should be administered to eliminate the malaria when (the malaria) has only launched a couple of attacks. This proves the best method. If attacks have caused vacuous and weak center qi, the disease evils having penetrated more deeply, or, if (the malaria) has lasted for several months or even over a year, a doctor, be he divine, is unable to offer a cure. Even if a treatment presumably achieves temporary relief, a relapse will occur once food and drink or some external evils cause damage. People of modern times are often plagued by this. (Therefore, one should) obtain 1 *liang* of quality Radix Dichroae Febrifugae (*Chang Shan*) and 5 *qian* of Semen Arecae Catechu (*Bing Lang*), powder, make into pills the size of Chinese parasol tree seeds with flour paste, and take 1 pill on the eve of the attack. Two doses will bring effect. *Chang Shan Yin Zi* (Dichroa Drink)[7] is equally good.

As a terminating method, use Mr. (Liu) Shou-zhen's[8] pills: Realgar (*Xiong Huang*), 1 *liang*, and Radix Panacis Ginseng (*Ren Shen*), 5 *qian*.

---

[7] There are at least three variants of this formula, all effective against malaria. For example, one is composed of Radix Dichroae Febrifugae (*Chang Shan*), Rhizoma Anemarrhenae (*Zhi Mu*), Fructus Amomi Tsao-ko (*Cao Guo*), Radix Glycyrrhizae (*Gan Cao*), Rhizoma Alpiniae Officinalis (*Gao Liang Jiang*), and Fructus Pruni Mume (*Wu Mei*).

[8] *I.e.*, Liu Wan-su or Liu He-jian. See Note 1, Ch.1, present Bk.

On the fifth day of the fifth month, with the tips of the *zong zi*[9] make into pills the size of Chinese parasol tree seeds. In the morning, when malaria is going to attack, face the east and take 1 pill with florid well water.[10] Hot flavors (*i.e.*, foods) are prohibited. [Radix Panacis Ginseng {*Ren Shen*} is replaced by Arsenolitum {*Ren Yan*} in a variant version {later editor}].

Another formula (is composed of) Semen Glycineae Hispidiae (*Da Hei Dou*), 7 *qian*, Realgar (*Xiong Huang*), 1 *qian*, Calomelas (*Qing Fen*), 5 *fen*, Radix Panacis Ginseng (*Ren Shen*), 1 *qian*, Herba Menthae (*Bo He*), 5 *fen*, and Radix Glycyrrhizae (*Gan Cao*), 1 *qian*. Powder the above, make into pills the size of red beans by means of dripping water. Take 1 pill with water fresh from the well at the cock-crow watch (*i.e.*, 1-3 AM) while facing the east. [*Ren Shen* is replaced by *Ren Yan* in a variant version. {later editor}].

In addition, Luo Qian-fu's[11] formula, *Zi He Che Wan* (Placenta Pills), is composed of Placenta Hominis (*Zi He Che*), 1 *liang*, Radix Glycyrrhizae (*Sheng Gan Cao*), 5 *qian*, Semen Phaseoli Radiati (*Lu Dou*), 1 *liang*, and Arsenolitum (*Ren Yan*), 1 *qian*, ground separately. Powder the above, 5 *fen* a dose. Take with a small amount of fresh water. For malaria attacking every other day, take these at night. For malaria attacking every day, take them deep at night in the middle of sleep. Refrain from pork and sea foods, fruits, wine, wheat food, fish and chicken, and raw and cold substances as well. Those with attacks every two or three days or suffering from deep (*i.e.*, recalcitrant) evil qi should take one dose only. Those above 10 years of age take one

---

[9] This is a pyramid-shaped dumpling made of glutinous rice wrapped in bamboo or reed leaves. The fifth of the fifth month of the Chinese lunar calendar is the anniversary of the death of the great patriotic poet, Qu Yuan, and *zong zi* are made on this day specially in honor of him.

[10] This refers to water obtained early in the morning from a spring or a well.

[11] A.k.a. Luo Tian-yi, a close pupil of Li Gao or Li Dong-yuan

character.[12] Those above 3 years take one half character. Pregnant women are not allowed to take these.

A person aged 60 who had been of strong constitution and took thick flavors (*i.e.*, ate rich foods) contracted malaria in the spring. Our master admonished him to abstain from sexual desire and to take (a diet of) bland flavors. He did not listen. A physician administered him 3-5 doses of a thwarting formula and he recovered. Ten days later, he had a relapse and was administered (the same formula) again. (The condition) persisted till the winter when he came for treatment. Our master learned that he had been suffering long from sweating; however, his stomach qi had not yet run out. What was more, it happened to be a season of severe cold, and, exposed to and offended (by the cold), he had contracted alternating cold and heat. The only choice was to apply supplementation. Two *jin* of one single flavor (*i.e.*, ingredient), Rhizoma Atractylodis Macrocephalae (*Bai Zhu*), was prescribed. This was to be powdered and made into pills with gruel. (The patient) was bid, when hungry, not to eat food but take 100-200 pills with hot boiled water. (He) was allowed to have only well-done rice gruel to nurture and regulate (the stomach). (He was told that) when the whole packet was finished, copious sweating ought to be induced and followed by recuperation. Since then, many (similar) cases have turned out successfully. The medicinals (in each case), however, varied in a small way.

A person had for long suffered from malaria with abdominal distention. His pulse was not rapid but moderately wiry and felt rough when pressure was applied but feeble when light pressure was

---

[12] In ancient times, coins were not only used as currency but also as measurements of weight. The commonly known *qian* is directly derived from a coin, referred to as cash in the Western literature. Such coins usually had four characters carved or cast on it. Therefore, 1 "character" equals 1/4 *qian*.

applied. He was prescribed *San He Tang* (Three Harmony Decoction)[13], the dosage being three times as much as Mr. Suo[14] prescribed. This (was boiled) with Rhizoma Atractylodis Macrocephalae (*Bai Zhu*) and taken brewed with Succus Zingiberis (*Jiang Zhi*). Several doses after, urination was disinhibited a little, and abdominal distention relieved a bit. Short voidings of scant urine, however, followed again. (The case) was then treated as a vacuity of both blood and qi. Radix Panacis Ginseng (*Ren Shen*), Radix Achyranthis Bidentatae (*Niu Xi*), and Radix Angelicae Sinensis (*Dang Gui Shen*) were introduced into the above formula and the dosage was large. Administration of a little more than 40 doses resulted in recovery.

A woman suffered from malaria attacking every third day with scant food intake and menstruation that did not come for three months running. The pulse was examined and it was found absent from both hands. Seeing that she was dressed as usual and did not show any fatigue in speaking or movement, the conclusion was reached that menstruation not coming was a result of phlegm obstruction rather than want of blood and that the absence of the pulse was not pulse expiry due to exhaustion or scant blood but merely an intangible pulse which was bound and hidden by accumulated phlegm generating heat. This should be treated as repletion heat and accordingly *San Hua*

---

[13] There are several different formulas surviving today with this name; however, none of them are indicated for malaria. The most likely one is composed of Herba Ephedrae Chinensis (*Ma Huang*), Pericarpium Citri Reticulatae (*Chen Pi*), Radix Linderae Strychnifoliae (*Wu Yao*), Rhizoma Ligustici Wallichii (*Chuan Xiong*), Bombyx Batryticatus (*Jiang Can*), Radix Angelicae (*Bai Zhi*), Radix Platycodi Grandiflori (*Jie Geng*), Fructus Citri Seu Ponciri (*Zhi Qiao*), Radix Glycyrrhizae (*Gan Cao*), dry Rhizoma Zingiberis (*Gan Jiang*), Sclerotium Poriae Cocoris (*Fu Ling*), Rhizoma Pinelliae Ternatae (*Ban Xia*), Rhizoma Cyperi Rotundi (*Xiang Fu*), Folium Perillae Frutescentis (*Zi Su Ye*), Rhizoma Atractylodis (*Cang Zhu*), and Radix Et Rhizoma Notopterygii (*Qiang Huo*).

[14] Today, little is known about this person except his name, Suo Ju.

Shen You Wan (Three Flowers God Bless Pills)[15] were administered. Ten days later, food intake increased a little and the pulse appeared to some extent. A month later, the six pulses all re-appeared and were only a little wiry.

(However,) the malaria yet remained to be overcome. Since the stomach qi was intact, when spring progressed deep, the channel blood would become effulgent of itself and (a complete) recovery would ensue. (Thus) there was no need to take any more medicinals. She was instructed to keep away from flavorful (*i.e.*, rich food) and go on an abstemious diet. Half a month later, her malaria was overcome and her menstrual flow recovered.

An old person who had suffered from malaria for half a year already had a rapid and forceful pulse in the *chi* section of both hands and a somewhat withered complexion. As a result of administration of *Si Shou Yin* (Four Animal Drink)[16] and other (such) formulas, damp heat in the middle burner had flown down and hidden and bound in the kidneys. Consequently, kidney fire had been transported up into the lungs. Thus coughing broke out with malaria. Radix Panacis Ginseng (*Ren Shen*), Rhizoma Atractylodis Macrocephalae (*Bai Zhu*), Radix Scutellariae Baicalensis (*Huang Qin*), Rhizoma Coptidis Chinensis (*Huang Lian*), Rhizoma Cimicifugae (*Sheng Ma*), and Radix Bupleuri (*Chai Hu*) were used to rectify the center and, one or two days later, *Huang Bai Wan* (Phellodendrum Pills)[17] were administered. (The patient) dreamed of sexual intercourse for two nights. This (showed

---

[15] This is composed of Radix Euphorbiae Kansui (*Gan Sui*), Radix Euphorbiae Pekinensis (*Da Ji*), Flos Daphnis Genkwae (*Yuan Hua*), Semen Pharbitidis (*Qian Niu Zi*), Radix Et Rhizoma Rhei (*Da Huang*), and Calomelas (*Qing Fen*).

[16] This is composed of Radix Panacis Ginseng (*Ren Shen*), Sclerotium Poriae Cocoris (*Fu Ling*), Rhizoma Pinelliae Ternatae (*Ban Xia*), Rhizoma Atractylodis Macrocephalae (*Bai Zhu*), Pericarpium Citri Reticulatae (*Chen Pi*), Fructus Pruni Mume (*Wu Mei*), and Fructus Amomi Tsao-ko (*Cao Guo*).

[17] This is composed of only one ingredient, Cortex Phellodendri (*Huang Bai*). This is powdered, stir-fried, and made into pills.

that) the heat was resolved in the kidneys which were freed of worry. On the following day, malaria and coughing both stopped abruptly.

A wealthy person in the prime of his life suffered from malaria with cold starting at the *mao* watch not yielding to heat till the *you* watch, and (the heat) ending early in the *yin* watch.[18] For one day and night, resurrection (*i.e.*, tranquil restitution, relaxation) lasted but one watch. Based on the consideration that this must be caused by contraction of cold in the process of sexual intercourse, Radix Panacis Ginseng (*Ren Shen*) and Rhizoma Atractylodis Macrocephalae (*Bai Zhu*) were used for great supplementation. Radix Praeparatus Aconiti Carmichaeli (*Fu Zi*, was used) to move the channels and at the same time to dissipate cold and secure perspiration. For several days no sweating was induced and the condition remained the same as before. This was because of failure to consider that, there being a (such) long way to reach the backs of the feet, the strength of the medicinals had difficult accessing these. Then Rhizoma Atractylodis (*Cang Zhu*), Rhizoma Ligustici Wallichii (*Chuan Xiong*), and Ramulus Pruni Persicae (*Tao Zhi*) were boiled and put in a (large) vessel. (The patient) was helped to sit up with his legs immersed in the decoction deep to the knees. About the time (it takes to eat) a meal later, he was made to take the formula he had previously taken. (Now) sweat exited profusely all over his body, and the disease was cured immediately.

Long-lasting malaria does not allow for termination directly. It is necessary to apply at once supplementation and effusion. Medicinals such as Arsenicum Album (*Pi Shuang*) which are poisonous should not be used without warrant. (Malaria) involving the yin phase is difficult to treat. That involving the yang phase is easy to treat. Malarial mother requires dispersing with poisonous medicinals. (In that case,) moving the qi and whittling hardness are the ruling (methods. Li) Dong-yuan explains that cold malaria is ascribed to the *tai yang*, thus necessitating diaphoresis. Heat malaria is ascribed to the *yang ming*, thus necessitat-

---

[18] These are the twelve earthly branches: *zi*, B1; *chou*, B2; *yin*, B3; *mao*, B4; *chen*, B5; *si*, B6; *wu*, B7; *wei*, B8; *shen*, B9; *you*, 10; *xu*, B11; *hai*, B12. The twelve earthly branches combine with the ten heavenly stems to create a sixty-day cycle.

ing precipitation. And cold and heat malaria is ascribed to the *shao yang*, thus necessitating harmonization. Malaria involving the three yin has no such classification and is generally (identified as) warm malaria. This explanation is quite right. In regard to the three yin channels, however, his explanation is not clear. That which attacks on the *zi, wu, mao*, and *you* days is *shao yin* malaria. (That which attacks on the) *yin, shen, si*, and *hai* days is *jue yin* malaria. (That which attacks on the) *chen, xu, chou*, and *wei* days is *tai yin* malaria.

The pulse (of malaria) is wiry. With heat, it is wiry and also rapid. With cold, it is wiry and also slow. Some (patients) with perduring malaria may have a pulse that is extremely vacuous, faint, and weak which is seemingly not wiry. Nonetheless, the pulse amidst being vacuous and faint must in fact be wiry, though not beating forcefully against the (palpating) fingers. This can be felt through careful examination.

Chapter Eighteen

Coughing

(This disease) is (further) classified into wind cold, fire, phlegm, taxation, and lung distention (types). In case of wind cold, move the phlegm and open the interstices with *Er Chen Tang* (Two Aged Decoction) plus Herba Ephedrae (*Ma Huang*), Semen Pruni Armeniacae (*Xing Ren*), Radix Platycodi Grandiflori (*Jie Geng*), and the like. In case of fire, the rule is to downbear fire, clear metal, and transform phlegm. In case of taxation, the rule is to supplement yin and clear metal with *Si Wu Tang* (Four Materials Decoction) plus Succus Zingiberis (*Jiang Zhi*), and Succus Bambusae (*Zhu Li*). For lung distention coughing, the rule is to astringe (qi) with Fructus Terminaliae Chebulae (*He Zi*), Pulvis Indigonis (*Qing Dai*), and Semen Pruni Armeniacae (*Xing Ren*). Fructus Terminaliae Chebulae is able to treat the lung qi when it is severely injured by fire and consequently depressed and confined, (thus) giving rise to distention. Its sour and bitter flavor is exploited to achieve the feat of astringing and downbearing fire. It should be assisted by Ovum Notarchi Leachii Freeri (*Hai Fen*), urine-soaked Rhizoma Cyperi Rotundi (*Xiang Fu Zi*), Fructus Trichosanthis Kirlowii (*Gua Lou*), Pulvis Indigonis (*Qing Dai*), Massa Medica Fermentata Cum Pinelliam (*Ban Xia Qu*), and Rhizoma Zingiberis (*Jiang*). These are mixed with honey and melted in the mouth. For phlegm rheum coughing, the rule is to sweep phlegm, and (the medicinals used) vary in accordance with signs.

Lung distention coughing with inability to sleep on either side is a disease due to phlegm embracing static blood, (thus) impeding qi. (One) should nourish the blood to downbear fire and course the liver to clear phlegm with *Si Wu Tang* plus Semen Pruni Persicae (*Tao Ren*), Fructus Terminaliae Chebulae (*He Zi*), Pericarpium Viridis Citri Reticulatae (*Qing Pi*), and Succus Bambusae (*Zhu Li*). Coughing caused by blood impeding the qi (requires) Semen Pruni Persicae (*Tao Ren*) and Radix Et Rhizoma Rhei (*Da Huang*). These are made into pills with Succus Zingiberis (*Jiang Zhi*).

For food accumulation and phlegm causing cough with fever (use) Rhizoma Pinelliae Ternatae (*Ban Xia*) and Rhizoma Arisaematis (*Nan Xing*) as the sovereigns, Fructus Trichosanthis Kirlowii (*Gua Lou*) and Semen Raphani Sativi (*Luo Bo Zi*) as the ministers, Pulvis Indigonis (*Qing Dai*) and Alkaloid (*Shi Jian*, mixture of starch with ash of wormwood or knotweed) as the envoys.

A thin woman suffering from occasional heat and coughing with phlegm at night and irregular menstruation (was given) Pulvis Indigonis (*Qing Dai*), Semen Trichosanthis Kirlowii (*Gua Lou Ren*), and urine-soaked Rhizoma Cyperi Rotundi (*Xiang Fu*) which were powdered, mixed with ginger and honey, and melted in the mouth.

Qing Jin Wan (Clear Metal Pills) treat food accumulation and depressed fire coughing. They consist of Rhizoma Anemarrhenae (*Zhi Mu*) and Bulbus Fritillariae (*Bei Mu*), each one half *liang*, and Pulvis Semenis Crotonis (*Ba Dou Shuang*), 5 *fen*. Powder and make into pills with

Succus Zingiberis (*Jiang Zhi*). Coat with Pulvis Indigonis (*Qing Dai*); 5-7 pills a dose taken with warm boiled water after a meal.

For taxation coughing with red (blood, use) Radix Panacis Ginseng (*Ren Shen*), Rhizoma Atractylodis Macrocephalae (*Bai Zhu*), Sclerotium Poriae Cocoris (*Fu Ling*), Bulbus Lilii (*Bai He*), Flos Carthami Tinctorii (*Hong Hua*), Herba Cum Radice Asari Sieboldi (*Xi Xin*), Fructus Schizandrae Chinensis (*Wu Wei Zi*), Cortex Cinnamomi (*Guan Gui*), Gelatinum Corii Asini (*E Jiao*), Radix Astragali Membranacei (*Huang Qi*), Rhizoma Pinelliae Ternatae (*Ban Xia*), Tuber Ophiopogonis Japonicae (*Mai Dong*), Semen Pruni Armeniacae (*Xing Ren*), Radix Albus Paeoniae Lactiflorae (*Bai Shao Yao*), and Radix Glycyrrhizae (*Gan Cao*). Take the above ingredients (orally). In case of heat, replace Cortex Cinnamomi and Radix Astragali Membranacei with Cortex Radicis Mori Albi (*Sang Bai Pi*), Herba Ephedrae (*Ma Huang*) with its joints preserved, and Semen Pruni Armeniacae (*Xing Ren*) with its skin preserved.

For fire depression coughing, (use) Fructus Terminaliae Chebulae (*He Zi*), Pumice (*Hai Shi*), Semen Trichosanthis Kirlowii (*Gua Lou Ren*), Pulvis Indigonis (*Qing Dai*), Rhizoma Pinelliae Ternatae (*Ban Xia*), and Rhizoma Cyperi Rotundi (*Xiang Fu*). Coughing with a hoarse voice is (due to) blood vacuity and (resultant) subjection to heat. (In this case,) it is necessary to use Pulvis Indigonis (*Qing Dai*) and Concha Mactrae Quadrangularis (*He Fen*) mixed with honey and melted in the mouth. For enduring coughing with wind having penetrated the lungs, it is appropriate to use the chimney method.[1] (Whereas) dry coughing is difficult to treat since this is a pattern of depressed fire. It is phlegm that has confined fire evils to the lungs. (For this, one) should use Radix Platycodi Grandiflori (*Ku Geng*) to open (depression) and precipitate (fire) with yin-supplementing and fire-downbearing medicinals. If not healed, (this condition) will become a consumptive

---

[1]   The ingredients in this formula are found in a later place in the present chapter.

(disease). The granary-emptying method[2] is good for it. In some cases, this pattern may be due to frustration. For lung depression phlegm coughing with disturbed sleep, (use) *Qing Hua Wan* (Clear & Transform Pills). These consist of Bulbus Fritillariae (*Bei Mu*) and Semen Pruni Armeniacae (*Xing Ren*). Powder and put in Succus Zingiberis (*Jiang Zhi*) mixed with granulated sugar, make into pills like cakes (*i.e.*, lozenges), and melt in the mouth.

A cough-settling, thwarting formula (consists of) Fructus Terminaliae Chebulae (*He Zi*), *Bai Yao Jian* (*i.e.*, fermented Galla Rhi Chinensis [*Wu Bei Zi*] and tea, sometimes with other additives such as rice and Fructus Pruni Mume [*Wu Mei*]), and Herba Seu Flos Schizonepetae Tenuifoliae [*Jie Sui*]). Powder, mix with ginger and honey, and melt in the mouth. Coughing with flank pain requires Pericarpium Viridis Citri Reticulatae (*Qing Pi*). In case of embraced phlegm, it is necessary to use Semen Sinapis Albae (*Bai Jie Zi*). Another formula (consists of) *Er Chen Tang* plus Rhizoma Arisaematis (*Nan Xing*), Rhizoma Cyperi Rotundi (*Xiang Fu*), Pulvis Indigonis (*Qing Dai*), and Succus Zingiberis (*Jiang Zhi*).

For asthma and coughing with phlegm, (use) stir-fried Semen Pruni Armeniacae (*Xing Ren*) and Semen Raphani Sativi (*Lai Fu Zi*) in equal amounts. Powder, make into pills with paste, and take. In (case of) coughing with dry mouth and throat, the existence of phlegm contraindicates (the use of) Rhizoma Pinelliae Ternatae (*Ban Xia*) and Rhizoma Arisaematis (*Nan Xing*) but indicates Fructus Trichosanthis

---

2   This method is believed to cure all sorts of accumulation in the stomach. Obtain in the summer months 20-30 kilos of beef from cow legs, slice thinly, strip away the tough membranes and sinews, boil in a ceramic vessel with river water till well done and then down to a gelatin. Remove the dregs and continue to heat this gelatin over a very small fire lest it gets cold. The patient must have abstained from pork for 3 days and fast in the evening before the following operation. He is placed in a bright room well protected from wind with a night stool and a jar ready at hand. The jar is to contain the urine he will void. Then he is made to drink the gelatin, cup after cup, till he cannot help but vomit. He must then vomit all he has out. Some time later, he will feel very thirsty, but no water should be given him. He is then made to drink the urine in the jar he has previously voided. After this operation, he is only allowed to eat thin gruel for several days.

Kirlowii (*Gua Lou*) and Bulbus Fritillariae (*Bei Mu*). In case of water rheum, do not use Fructus Trichosanthis Kirlowii or Bulbus Fritillariae for fear that they may make (water rheum) sluggish and retarded.

To treat vexation of the heart and coughing, add Cinnabar (*Chen Sha*) to *Liu Yi San* (Six To One Powder).[3] Coughing more common in the morning is due to existence of stomach fire. (For this use) Rhizoma Anemarrhenae (*Zhi Mu*) and Gypsum (*Shi Gao*). Coughing more common in the afternoon is due to yin vacuity. (This requires) *Si Wu Tang* plus stir-fired Cortex Phellodendri (*Huang Bai*) and Rhizoma Anemarrhenae (*Zhi Mu*). Coughing more common at the fifth watch (or early morning) is due to food accumulation in the stomach. At that moment, (the fire of food) is flowing into the lung channel. (For this) use Rhizoma Anemarrhenae (*Zhi Mu*) and Cortex Radicis Lycii (*Di Gu Pi*) to downbear lung fire. (Whereas) coughing more common in the evening is due to fire qi floating in the lungs. It is inappropriate to use cool medicinals but appropriate to use Fructus Schizandrae Chinensis (*Wu Wei Zi*) to astringe and downbear fire. If phlegm ascension counterflow is the result of stirring fire, treat the fire first and the phlegm later.

For cough due to severe lung vacuity, use *Ren Shen Gao* (Ginseng Paste)[4] plus Pericarpium Citri Reticulatae (*Chen Pi*) and fresh Rhizoma Zingiberis (*Sheng Jiang*) as assistants. This is most often seen in lustful persons with kidney vacuity. In the presence of phlegm, add phlegm (removing) medicinals.

Rhizoma Anemarrhenae (*Zhi Mu*) stops coughing and clears the lungs as well as enriches yin and downbears fire. It is appropriate when used (to treat) cough in the night. For phlegm coughing due to the lungs having been damaged by drinking wine, boil Fructus Perillae Frutescentis (*Zi Su*) in Succus Bambusae (*Zhu Li*), put in Succus Allii Tuberosi (*Jiu Zhi*), and take with Fructus Trichosanthis Kirlowii (*Gua*

---

[3]   This is composed of Talcum (*Hua Shi*) and Radix Glycyrrhizae (*Gan Cao*).

[4]   This refers to a thick decoction of Radix Panacis Ginseng (*Ren Shen*).

Lou), Semen Pruni Armeniacae (*Xing Ren*), and Rhizoma Coptidis Chinensis (*Huang Lian*), which, after powdering, prepare in the shape of pills.

For vomiting of blood and coughing with blood (use) Flos Carthami Tinctorii (*Hong Hua*), skinned and tip-nipped Semen Pruni Armeniacae (*Xing Ren*), Radix Asteris Tatarici (*Zi Wan*), Cornu Cervi Parvum (*Lu Rong*), hair-stripped Folium Eriobotryae Japonicae (*Pi Ba Ye*), Cortex Radicis Mori Albi (*Sang Bai Pi*), Caulis Akebiae Mutong (*Mu Tong*), 1 *liang* for each of the above, and Radix Et Rhizoma Rhei (*Da Huang*), one half *liang*. Powder the above, make into pills with heated honey, and melt in the mouth. For enduring cough and phlegm asthma (use) skinned and tip-nipped Semen Pruni Armeniacae (*Xing Ren*) stir-fried with an equal amount of *Lai Fu Dan* (Return & Recover Elixir).[5] Powder and make into pills the size of Semen Cannabis Sativae (*Ma Zi*) with gruel. Take 15 pills per dose with boiled water. For yin vacuity qi asthma, add Pericarpium Citri Reticulatae (*Chen Pi*) and a small amount of Radix Glycyrrhizae (*Gan Cao*) to *Si Wu Tang* to downbear qi and supplement yin. The Radix Albus Paeoniae Lactiflorae (*Bai Shao Yao*) introduced must have undergone wine-soaking and drying in the sun.

Asthma and cough with damp phlegm complicated by wind does not allow for (the use of) exclusively bitter and cold ingredients. It is appropriate to administer *Qian Min Tang* (Thousand Strings of Coins Decoction)[6] and *Zhui Tan Wan* (Drop Phlegm Pills). Another formula (is composed of) Fructus Gleditschiae Sinensis (*Zao Jiao*), Semen Raphani Sativi (*Fu Zi*), Semen Pruni Armeniacae (*Xing Ren*), and *Bai Yao Jian*. Powder together, make into pills with ginger and honey, and melt in the mouth.

---

[5] This is composed of Mirabilitum (*Xiao Shi*), Sulphur (*Liu Huang*), Glaubertum (*Xuan Jing Shi, i.e.,* Gypsum ore), Feces Trogopterori Seu Pteromi (*Wu Ling Zhi*), Pericarpium Viridis Citri Reticulatae (*Qing Pi*), and Pericarpium Citri Reticulatae (*Chen Pi*).

[6] This consists of Rhizoma Pinelliae Ternatae (*Ban Xia*), Fructus Gleditschiae Sinensis (*Zao Jiao*), Radix Glycyrrhizae (*Gan Cao*), and Rhizoma Zingiberis (*Jiang*).

A formula for phlegm coughing (consists of) wine-washed Radix Scutellariae Baicalensis (*Huang Qin*), 1.5 *liang*, Talcum (*Hua Shi*), 5 *qian*, Bulbus Fritillariae (*Bei Mu*), Rhizoma Arisaematis (*Nan Xing*), 1 *liang* each, husked Semen Sinapis Albae (*Bai Jie Zi*), 5 *qian*, and Sodium Sulphate (*Feng Hua Xiao*), 2.5 *qian* [Its light and floating nature is exploited to chase and downbear {fire. later editor}]. Powder the above and make into pills with watersoaked cake. Coat with Pulvis Indigonis (*Qing Dai*).

To treat coughing with dysentery, Pericarpium Papaveris Somnoferi (*Su Ke*) is commonly used. There is no reason for disbelief (about using this). However, the root of the disease must be exterminated before using it. This is a medicinal to close up (*i.e.*, complete a cure). Cough involving the yin phase is usually impugned to yin vacuity. Desire but inability to cough due to lung distension with congestion and obstruction is difficult to treat. To treat cough with phlegm, moxa at the two points, *Tian Tu* (CV 22) and *Fei Shu* (Bl 13).[7] This (method) is able to drain fire heat and greatly drain qi. A (variant) version gives drain fire. The point for lung heat is located below the third vertebra (*i.e.*, T2), 1.5 *cun* bilateral to (the spine). Moxa (this point) as many cones as possible.

Phlegm accumulation cough cannot be eliminated except with Pulvis Indigonis (*Qing Dai*) and Fructus Trichosanthis Kirlowii (*Gua Lou*). Persons with food accumulation have a green-blue, white, and yellow facial complexion usually with crab-leg shaped reticulation on the face, (*i.e.*), yellow and a white (striae). Counterflow coughing cannot be eliminated except with Concha Mactrae Quadrangularis (*He Fen*), Pulvis Indigonis (*Qing Dai*), Fructus Trichosanthis Kirlowii (*Gua Lou*), and Bulbus Fritillariae (*Bei Mu*).

The chimney method for treating cough (is composed of) Herba Saxifragae Stoloniferae (*Fo Er Cao*), 1 *qian*, Flos Tussilagi Farfarae (*Kuan Dong Hua*), 1 *qian*, and Stalactitum Seu Os Balonophylliae (*E Guan Shi*) and Realgar (*Xiong Huang*), 5 *qian* each. Roll Folium Artemisiae Argyii

---

[7] Heaven's Prominence and Lung Transport respectively

(*Ai*), burn and inhale the smoke and take (the above medicinals) with tea water.

A thwarting formula that treats cough (consists of) Galla Rhi Chinensis (*Wu Bei Zi*), 1 *qian*, Fructus Schizandrae Chinensis (*Wu Wei Zi*), 5 *qian*, Radix Glycyrrhizae (*Gan Cao*), 2.5 *qian*, and Sodium Sulphate (*Feng Hua Xiao*), 1 *qian*. Powder the above finely, make into pills with honey, and melt in the mouth. For qi vacuity asthma and cough or (for) fat persons with a white facial complexion and a thin and weak pulse, weak qi, low food intake, and sweating, (use) *Cang Zhu Tiao Zhong Tang* (Atractylodes Rectify the Center Decoction).[8] In case of a heat pattern, add Radix Scutellariae Baicalensis (*Huang Qin*) and Fructus Perillae Frutescentis (*Zi Su*). In case of copious phlegm, add Rhizoma Pinelliae Ternatae (*Ban Xia*), Bulbus Fritillariae (*Bei Mu*), and Fructus Trichosanthis Kirlowii (*Gua Lou*).

For lung atony cough, (use) *Ren Shen Ping Fei San* (Ginseng Level the Lungs Powder).[9] It is a ruling formula for blood vacuity asthma and cough and for thin persons with a red facial complexion and a wiry, rapid pulse, enduring cough with yin vacuity, low food intake with sticky nasal mucus and spittle, incipient consumptive (disease) developing from coughing, and for red phlegm tassels. In case of severe heat, add Radix Scutellariae Baicalensis (*Huang Qin*), Fructus Perillae Frutescentis (*Zi Su*), and Rhizoma Pinelliae Ternatae (*Ban Xia*).

---

[8] This consists of Rhizoma Atractylodis (*Cang Zhu*), Pericarpium Citri Reticulatae (*Chen Pi*), Fructus Amomi (*Sha Ren*), Herba Agastachis Seu Pogostemi (*Huo Xiang*), Radix Paeoniae Lactiflorae (*Shao Yao*), Radix Glycyrrhizae (*Gan Cao*), Radix Platycodi Grandiflori (*Jie Geng*), Rhizoma Pinelliae Ternatae (*Ban Xia*), Radix Angelicae (*Bai Zhi*), Radix Et Rhizoma Notopterygii (*Qiang Huo*), and Fructus Citri Seu Ponciri (*Zhi Qiao*).

[9] This consists of Cortex Radicis Mori Albi (*Sang Bai Pi*), Rhizoma Anemarrhenae (*Zhi Mu*), Radix Glycyrrhizae (*Gan Cao*), Cortex Radicis Lycii (*Di Gu Pi*), Pericarpium Citri Reticulatae (*Chen Pi*), Fructus Schizandrae Chinensis (*Wu Wei Zi*), Sclerotium Poriae Cocoris (*Fu Ling*), Pericarpium Viridis Citri Reticulatae (*Qing Pi*), Radix Panacis Ginseng (*Ren Shen*), and Tuber Asparagi Cochinensis (*Tian Men Dong*).

For qi vacuity asthma and cough with fatigue and lassitude or inability to take in food, insomnia, spontaneous sweating, fever, a large, surging yet vacuous or a deep, thin, and weak pulse with asthma or coughing, (use) *Bu Zhong Yi Qi Tang* (Supplement the Center & Boost the Qi Decoction). For a severe case, add Fructus Schizandrae Chinensis (*Wu Wei Zi*), Rhizoma Anemarrhenae (*Zhi Mu*), and Tuber Ophiopogonis Japonicae (*Mai Men Dong*). In case of copious sweating, delete Rhizoma Cimicifugae (*Sheng Ma*) and Radix Bupleuri (*Chai Hu*). In case of severe asthma and cough, add Cortex Radicis Mori Albi (*Sang Bai Pi*) and Cortex Radicis Lycii (*Di Gu Pi*).

For yin vacuity asthma and cough or vomiting of blood, (use) *Si Wu Tang* plus Rhizoma Anemarrhenae (*Zhi Mu*), Cortex Phellodendri (*Huang Bai*), Fructus Schizandrae Chinensis (*Wu Wei Zi*), Radix Panacis Ginseng (*Ren Shen*), Tuber Ophiopogonis Japonicae (*Mai Men Dong*), Cortex Radicis Mori Albi (*Sang Bai Pi*) and Cortex Radicis Lycii (*Di Gu Pi*). In case of a thin, rapid pulse with exuberant phlegm, add Fructus Trichosanthis Kirlowii (*Gua Lou*) to drain (the phlegm). In case of low food intake, add Rhizoma Atractylodis Macrocephalae (*Bai Zhu*) and Pericarpium Citri Reticulatae (*Chen Pi*).

For coughing in the night due to wind cold depressed into heat in the lungs (use) *San Niu Tang* (Three Negatives Decoction)[10] plus Rhizoma Anemarrhenae (*Zhi Mu*). In case of a large, floating pulse with heat, add Radix Scutellariae Baicalensis (*Huang Qin*) and fresh Rhizoma Zingiberis (*Sheng Jiang*). For cough and vomiting of red (blood) with vacuity of both qi and blood, (use) *Ba Wu Tang* (Eight Materials

---

[10] This consists of Radix Glycyrrhizae (*Gan Cao*), Herba Ephedrae (*Ma Huang*), root and joint not removed, and Semen Pruni Armeniacae (*Xing Ren*), skin and tip not removed. It is so named because there are three ingredients which are required not to be prepared as usual in the formula.

Decoction)[11] plus Tuber Ophiopogonis Japonicae (*Mai Men Dong*), Rhizoma Anemarrhenae (*Zhi Mu*), and lung qi draining medicinals.

Asthma and cough that never fail to arise in winter are (due to) cold wrapping heat. When the exterior is resolved, the heat is naturally eliminated. Use *Jie Geng Zhi Qiao Tang* (Platycodon & Aurantium Decoction): Fructus Citri Seu Ponciri (*Zhi Qiao*), Radix Platycodi Grandiflori (*Jie Geng*), Pericarpium Citri Rubri (*Ju Hong*), and Rhizoma Pinelliae Ternatae (*Ban Xia*) plus Radix Ledebouriellae Sesloidis (*Fang Feng*), Herba Ephedrae (*Ma Huang*), Fructus Perillae Frutescentis (*Zi Su*), Caulis Akebiae Mutong (*Mu Tong*), and Radix Scutellariae Baicalensis (*Huang Qin*). In case of severe cough in cold winter, add Semen Pruni Armeniacae (*Xing Ren*) and subtract Radix Scutellariae Baicalensis.

For cough which never fails to arise on exposure to cold with abundant phlegm above the diaphragm, (use) *Er Chen Tang* plus stir-fried Fructus Citri Seu Ponciri (*Zhi Qiao*), Radix Scutellariae Baicalensis (*Huang Qin*), Radix Platycodi Grandiflori (*Jie Geng*), Rhizoma Atractylodis (*Cang Zhu*), Herba Ephedrae (*Ma Huang*), and Caulis Akebiae Mutong (*Mu Tong*). Boil with ginger in water. (However, for) enduring heat cough in persons with a sturdy constitution, qi repletion, ability to eat, exuberant wine heat, and a replete, rapid pulse (use) *Liang Ge San* (Cool the Diaphragm Powder). In case of heat cough with sore throat in summer months, add Radix Platycodi Grandiflori (*Jie Geng*), Herba Seu Flos Schizonepetae Tenuifoliae (*Jing Jie*), and Fructus Citri Seu Ponciri (*Zhi Qiao*).

For vacuity cough, add Radix Angelicae Sinensis (*Dang Gui*), Radix Paeoniae Lactiflorae (*Shao Yao*), and mix-fried Radix Glycyrrhizae (*Zhi Gan Cao*) to *Si Jun Zi Tang* (Four Gentlemen Decoction. (But for) alternating cold and heat with phlegm-coughing, (use) *Xiao Chai Hu*

---

[11] This consists of Cortex Cinnamomi (*Gui Xin*), Radix Angelicae Sinensis (*Dang Gui*), Rhizoma Ligustici Wallichii (*Chuan Xiong*), Radix Peucedani (*Qian Hu*), Radix Ledebouriellae Sesloidis (*Fang Feng*), Radix Paeoniae Lactiflorae (*Shao Yao*), Radix Glycyrrhizae (*Gan Cao*), and Sclerotium Poriae Cocoris (*Fu Ling*).

Tang (Minor Bupleurum Decoction) plus Rhizoma Anemarrhenae (*Zhi Mu*), etc. In a (variant) formula, Radix Albus Paeoniae Lactiflorae (*Bai Shao Yao*), Fructus Schizandrae Chinensis (*Wu Wei Zi*), and Cortex Radicis Mori Albi (*Sang Bai Pi*) are added.

Shen Su Wen Fei Tang (Ginseng & Perilla Warm the Lungs Decoction) is a formula that treats asthma and cough due to the lungs being damaged by cold form and cold drinks with vexation of the heart, chest fullness and inhibited breathing: Pericarpium Citri Reticulatae (*Chen Pi*), Fructus Perillae Frutescentis (*Zi Su*), Radix Panacis Ginseng (*Ren Shen*), Cortex Radicis Mori Albi (*Sang Bai Pi*), and fresh Rhizoma Zingiberis (*Sheng Jiang*). Another formula consists of *Si Jun Zi Tang* plus Fructus Perillae Frutescentis (*Zi Su*), Cortex Radicis Mori Albi (*Sang Pi*), Pericarpium Citri Reticulatae (*Chen Pi*), Rhizoma Pinelliae Ternatae (*Ban Xia*), Cortex Cinnamomi (*Rou Gui*), Fructus Schizandrae Chinensis (*Wu Wei Zi*), and Radix Saussureae Seu Vladimiriae (*Mu Xiang*). In cold winter, add joint-stripped Herba Ephedrae (*Ma Huang*) and Rhizoma Atractylodis (*Cang Zhu*).

For coughing, retching and vomiting, and distressed rapid breathing with yin qi in the lower and yang qi in the upper, use *Xie Bai San* (Drain the White Powder): stir-fried Cortex Radicis Mori Albi (*Sang Bai Pi*), 3 *liang*, Radix Scutellariae Baicalensis (*Huang Qin*), 3 *liang*, Cortex Radicis Lycii (*Di Gu Pi*), 1 *liang*, and mix-fried Radix Glycyrrhizae (*Zhi Gan Cao*), 5 *qian*, plus Pericarpium Citri Reticulatae (*Chen Pi*), Pericarpium Viridis Citri Reticulatae (*Qing Pi*), Fructus Schizandrae Chinensis (*Wu Wei Zi*), Radix Panacis Ginseng (*Ren Shen*), and Sclerotium Poriae Cocoris (*Fu Ling*), and 21 grains of Semen Oryzae Sativae (*Jing Mi*).

Inability to lie down in asthma or asthma arising upon lying down (is caused by) diminished qi[12] ascension counterflow overwhelming the lungs. The lungs float in the presence of water, (thus) making qi

---

[12] The translator believes that water qi should be read for diminished qi. If he is right, the relevant part should be retranslated as follows: "... asthma arising upon lying is caused by water qi ascension counterflow..." This alternate translation is supported by the similarity in writing between *shao qi* (diminished qi) and *shui qi* (water qi) in Chinese.

unable to flow freely. (For this) prescribe *Shen Mi Tang* (Divine Subtle Decoction): Sclerotium Poriae Cocoris (*Bai Fu Ling*), 5 *qian*, Radix Saussureae Seu Vladimiriae (*Mu Xiang*), 5 *qian*, and Cortex Radicis Mori Albi (*Sang Bai Pi*), Folium Perillae Frutescentis (*Zi Su Ye*), stir-fried Pericarpium Citri Reticulatae (*Ju Pi*), and Radix Panacis Ginseng (*Ren Shen*), 7 *qian* for each of the above. In case of asthma and cough with a deep yet large pulse, add fresh Rhizoma Zingiberis (*Sheng Jiang*).

In case of internal vacuity or contraction of wind cold, complicated in addition by excessive bedroom affairs with coughing and aversion to wind due to taxation, (use) Radix Panacis Ginseng (*Ren Shen*), 4 *qian*, and Herba Ephedrae (*Ma Huang*) with root and joints preserved, 1.5 *qian*. Two or three doses offer a cure. This is a miraculous formula of Master Dan-xi's.

To treat cough with vacuity of both qi and blood or any other kind of cough, (use) Radix Panacis Ginseng (*Ren Shen*), Flos Tussilagi Farfarae (*Kuan Dong Hua*), Cortex Radicis Mori Albi (*Sang Bai Pi*), Radix Platycodi Grandiflori (*Jie Geng*), Fructus Schizandrae Chinensis (*Wu Wei Zi*), Gelatinum Corii Asini (*E Jiao*), Fructus Pruni Mume (*Wu Mei*), 1 *liang* for each of the above, Bulbus Fritillariae (*Bei Mu*), 5 *qian*, and Pericarpium Papaveris Somnoferi (*Yu Mi Ke*), 8 *liang*, which is nipped and fried to yellow with honey. This (formula) is called *Jiu Xian San* (Nine Immortals Powder).

For phlegm drool coughing with spleen vacuity and cold lungs, (use) *Zi Su Yin Zi* (Perilla Drink). This consists of) *San Niu Tang* (Three Negatives Decoction) plus Fructus Perillae Frutescentis (*Zi Su*), Cortex Radicis Mori Albi (*Sang Bai Pi*), Pericarpium Viridis Citri Reticulatae (*Qing Pi*), Pericarpium Citri Reticulatae (*Chen Pi*), Fructus Schizandrae Chinensis (*Wu Wei Zi*), Radix Panacis Ginseng (*Ren Shen*), and Rhizoma Pinelliae Ternatae (*Ban Xia*). Boil with fresh Rhizoma Zingiberis (*Sheng Jiang*).

For heat cough with chest fullness, (use) *Xiao Xian Xiong Tang* (Minor Sunken Chest Decoction).[13] In lustful persons whose original qi tends to be vacuous with enduring and persisting cough, (use) *Qiong Yu Gao* (Fine Jade Paste).[14] For coughing in alcoholics, (use) Pulvis Indigonis (*Qing Dai*) and Fructus Trichosanthis Kirlowii (*Gua Lou*, made) in the shape of pills with ginger and honey and melted in the mouth to succor the lungs. Generally speaking, Succus Zingiberis (*Jiang Zhi*) with its acridity is usually used to dissipate in the treatment of cough.

A male, aged 20, suffered from affection of cold and coughing with phlegm as a result of taxation fatigue and inability to sleep through the night. The phlegm was like yellow and white pus and the coughing sound failed to exit (*i.e.*, was like hissing and puffing). It was early spring with great cold. He was given four doses of *Xiao Qing Long Tang* (Minor Green-Blue Dragon Decoction).[15] He then felt a thread in his throat and bloody qi counterflowing up. With a thread of blood flowing out on the left side of his mouth, (the fit) came to an end after a while. This happened more than 10 times each night. His pulse was wiry, large, scattered, and weak and was particularly large on the right hand. The person was exhausted and felt bitter (*i.e.*, tormented) about the cough. I determined this was a contraction of cold in taxation fatigue. Since a sweet, acrid, dry, hot formula had been used unwarrantedly, resulting in stirring up his blood, there was a fear that (his condition) might develop into lung atony unless an (appropriate) treatment was given without delay. Therefore, he was treated with Radix Panacis Ginseng (*Ren Shen*), Radix Astragali Membranacei (*Huang Qi*), Radix Angelicae Sinensis (*Dang Gui Shen*),

---

[13] This consists of Rhizoma Coptidis Chinensis (*Huang Lian*), Rhizoma Pinelliae Ternatae (*Ban Xia*), and Fructus Trichosanthis Kirlowii (*Gua Lou*).

[14] This consists of Radix Panacis Ginseng (*Gao Li Shen*), Succus Radicis Rehmanniae (*Di Huang Zhi*), and Sclerotium Poriae Cocoris (*Fu Ling*).

[15] This consists of Radix Paeoniae Lactiflorae (*Shao Yao*), Herba Cum Radice Asari Sieboldi (*Xi Xin*), dry Rhizoma Zingiberis (*Gan Jiang*), Radix Glycyrrhizae (*Gan Cao*), Ramulus Cinnamomi (*Gui Zhi*), Fructus Schizandrae Chinensis (*Wu Wei Zi*), and Rhizoma Pinelliae Ternatae (*Ban Xia*).

Rhizoma Atractylodis Macrocephalae (*Bai Zhu*), Radix Paeoniae Lactiflorae (*Shao Yao*), Pericarpium Citri Reticulatae (*Chen Pi*), mix-fried Radix Glycyrrhizae (*Zhi Gan Cao*), Radix Glycyrrhizae (*Sheng Gan Cao*), and Herba Ephedrae (*Ma Huang*) with joints preserved. These were boiled well and then Succus Rhizomatis Nelumbinis Nuciferae (*Ou Zhi*) was put in. After two months, his condition improved and his cough stopped. Then the same formula was prescribed but with Herba Ephedrae removed. Another four doses were administered, and bleeding was stopped. His pulse, (however,) was still large and scattered, remaining to be contracted and astringed. Moreover, the patient was still fatigued with very low food intake. Accordingly, Succus Rhizomatis Nelumbinis Nuciferae was removed and Radix Scutellariae Baicalensis (*Huang Qin*), Fructus Amomi (*Suo Sha*), and Rhizoma Pinelliae Ternatae (*Ban Xia*) were added to the preceding formula. Half a month later, (he) recovered.

Dai comments: Wind cold cough (is characterized by) nasal congestion, heavy (*i.e.*, hoarse) voice, and fear of cold. Fire cough (is characterized by) sonorousness, scant phlegm, and a red facial complexion; taxation cough (by) thief sweating; complication of phlegm usually (by alternating) cold and heat; distended lung cough (by) cough arising on slight movement with panting and fullness, and distressed rapid breathing; and phlegm cough (by) rale heard once on coughing and cough stopping immediately after phlegm is discharged. (One) should first be able to identify these five types before (one) can administer an (appropriate) treatment.

A female suffered from accumulation cough with a lump in her abdomen and steaming heat in the internal. (Therefore, she was given) Bulbus Fritillariae (*Bei Mu*), Fructus Trichosanthis Kirlowii (*Gua Lou*), Rhizoma Arisaematis (*Nan Xing*), and Rhizoma Cyperi Rotundi (*Xiang Fu*), 1 *liang* for each of the above, Rhizoma Curcumae (*Jiang Huang*), and Fructus Polygoni Tinctorii (*Lan Shi*), 2.5 *qian* each, and Rhizoma Atractylodis Macrocephalae (*Bai Zhu*), 1 *liang*.

(Another) female suffered from accumulated phlegm cough. (She was given) Radix Scutellariae Baicalensis (*Huang Qin*), Rhizoma Coptidis Chinensis (*Huang Lian*), Rhizoma Cyperi Rotundi (*Xiang Fu*), Bulbus

Fritillariae (*Bei Mu*), Fructus Trichosanthis Kirlowii (*Gua Lou*), Radix Glycyrrhizae (*Sheng Gan Cao*), Pericarpium Citri Reticulatae (*Chen Pi*), Sclerotium Poriae Cocoris (*Fu Ling*), Rhizoma Atractylodis Macrocephalae (*Bai Zhu*), Rhizoma Anemarrhenae (*Zhi Mu*), Semen Pruni Armeniacae (*Xing Ren*), and Cortex Radicis Mori Albi (*Sang Bai Pi*).

A person suffered from phlegm accumulation and depression cough. (This person was given) Bulbus Fritillariae (*Bei Mu*), Radix Scutellariae Baicalensis (*Huang Qin*), Rhizoma Cyperi Rotundi (*Xiang Fu*), Fructus Trichosanthis Kirlowii (*Gua Lou*), and Pericarpium Viridis Citri Reticulatae (*Qing Pi*), 1.5 *liang* for each of the above.

A fat person who had had fat meat and fine grain and drunk wine had attacks of sore throat, congested nose, and phlegm cough arising at once upon taxation fatigue. (This person was given) *Liang Ge San* (Cool the Diaphragm Powder) plus Radix Platycodi Grandiflori (*Jie Geng*), Herba Seu Flos Schizonepetae Tenuifoliae (*Jing Jie*), Rhizoma Arisaematis (*Nan Xing*), and Fructus Immaturus Citri Seu Ponciri (*Zhi Shi*).

Book Two

Chapter Nineteen

Phlegm

(This condition) is (further) classified into damp, heat, cold, wind, old, and food accumulation (types of phlegm). A floating pulse usually justifies ejection, (whereas) phlegm existing above the diaphragm invariably requires ejection. (And) phlegm existing in the channels and connecting vessels cannot be driven out except by ejection. Ejection also means effusion and dissipation. Epilepsy, for instance, may be caused by fright. Because of fright, the spirit leaves its abode, and, when its abode is left vacant, phlegm may enter. Occupying this abode, phlegm repulses the spirit. Thus it is impossible for the spirit to return (to its abode).

Phlegm existing in the stomach and intestines (on the other hand) can be cured by precipitation. For damp phlegm, (use) Rhizoma Atractylodis (*Cang Zhu*), Rhizoma Atractylodis Macrocephalae (*Bai Zhu*), and the like. For heat phlegm, (use) Pulvis Indigonis (*Qing Dai*), Radix Scutellariae Baicalensis (*Huang Qin*), Rhizoma Coptidis Chinensis (*Huang Lian*), etc. For cold phlegm (use) *Er Chen Tang* (Two Aged Decoction). For wind phlegm, (use) Rhizoma Arisaematis (*Nan Xing*), Radix Aconiti Coreani (*Bai Fu*), and the like. For old phlegm, (use) Pumice (*Hai Shi*), Fructus Trichosanthis Kirlowii (*Gua Lou*), etc, and for food accumulation phlegm, (use) Massa Medica Fermentata (*Shen Qu*), Fructus Germinatus Hordei Vulgaris (*Mai Ya*) and the like.

Qi repletion with hot, bound phlegm which is difficult to spit out (due to) forming into lumps or simply refusing to come out with coughing or hacking with qi stagnation are difficult to treat. Phlegm existing in the upper that is sticky, solid, thick, and turbid invariably requires ejection. Emetics include Folium Camelliae Sinensis (*Ya Chai*), pickle, Succus Zingiberis (*Jiang Zhi*), a small amount of vinegar, and a small dose of *Lu Gua Di San* (Stem-preserved Melon Pedicle Powder) plus

Radix Platycodi Grandiflori (*Jie Geng*) and Radix Ledebouriellae Sesloidis (*Fang Feng*). All of these are able to uplift and stir the qi and therefore provoke vomiting. Another method is to use Apex Radicis Praeparati Aconiti Carmichaeli (*Fu Zi Jian*), Radix Platycodi Grandiflori (*Jie Geng*), stem-preserved Radix Panacis Ginseng (*Lu Ren Shen*), Pediculus Melonis (*Gua Di*), and Radix Veratri Nigri (*Li Lu*). Arsenic (*Pi*) is rarely used except in emergencies. Whether in the form of decoctions or not, Folium Artemisiae Argyii (*Ai*) and Pulvis Folii Camelliae Sinensis (*Mo Cha*) both can induce vomiting without applying any (other) operation or maneuver.

Another method of (inducing) vomiting is to first gird the waist tightly with a strip of cloth and then perform the operation in a wind-tight place. Pound one half *sheng* of Semen Raphani Sativi (*Luo Bo Zi*), mix well with one bowl of fermented sorghum and flour water (*Jiang Shui*), filter out the dregs, and put in a little oil and honey. Then simmer till lukewarm and take. Next, probe (the throat) with a goose quill to provoke vomiting. The goose quill should be dipped in tung oil which is washed away again with water of Fructus Gleditschiae Sinensis (*Zao Jiao*) and then dried in the sun for use. In addition, the shrimp soup ejection method is also a good method.

Uncheckable vomiting necessitates resolving medicinals. Secretio Moschi Moschiferi (*She Xiang*) resolves Radix Veratri Nigri (*Li Lu*) and Pediculus Melonis (*Gua Di*). Bulbus Allii Fistulosi (*Cong Bai*, also) resolves Pediculus Melonis (*Gua Di*). Water and Radix Glycyrrhizae (*Gan Cao*) resolve all kinds (of medicinal toxins able to provoke vomiting).

Non-erythematous tubercles anywhere on the body which are painless and not festering are all (a result of) streaming phlegm. Those patients for whom no medicinals can bring effect and who have a hidden yet large pulse in the *guan* section are suffering from phlegm. Soot black eyelids and suborbital regions also indicate phlegm. Lumps existing in the upper, the middle, or lower body are phlegm. After finding out what kind of substance (the patient) is fond of (eating), disperse (the lumps) with medicinals counteracting (that food) after ejection and precipitation. Solidifying spleen earth and drying spleen dampness are the fundamental methods for treating phlegm.

Master Xue instructs: To treat phlegm rheum developing into a gathering lump, use Rhizoma Atractylodis (*Cang Zhu*). It is extremely efficacious in moving phlegm. Phlegm, if embracing blood, may develop into gathering lumps. If phlegm disease has persisted long enough to make the pulse choppy/astringent, it is difficult to open (the bound phlegm) in a short time. This must take a long time to rectify and treat. *Er Chen Tang* (Two Aged Decoction) plus Rhizoma Cimicifugae (*Sheng Ma*) and Radix Bupleuri (*Chai Hu*) can moisten the stools, make the voiding of urine long, and loosen the chest and diaphragm.

Internal damage embracing phlegm invariably requires the use of Radix Panacis Ginseng (*Ren Shen*), Radix Astragali Membranacei (*Huang Qi*), and Rhizoma Atractylodis Macrocephalae (*Bai Zhu*). Succus Zingiberis (*Jiang Zhi*) should be used in large quantities to transport these, or add Rhizoma Pinelliae Ternatae (*Ban Xia*) and the like. In case of severe vacuity, add Succus Bambusae (*Zhu Li*). Phlegm heat usually embraces wind and, hence, manifests as an external pattern. In some cases, (the hot phlegm) may form into lumps refusing to come out with spitting and hacking. If complicated by depression, it is difficult to treat. Damp phlegm (on the other hand) tends to give rise to softening, for example, fatigue and heavy body.

Wind phlegm often displays strange patterns. Food accumulation phlegm invariably requires extra attacking. (While) in case of qi vacuity, qi-supplementing medicinals must be used to send off (the phlegm). If (phlegm) is caused by exuberant fire counterflowing up, the treatment of fire is given priority with Rhizoma Atractylodis Macrocephalae (*Bai Zhu*), Radix Scutellariae Baicalensis (*Huang Qin*), Gypsum (*Shi Gao*), and the like. In case of insufficient center qi, add Rhizoma Atractylodis Macrocephalae (*Bai Zhu*) and Radix Panacis Ginseng (*Ren Shen*, to supplement the qi) before treating the phlegm. As a substance, phlegm can follow qi up and down in the human body. Everywhere is accessible to it, and nothing is beyond its capability. (Further,) phlegm complicates the majority of the hundreds of diseases. Of this the world is unaware. In case of spleen vacuity, clear the center qi to convey phlegm down with *Er Chen Tang* plus Rhizoma Atractylodis Macrocephalae (*Bai Zhu*) and the like, and in addition, employ Rhizoma Cimicifugae (*Sheng Ma*) to upraise qi. One cannot use simply the attacking method on vacuous persons with phlegm in the middle burner since even the stomach qi depends (upon the middle burner) for nourishment. If one only uses attacking, the vacuity will be made (all) the more serious.

Dizziness and clamoring stomach are (due to) phlegm being stirred by fire. (For this) administer *Er Chen Tang* plus Fructus Gardeniae Jasminoidis (*Zhi Zi*), Radix Scutellariae Baicalensis (*Huang Qin*), Rhizoma Coptidis Chinensis (*Huang Lian*), etc. For phlegm formed into tubercles in the throat which is dry and unable to exit when the throat is open, (one should use) phlegm-transforming medicinals plus salty ingredients to soften the hard (such as) Fructus Trichosanthis Kirlowii (*Gua Lou*), Semen Pruni Armeniacae (*Xing Ren*), Pumice (*Hai Shi*), Radix Platycodi Grandiflori (*Jie Geng*), and Fructus Forsythiae Suspensae (*Lian Qiao*) plus a small amount of Sodium Sulfate (*Feng Xiao*) as assistants. Make into pills with ginger and honey and melt in the mouth.

Phlegm existing beneath the skin but above the membrane or in the channels and connecting vessels cannot be cured except with Succus Zingiberis (*Jiang Zhi*), Succus Bambusae (*Zhu Li*), and Succus Viticis Negundi (*Jing Li*). Phlegm existing in the limbs can be moved by nothing else than Succus Bambusae (*Zhu Li*. If there is the feeling as if) something were stuck in the throat which is impossible to hack out or swallow down, this is phlegm. A severe case requires ejection and a moderate case requires such medicinals as Fructus Trichosanthis Kirlowii (*Gua Lou*). Qi repletion makes it necessary to use Succus Viticis Negundi (*Jing Li*). In case of obstructed, stagnated blood, and rheum existing in the middle burner, drink 3-4 winecups of cold Succus Allii Tuberosi (*Jiu Zhi*). This must be followed by vexation, agitation, and disquietude in the chest. (However,) there is nothing to worry about. Just keep administering and recuperation will presently follow.

Ovum Notarchi Leachii Freeri (*Hai Fen*) is capable of downbearing hot phlegm, drying damp phlegm, softening bound phlegm, and dispersing stubborn phlegm. It can be introduced into pills but not into decoctions. Radix Scutellariae Baicalensis (*Huang Qin*) is able to treat phlegm heat since it is easy for it to downbear fire. Fructus Immaturus Citri Seu Ponciri (*Zhi Shi*) drains phlegm and is even able to butt (down) walls.[1] Radix Trichosanthis Kirlowii (*Tian Hua Fen*) greatly treats hot phlegm above the diaphragm. With the assistance of other medicinals, Galla Rhi Chinensis (*Wu Bei Zi*) greatly treats stubborn phlegm. Fructus Trichosanthis Kirlowii (*Gua Lou*) and Talcum (*Hua Shi*) greatly treat food accumulation phlegm. They flush the viscera and bowels. Oil-fried Rhizoma Pinelliae Ternatae (*Ban Xia*) greatly treats damp phlegm and also treats asthma and cough with heart pain. (For this,) it is made into pills with gruel and taken with ginger soup, 30 pills (per dose). Because *Xiao Wei Dan* (Minor Stomach Elixir)[2] is capable of causing detriment to the stomach qi, it can also be used, but not in large quantities (in the treatment of) food accumulation phlegm.

A formula to treat damp phlegm (consists of) Radix Scutellariae Baicalensis (*Huang Qin*), Rhizoma Pinelliae Ternatae (*Ban Xia*), Rhizoma Cyperi Rotundi (*Xiang Fu*), and Bulbus Fritillariae (*Bei Mu*). If Fructus Trichosanthis Kirlowii (*Gua Lou*) and Pulvis Indigonis (*Qing Dai*) are added, it can treat hot phlegm. Take it in the shape of pills. (However, to treat) clear phlegm, (use a formula) such as *Er Chen Tang*. To treat wind phlegm, it is always necessary to use Radix Aconiti Coreani (*Bai Fu Zi*), Rhizoma Gastrodiae Elatae (*Tian Ma*), Realgar (*Xiong Huang*), Calculus Bovis (*Niu Huang*), Bombyx Batryticatus (*Jiang Can*), and Fructus Gleditschiae Sinensis (*Zhu Ya Zao Jiao*).

Zhong He Wan (Center Harmony Pills) treat damp phlegm qi heat. (They consist of) Rhizoma Atractylodis (*Cang Zhu*), Radix Scutellariae Baicalensis (*Huang Qin*), Rhizoma Pinelliae Ternatae (*Ban Xia*), and Rhizoma Cyperi Rotundi (*Xiang Fu*), all in equal amounts. Powder and make into pills with gruel. A formula to dry damp phlegm (consists of) Rhizoma Arisaematis (*Nan Xing*), 1 *liang*, Rhizoma Pinelliae Ternatae (*Ban Xia*), 2 *liang*, and Concha Mactrae Quadrangularis (*He Fen*), 3 *liang*. Powder the above, make into pills with steamed cake, and coat

---

[1] This implies that the medicinal is so powerful that it opens all kinds of depression and breaks all kinds of binds. Muscles and flesh are often spoken of as walls in TCM.

[2] This consists of Rhizoma Coptidis Chinensis (*Huang Lian*), Radix Scutellariae Baicalensis (*Huang Qin*), and Cortex Phellodendri (*Huang Bai*).

with Pulvis Indigonis (*Qing Dai*). A formula to treat yin vacuity with abundant food accumulation phlegm in the internal (consists of) true Rhizoma Ligustici Wallichii (*Chuan Xiong*), 7 *qian*, Rhizoma Coptidis Chinensis (*Huang Lian*), Semen Trichosanthis Kirlowii (*Gua Lou Ren*), Rhizoma Atractylodis Macrocephalae (*Bai Zhu*), Massa Medica Fermentata (*Shen Qu*), and Fructus Germinatus Hordei Vulgaris (*Mai Ya*), 1 *liang* for each of the above, Pulvis Indigonis (*Qing Dai*), 5 *qian*, and crystallized urine (*Ren Zhong Bai*), 3 *qian*. Powder the above and make into pills with steamed cake and Succus Zingiberis (*Jiang Zhi*).

Succus Bambusae (*Zhu Li*) treats phlegm existing around the diaphragm with mania or withdrawal, impaired memory, or wind phlegm. It is also able to nurture blood. Its use is the same as Succus Viticis Negundi (*Jing Li*). *Xiao Wei Dan* (on the other hand) treats damp hot phlegm accumulation and also white vaginal discharge. Coat Radix Euphorbiae Kansui (*Gan Sui*) with water-dampened flour, boil in river water till the flour is well-done, wash with water, and then dry in the sun. Boil Radix Euphorbiae Pekinensis (*Da Ji*) in river water for one watch, wash with water, and then dry it in the sun. Mix Flos Daphnis Genkwae (*Yuan Hua*) evenly with good quality vinegar and, after (allowing it to sit) overnight, fry in a ceramic vessel, stirring all the while till it turns black but without charring. Wrap Radix Et Rhizoma Rhei (*Da Huang*) with paper which is wet with water, roast in live ash fire without charring it, remove the paper, cut, bake dry, moisten with wine, and stir-fry till hot. Its quantity is double (that of each) of the preceding medicinals. Stir-fry Cortex Phellodendri (*Huang Bai*), double the quantity of Radix et Rhizoma Rhei. Grind (all) the above separately, weigh out each, and make them into pills with gruel the size of Semen Cannabis Sativae (*Ma Zi*); 12 pills per dose. A (variant) formula consists of reducing Radix Euphorbiae Kansui (*Gan Sui*) and Radix Euphorbiae Pekinensis (*Da Ji*) by one third in quantity and coat (the pills) with Cinnabar (*Zhu Sha*). This is called *Chen Sha Hua Tan Wan* (Cinnabar Transform Phlegm Pills).

Another formula for phlegm (consists of) Rhizoma Arisaematis (*Nan Xing*) and Rhizoma Pinelliae Ternatae (*Ban Xia*), 1 *liang* each, and Concha Mactrae Quadrangularis (*He Fen*), 2 *liang*. This specifically treats damp phlegm. (In case of) heat, add Pulvis Indigonis (*Qing Dai*.

In case of) dampness, add Rhizoma Atractylodis (*Cang Zhu*. In case of) food accumulation, add Massa Medica Fermentata (*Shen Qu*), Fructus Germinatus Hordei Vulgaris (*Mai Ya*), and Fructus Crataegi (*Shan Zha*). Another formula (consists of) Radix Scutellariae Baicalensis (*Huang Qin*), Rhizoma Cyperi Rotundi (*Xiang Fu*), Rhizoma Pinelliae Ternatae (*Ban Xia*), Fructus Trichosanthis Kirlowii (*Gua Lou*), Bulbus Fritillariae (*Bei Mu*), and Pulvis Indigonis (*Qing Dai*). Powder and make into pills.

(A formula) that treats food accumulation phlegm fire and is also able to greatly drain stomach fire is made by powdering Gypsum (*Ruan Shi Gao*) finely and making into pills the size of Semen Phaseoli Radiati (*Lu Dou*) with vinegar; 10 pills per dose, (while) *Qing Meng Shi Wan* (Chlorite Schist Pills) resolve food accumulation and eliminate damp phlegm. This may also be administered in the form of decoction depending on whether (the condition) is cold or hot, vacuity or repletion.(The formula consists of) Chlorite Schist (*Qing Meng Shi*), one half *liang*, calcined in the conventional way, Rhizoma Pinelliae Ternatae (*Ban Xia*), 7 *qian*, Rhizoma Arisaematis (*Nan Xing*), Sclerotium Poriae Cocoris (*Fu Ling*), and Radix Scutellariae Baicalensis (*Pian Qin*), one half *liang* for each of the above, and slaked lime (*Xiao*), 3 *qian*. (Slaked lime is processed as follows:) Boil Mirabilitum (*Mang Xiao*) together with Rhizoma Raphani Sativi (*Luo Bo*) in water to melt it, remove the radish, filter (the solution) with cloth, and let crystalize. Powder (all the ingredients) and make into pills with flour paste. A (variant) version adds Rhizoma Atractylodis (*Cang Zhu*) and Talcum (*Hua Shi*). Another formula (consists of) Rhizoma Pinelliae Ternatae (*Ban Xia*), 2 *liang*, Rhizoma Atractylodis Macrocephalae (*Bai Zhu*), 1 *liang*, Sclerotium Poriae Cocoris (*Fu Ling*), and Pericarpium Citri Reticulatae (*Chen Pi*), 7.5 *qian* each, Radix Scutellariae Baicalensis (*Huang Qin*), and Chlorite Schist (*Meng Shi*), one half *liang* each, and Sodium Sulfate (*Feng Hua Xiao*), 2 *qian*.

A formula for phlegm asthma (consists of) carbonized Fructus Gleditschiae Sinensis (*Zao Jiao Hui*), one half *liang*, Ovum Notarchi Leachii Freeri (*Hai Fen*), steamed Semen Raphani Sativi (*Luo Bo Zi*), Rhizoma Arisaematis (*Nan Xing*), soaked in a solution of 1.5 *qian* of Alum (*Bai Fan*) and then dried in the sun, 1 *liang* for each of the above, and Semen Trichosanthis Kirlowii (*Gua Lou Ren*), 1 *liang*. Powder the above, make into pills with ginger and honey, and melt in the mouth. Another formula (consists of) Rhizoma Arisaematis (*Nan Xing*), Rhizoma Pinelliae Ternatae (*Ban Xia*), Semen Pruni Armeniacae (*Xing Ren*), Fructus Trichosanthis Kirlowii (*Gua Lou*), Semen Raphani Sativi (*Luo Bo Zi*), Pulvis Indigonis (*Qing Dai*), and Rhizoma Cyperi Rotundi (*Xiang Fu*). Make into pills with Massa Medica Fermentata (*Shen Qu*) paste.

Qing Jin Wan (Clear Metal Pills) eliminate lung fire and precipitate hot phlegm above the diaphragm. Use in combination with *Qing Hua Wan* (Clear & Transform Pills. *Qing Hua Wan*) are composed of stir-fried Radix Scutellariae Baicalensis (*Huang Qin*). Powder and make into pills with water. This *Qing Hua Wan* formula can dry damp heat by strength of its bitterness and treat (conditions) in the upper by the strength of its lightness, (thus) offering a specific remedy for heat cough. It also treats sore throat when ground finely, mixed with vinegar, and applied to the throat. (It is composed of) stir-fried Herba Physalis Peruvianae (*Deng Long Cao Ye*). Powder and make into pills with steamed cake.

Fu Ling Wan (Poria Pills) treat phlegm. (They consist of) Rhizoma Pinelliae Ternatae (*Ban Xia*), 4 *liang*, Sclerotium Poriae Cocoris (*Fu Ling*), 2 *liang*, Fructus Citri Seu Ponciri (*Zhi Qiao*), 1 *liang*, and Sodium Sulfate (*Feng Hua Xiao*), 5 *qian*. To treat depressive phlegm, (use) Bombyx Batryticatus (*Bai Jiang Can*), Semen Pruni Armeniacae (*Xing Ren*), Semen Trichosanthis Kirlowii (*Gua Lou Ren*), Fructus Terminaliae Chebulae (*He Zi*), Bulbus Fritillariae (*Bei Mu*), and Galla Rhi Chinensis (*Wu Bei Zi*). *Dao Yin Wan* (Conduct Rheum Pills consist of) Fructus Evodiae Rutecarpae (*Wu Zhu Yu*), processed, 3 *qian*, Sclerotium Poriae Cocoris (*Fu Ling*), 1 *liang*, Rhizoma Coptidis Chinensis (*Huang Lian*), 5 *qian*, Talcum (*Hua Shi*), 7.5 *qian*, and Rhizoma Atractylodis (*Cang Zhu*), 1.5 *liang*, soaked in rice water. Powder the above and make into pills with Massa Medica Fermentata (*Shen Qu*) paste. Take 100 pills per dose with ginger soup.

Bai Yu Wan (White Jade Pills) consist of Semen Crotonis (*Jiang Zi*), 30 pieces, Rhizoma Arisaematis (*Nan Xing*), Rhizoma Pinelliae Ternatae (*Ban Xia*), Talcum (*Hua Shi*), and Calomelas (*Qing Fen*), 3 *qian* for each of the above. Powder and make into pills with a thick extraction from soaked Semen Gleditschiae Sinensis (*Zao Jiao Ren*), the size of Semen Cannabis Sativae (*Ma Zi*); 5-7 pills a dose. *Gua Lou Wan* (Trichosanthes Pills) treat food accumulation and phlegm congestion and stagnation asthma. (They consist of) Semen Trichosanthis Kirlowii (*Gua Lou Ren*), Rhizoma Pinelliae Ternatae (*Ban Xia*), Fructus Crataegi (*Shan Zha Rou*), and Massa Medica Fermentata (*Shen Qu*), all in equal amounts. Powder the above and make into pills with Succus Fructi Trichosanthis Kirlowii (*Gua Lou Shui*). Take 20 pills with Succus Bambusae (*Zhu Li*) mixed in ginger soup. Another formula (consists of) Rhizoma Pinelliae Ternatae (*Ban Xia*), 1 *liang*, Rhizoma Atractylodis (*Cang Zhu*), 2 *liang*, Rhizoma Cyperi Rotundi (*Xiang Fu*), 2.5 *liang*, and Radix Scutellariae Baicalensis (*Huang Qin*), Rhizoma Coptidis Chinensis (*Huang Lian*), and Fructus Trichosanthis Kirlowii (*Gua Lou*), 1 *liang* for each of the above. Powder the above and make into pills with Massa Medica Fermentata (*Shen Qu*) paste.

Qing Ge Hua Tan Fang (Clear the Diaphragm & Transform Phlegm Formula) consist of Rhizoma Coptidis Chinensis (*Huang Lian*), 1 *liang*, Radix Scutellariae Baicalensis (*Huang Qin*), 1 *liang*, Cortex Phellodendri (*Huang Bai*), 5 *qian*, Fructus Gardeniae Jasminoidis (*Shan Zhi*), 5 *qian*, Rhizoma Cyperi Rotundi (Xiang Fu), 2.5 *qian*, and Rhizoma Atractylodis (*Cang Zhu*), 2 *liang*. Powder the above and make into pills with Massa Medica Fermentata (*Shen Qu*) paste.

Sou Feng Hua Tan Wan (Track Wind & Transform Phlegm Pills) consist of Radix Panacis Ginseng (*Ren Shen*), Bombyx Batryticatus (*Jiang Can*), Fructus Sophorae Japonicae (*Huai Jiao Zi*), Alum (*Bai Fan*), Rhizoma Gastrodiae Elatae (*Tian Ma*), Pericarpium Citri Reticulatae (*Chen Pi*) stripped of its white inner skin, Herba Seu Flos Schizonepetae Tenuifoliae (*Jing Jie*), 1 *liang* (for each of the above), Rhizoma Pinelliae Ternatae (*Ban Xia*), 4 *liang*, soaked with Succus Zingiberis (*Jiang Zhi*), and Cinnabaris (*Chen Sha*), one half *liang*. Powder the above, make into pills with cake of Succus Zingiberis (*Jiang Zhi*), dry in the shade, and coat with one half *liang* of Cinnabar. Take 40 pills with ginger soup.

Zhui Tan Wan (Drop Phlegm Pills) treat phlegm rheum effectively. (They consist of) Fructus Immaturus Citri Seu Ponciri (*Zhi Shi*) and Fructus Citri Seu Ponciri (*Zhi Qiao*), stir-fried and stripped of the pulp, one half *liang* each, Semen Pharbitidis (*Hei Qian Niu*), one half *jin*, with bran and husk removed after being ground, Fructus Gleditschiae Sinensis (*Zhu Ya Zao Jiao*), 2 *qian*, stir-fried with wine, Alum (*Ming Fan*), 3 *qian*, half waterground, and slaked lime (*Po Xiao*), 3 *qian*, powdered by exposure to air. Powder the above and make into pills with Succus Rhizomae Raphani Sativi (*Luo Bo Zhi*); 40 pills per dose taken at the cock-crow watch. (After taking it), first stool will be evacuated and then phlegm will be discharged.

To treat damp phlegm, (use) Rhizoma Atractylodis (*Cang Zhu*), 1 *qian*, Rhizoma Atractylodis Macrocephalae (*Bai Zhu*), 6 *qian*, Rhizoma Cyperi Rotundi (*Xiang Fu*), 1 *qian*, and wine-processed Radix Albus Paeoniae Lactiflorae (*Bai Shao Yao*), 2 *qian*. Powder the above and make into pills with cake. (However,) to treat damp phlegm in fat persons, (use) Radix Sophorae Flavescentis (*Ku Shen*) and Rhizoma Pinelliae Ternatae (*Ban Xia*), each 1.5 *qian*, Rhizoma Atractylodis Macrocephalae (*Bai Zhu*), 2.5 *qian*, and Pericarpium Citri Reticulatae (*Chen Pi*), 1 *qian*, all as one dose. Boil together with 3 slices of Rhizoma Zingiberis (*Jiang*) in one cupful of mixture of Succus Bambusae (*Zhu Li*) and water, and take between meals with 15 pills of *San Bu Wan* (Three Supplementations Pills).[2]

To treat wind phlegm in the upper burner, (use) Semen Trichosanthis Kirlowii (*Gua Lou Ren*), Rhizoma Coptidis Chinensis (*Huang Lian*), Rhizoma Pinelliae Ternatae (*Ban Xia*), and Fructus Gleditschiae Sinensis (*Zhu Ya Zao Jiao*), all in equal amounts. Powder the above and make into pills with Succus Zingiberis (*Jiang Zhi*) cake. (But) to treat phlegm qi, (use) Radix Scutellariae Baicalensis (*Pian Huang Qin*), Pericarpium Citri Reticulatae (*Chen Pi*), and Rhizoma Pinelliae Ternatae (*Ban Xia*), 5 *qian* for each of the above, Rhizoma Atractylodis Macrocephalae (*Bai Zhu*) and Radix Albus Paeoniae Lactiflorae (*Bai Shao Yao*), 1 *liang* each, and Sclerotium Poriae Cocoris (*Fu Ling*), 3 *qian*. Powder the above and make into pills with Succus Zingiberis (*Jiang Zhi*) cake. To dispel wind phlegm and move turbid qi, (use) Radix Ledebouriellae Sesloidis (*Fang Feng*), Rhizoma Ligustici Wallichii (*Chuan Xiong*), Fructus Gleditschiae

---

[2] This consists of Rhizoma Coptidis Chinensis (*Huang Lian*), Radix Scutellariae Baicalensis (*Huang Qin*), and Cortex Phellodendri (*Huang Bai*).

Sinensis (*Ya Zao*), Alum (*Bai Fan*), and Tuber Curcumae (*Yu Jin*), 1 *liang* for each of the above, and Scolopendra Subspinipes (*Wu Gong*), a red and a white piece. Powder the above and make into pills as big as Semen Cannabis Sativae (*Ma Zi*) with cake; 25 pills a dose taken with tea water before a meal. In spring, take with Radix Musae Basjooris (*Ba Jiao*) soup and perform mechanical emesis for phlegm.

Li Ge Hua Tan Wan (Disinhibit the Diaphragm & Transform Phlegm Pills) treat phlegm qi in the chest and diaphragm with most wonderful results. (They consist of) Bulbus Fritillariae (*Bei Mu*) and Rhizoma Pinelliae Ternatae (*Ban Xia*), each one half *liang*, Rhizoma Arisaematis (*Tian Nan Xing*) and Concha Mactrae Quadrangularis (*He Fen*), 1 *liang* each, and Semen Trichosanthis Kirlowii (*Gua Lou Ren*) and Rhizoma Cyperi Rotundi (*Xiang Fu*), soaked with child's urine, one half *liang* each. Powder the above finely together. Break 14 pieces of Fructus Gleditschiae Sinensis (*Zhu Ya Zao Jiao*), and boil in 1.5 bowls of water with 1 *liang* of skinned and tip-nipped Semen Pruni Armeniacae (*Xing Ren*) till the water is nearly dried up. (Then) remove Fructus Gleditschiae Sinensis, smash Semen Pruni Armeniacae by pounding, and put this in and mix with the above ingredients. Next put in Succus Zingiberis (*Jiang Zhi*), make into pills the size of Semen Phaseoli Radiati (*Lu Dou*) with cake, coat with Pulvis Indigonis (*Qing Dai*), and then dry in the sun; 50-60 pill per dose.

A (variant) version of *Qing Tan Wan* (Clear Phlegm Pills) are specific against phlegm accumulation in the chest or phlegm accumulation in the central palace. (They are composed of) Fructus Pruni Mume (*Wu Mei*), 5 *qian*, Alum (*Ku Ming Fan*), 5 *qian*, Rhizoma Arisaematis (*Nan Xing*), and Rhizoma Pinelliae Ternatae (*Ban Xia*), 1 *liang* each, Radix Scutellariae Baicalensis (*Huang Qin*), 5 *qian*, Rhizoma Atractylodis (*Cang Zhu*), 5 *qian*, Massa Medica Fermentata (*Shen Qu*), 1 *liang*, Fructus Crataegi (*Tang Qiu*), 1 *liang*, Pericarpium Viridis Citri Reticulatae (*Qing Pi*), Pericarpium Citri Reticulatae (*Chen Pi*), 5 *qian* each, Rhizoma Cyperi Rotundi (*Xiang Fu*), 1 *liang*, stir-fried Talcum (*Hua Shi*), 5 *qian*, dry fresh Rhizoma Zingiberis (*Gan Sheng Jiang*), 1 *liang*, and Fructus Immaturus Citri Seu Ponciri (*Zhi Shi*), 1 *liang*. Powder the above and make into pills with cake.

A male, aged 79, suffered from clouding and heaviness of the head and eyes, weakness in the limbs, and spitting after spitting of phlegm. His pulse was scattered, large, and retarded on the left hand and retarded and large on the right but less so than on the left. (It also) felt weak on the both (hands) when pressure was applied. (In addition, he suffered from) slightly reduced food intake, moderate thirst, and one bowel movement every 3-4 days. (In this case,) if wind(-dispelling) medicinals were administered, death would be bound to come when spring advanced deep. This was a pattern of great vacuity and required a large dose of a supplementing formula. (Therefore, he) was prescribed Radix Astragali Membranacei (*Huang Qi*), Radix Panacis Ginseng (*Ren Shen*), Radix Angelicae Sinensis (*Dang Gui Shen*), Radix Paeoniae Lactiflorae (*Shao Yao*), Rhizoma Atractylodis Macrocephalae (*Bai Zhu*), and Pericarpium Citri Reticulatae (*Chen Pi*). These were boiled down to a thick decoction. (He) was made to take this with 30 pills of *Lian Bai Wan* (Coptis & Phellodendron Pills). One and half years of administration (of this regime) restored his energy as in the prime of his life. *Lian Bai Wan* should be expanded by a small amount of dry Rhizoma Zingiberis (*Gan Jiang*) in winter as a seasonal medicinal. In the other three seasons, it is composed as follows: Rhizoma Coptidis Chinensis (*Huang Lian*) and Cortex Phellodendri (*Huang Bai*), both stir-fried with Succus Zingiberis (*Jiang Zhi*). Powder and make into pills with Succus Zingiberis (*Jiang Zhi*) paste.

In the autumn, a male nearly 30 years of age, who used to have (a diet) of thick flavors (*i.e.*, rich foods) and was irascible, began to suffer pain in the hip joints on both sides. This spread from these small areas gradually to his knees and shins. (This pain) was relieved by day but exacerbated by night, and the painful parts were averse to cold. (Further, he was) thirsty sometimes but not thirsty at other (times). A doctor prescribed him wind-treating and some blood-supplementing medicinals as well. Towards the next spring, his knees gradually became swollen with severe pain, his food intake gradually decreased, and his form became markedly emaciated. Late in the spring, his knees became so swollen that they were as large as bowls and he was not able to flex or extend (them). His pulse was bowstring, large, and rather replete. In addition, (it was) rapid and short in all (sections), presumably with frequent, short voidings of urine. He was treated for food and drink (accumulation) and phlegm accumulation in the *tai yin* and *yang ming* (with) Rhizoma Pinelliae Ternatae (*Ban Xia*), 5 *qian*, Cortex Phellodendri (*Huang Bai*), 1 *liang*, stir-fried with wine, Apex Radicis Glycyrrhizae (*Sheng Gan Cao Shao*), 3 *qian*, Rhizoma Atractylodis (*Cang Zhu*), 3 *qian*, stir-fried with salt, Rhizoma Ligustici Wallichii (*Chuan Xiong*), 3 *qian*, dust of Cornu Rhinocerori (*Sheng Xi Niu Jiao*), 3 *qian*, Pericarpium Citri Reticulatae (*Chen Pi*), Achyranthes Bidentata (*Niu Xi*), Caulis Akebiae Mutong (*Mu Tong*), and Radix Paeoniae Lactiflorae (*Shao Yao*), 5 *qian* for each of the above. In case of superficial heat, add 2 *qian* of Radix Scutellariae Baicalensis (*Tiao Qin*). Powder the above; 3 *qian* per dose. After grinding together with Succus Zingiberis (*Jiang Zhi*) to an appropriate fineness, heat in water just to a boil and then take before a meal while hot. Four doses were administered in a day and night.

Half a month later, his pulse gradually slowed down and his pain improved. (The formula's) administration was continued in the same way as before (but) with Cornu Rhinocerori subtracted and (one half *liang* of) Achyranthes Bidentata (*sic, Niu Xi*), Plastrum Praeparatum Testudinis (*Bai Gui Ban*), one half *liang*, and Radix Angelicae Sinensis (*Dang Gui*), one half *liang*, added. In another half month, the swelling gradually abated, food intake gradually increased, and there was no more aversion to cold. Only his knees were (still) atonic and weak, and he was unable to stand or walk for long. Rhizoma Atractylodis and Radix Scutellariae Baicalensis were (then) deducted, and, because it was a summer month, stir-fried Cortex Phellodendri was increased to 1.5 *liang*. The other (ingredients) were the same as in the original formula. As to Achyranthes Bidentata, in spring and summer, Ramus (*Geng*) is used, while in autumn and winter, Radix (*Gen*) is used. However, the juice of the leaves is most efficacious. (One) must cut off (eating and drinking) wine, meat, sodden wheat food, and pepper. For a middle-aged person, one half *liang* of Radix Rehmanniae (*Sheng Di*) should be added, (but) in winter, add Fructus Evodiae Rutecarpae (*Zhu Yu*) and Ramulus Cinnamomi (*Gui Zhi*).

A person felt a scraping (pain) in the face whenever exposed to the lightest wind with neither the front nor the back of the body (*i.e.,* trunk) averse to cold. (He was) able to eat, (had) a bowstring pulse, and his daily life activities were normal. He was first administered

Rhizoma Ligustici Wallichii (*Chuan Xiong*), Radix Platycodi Grandiflori (*Jie Geng*), fresh Rhizoma Zingiberis (*Sheng Jiang*), Fructus Gardeniae Jasminoidis (*Shan Zhi*), and powdered Folium Camelliae Sinensis (*Cha*). After ejection of phlegm, he was administered *Huang Lian Dao Tan Tang* (Coptis Conduct Phlegm Decoction).[3]

One day, my brother-in-law, drunk and overeating, uttered nonsense and had confused vision, giving a blasphemous account of his dead brother (when alive). His uncle scolded him, saying that all this was due to eating too many fish and drinking too much wine. This was a trouble made by phlegm. A large bowl of salt water was poured down (his throat) and then one *sheng* of phlegm was vomited. Subsequently sweat broke out heavily. After a sound night's sleep, he recovered.

A woman, (known) by her husband's surname Jin, was in the prime of her life. In a summer month, after she returned from a banquet, her sister-in-law enquired about her *faux pas* of taking the wrong seat. (At this) she felt ashamed and subsequently fell ill. She uttered nonsense, particularly full of self-reproach, with the pulse bowstring and rapid at the both sides. I argued that this was an illness rather than an obsession by ghost evil and that, if only the spleen were supplemented, phlegm conducted, and heat cleared, she would recover for sure in a few days. Her family, however, did not believe (this). Several witches were invited to spray water (which) only frightened her. (After) a little more than 10 days, she died.

One evening, a woman more than 50 years of age and in a raging mood ate roasted pork. The next morning her face was distended and she was unable to take in food. (She was also) bodily fatigued, and her

---

[3] This consists of ginger-processed Rhizoma Pinelliae Ternatae (*Ban Xia*), Sclerotium Poria Cocoris (*Fu Ling*), Pericarpium Citri Reticulatae (*Chen Pi*), Radix Glycyrrhizae (*Gan Cao*), Succus Zingiberis (*Sheng Jiang Zhi*), Fructus Pruni Mume (*Wu Mei*), Rhizoma Arisaematis (*Tian Nan Xing*), Fructus Immaturus Citri Seu Ponciri (*Zhi Shi*), Radix Panacis Ginseng (*Ren Shen*), Rhizoma Atractylodis Macrocephalae (*Bai Zhu*), Radix Scutellariae Baicalensis (*Huang Qin*), Rhizoma Coptidis Chinensis (*Huang Lian*), powdered Fructus Trichosanthis Kirlowii (*Gua Lou*), Radix Platycodi Grandiflori (*Jie Geng*), Succus Bambusae (*Zhu Li*), and Fructus Zizyphi Jujubae (*Zao*).

six pulses were deep and choppy, yet hollow and large. This was a vacuous body with phlegm obstructed and unable to descend and required supplementation of vacuity and disinhibition of phlegm. Every morning, she was made to take a large dose of *Er Chen* (Two Aged [Decoction]) plus Radix Panacis Ginseng (*Ren Shen*) and Rhizoma Atractylodis Macrocephalae (*Bai Zhu*), and after that, mechanical emesis was performed to send out the medicinals again. After the *chen* watch (7-9 AM), she was made to take two doses of *San He Tang* (Three Harmonies Decoction) with Rhizoma Atractylodis Macrocephalae (*Bai Zhu*) in triple amount, and, before sleeping, she took seven pills of *Shen You Wan* (God Bless Pills) to dispel phlegm. With Semen Pharbitidis (*Qian Niu*) deleted, this was administered for one month and she recovered.

In a summer month, the son of Fu, an assistant at the Procurator's yeomen, felt thirsty because of taxation and drank quantities of plum juice to his heart's content. In addition, he experienced terrible fright 3-4 times in succession. With confused speech and vision, the disease looked like an obsession by ghost evil. His pulse at both sides was vacuous and wiry as well as deep and rapid. I concluded that a rapid pulse indicated existence of heat, (while) a vacuous, wiry pulse revealed terrible fright, and that sour juice was retained in the middle venter. If vacuity was supplemented, heat cleared, and stagnated phlegm led out, the disease would be overcome. (I) prescribed Radix Panacis Ginseng (*Ren Shen*), Rhizoma Atractylodis Macrocephalae (*Bai Zhu*), Pericarpium Citri Reticulatae (*Chen Pi*), Radix Scutellariae Baicalensis (*Huang Qin*), Rhizoma Coptidis Chinensis (*Huang Lian*), and Sclerotium Poriae Cocoris (*Fu Ling*). These were boiled to a thick decoction and taken with Succus Bambusae (*Zhu Li*) and Succus Zingiberis (*Jiang Zhi*) put in. More than 10 days passed with no effect. Everyone grumbled that the prescription was not correct. I was aware that his vacuity was yet to be overcome and his phlegm was yet to be led out. (I) continued the same formula but with Succus Viticis Negundi (*Jing Li*) added, and, in another 10 days, recovery ensued.

A person with yin vacuity suffered from phlegm. (Therefore, I gave them) Massa Medica Fermentata (*Shen Qu*), Fructus Germinatus Hordei Vulgaris (*Mai Ya*), Rhizoma Coptidis Chinensis (*Huang Lian*), and

Rhizoma Atractylodis Macrocephalae (*Bai Zhu*), 1 *liang* for each of the above, Rhizoma Ligustici Wallichii (*Chuan Xiong*), 7 *qian*, Semen Trichosanthis Kirlowii (*Gua Lou Ren*), Pulvis Indigonis (*Qing Dai*), and crystallized human urine (*Ren Zhong Bai*), one half *liang* each. The above were powdered, pounded with Succus Zingiberis (*Jiang Zhi*), and made into pills with cake.

A person suffered from damp heat and taxation fatigue. Shortly after his wedding, he felt a discomfort in his chest and diaphragm, feeling there the existence of cold rheum. The pulse was choppy and large. He had previously been administered quantities of acrid, warm, dissipating medicinals with the result that both blood and qi had been damaged. (Now he was prescribed) Rhizoma Atractylodis (*Cang Zhu*), Rhizoma Pinelliae Ternatae (*Ban Xia*), Rhizoma Atractylodis Macrocephalae (*Bai Zhu*), Pericarpium Citri Reticulatae (*Chen Pi*), 5 *qian* for each of the above, Radix Albus Paeoniae Lactiflorae (*Bai Shao Yao*), 6 *qian*, Plastrum Testudinis (*Gui Ban*), 7.5 *qian*, stir-fried Cortex Phellodendri (*Huang Bai*), 1.5 *qian*, Radix Scutellariae Baicalensis (*Huang Qin*), 3 *qian*, and Fructus Amomi (*Sha Ren*) and Radix Glycyrrhizae (*Gan Cao*), 1 *qian* each. The above were powdered, made into pills with cake, and taken with Succus Zingiberis (*Jiang Zhi*) before meals; 40-50 pills (each time). After administration, the cold phlegm around the diaphragm remained uneliminated. Then *Xiao Xian Xiong Tang* (Minor Sunken Chest Decoction) was administered in the shape of pills with a small amount of Fructus Evodiae Rutecarpae (*Wu Zhu Yu*) added as the conductor.

An(other) person with replete qi and a sturdy form often felt an unsoothed qi in the chest and diaphragm. *San Yi Cheng Qi Tang* (Three to One Support the Qi Decoction was used) to precipitate (the qi), and certain phlegm-conducting (medicinals) were administered in addition.

A person suffered from food accumulation, phlegm qi, and a weak spleen. (They were given) Bulbus Fritillariae (*Bei Mu*), Fructus Forsythiae Suspensae (*Lian Qiao*), Fructus Germinatus Hordei Vulgaris (*Mai Ya*), Pericarpium Citri Reticulatae (*Chen Pi*), one half *liang* for each of the above, Rhizoma Arisaematis (*Nan Xing*), Radix Scutellariae Baicalensis (*Huang Qin*), Rhizoma Atractylodis Macrocephalae (*Bai Zhu*), 1 *liang* for each of the above, and Semen Raphani Sativi (*Lai Fu*

Zi), 2.5 *qian*. The above were powdered and made into pills with cake.

An old person suffered from retching of phlegm, chest fullness, and (alternating) cold and heat as a result of food damage. *Er Chen* (Two Aged [Decoction]) was used to conduct rheum; Rhizoma Atractylodis Macrocephalae (*Bai Zhu*) to supplement the spleen; Radix Bupleuri (*Chai Hu*) and Radix Scutellariae Baicalensis (*Huang Qin*) to abate cold and heat; Rhizoma Atractylodis (*Cang Zhu*) to resolve the exterior cold; and Fructus Amomi (*Sha Ren*) to settle retching and precipitate (counterflow) qi.

A female had thick fur over the tongue with pain and frequent hardness appearing below the heart. (This was a case of) phlegm heat in the *yang ming*. (For this, she was given) Cortex Phellodendri (*Huang Bai*), Rhizoma Anemarrhenae (*Zhi Mu*), both fried with honey, Bulbus Fritillariae (*Bei Mu*), 2 *liang* for each of the above, Fructus Trichosanthis Kirlowii (*Gua Lou*), Fructus Immaturus Citri Seu Ponciri (*Zhi Shi*), Fructus Germinatus Hordei Vulgaris (*Mai Ya*), Rhizoma Curcumae (*Jiang Huang*), and Radix Achyranthis Bidentatae (*Niu Xi*), one half *liang* for each of the above. (The above) are powdered and can be applied by retaining on the tongue. In addition, prescribe Rhizoma Atractylodis Macrocephalae (*Bai Zhu*), 2 *liang*, Fructus Piperis Cubebae (*Bi Cheng Qie*), Semen Raphani Sativi (*Lai Fu Zi*), Fructus Forsythiae Suspensae (*Lian Qiao*), and Gypsum (*Shi Gao*), one half *liang* for each of the above, Fructus Canarii Albi (*Qing Zi*), Sodium Sulfate (*Feng Hua Xiao*), and Rhizoma Cimicifugae (*Sheng Ma*), 3 *qian* for each of the above. Powder the above, make into pills with cake, and take.

Er Chen (Tang) is a very important formula for treating phlegm, but many people tend to neglect it. Since even *Ping Wei San* (Level the Stomach Powder)[4] is in constant use, why should not *Er Chen Tang* be administered? If only (one) is able to make (appropriate) additions and subtractions in accordance with signs, (one) will never use it but with effect. This is but one example that people do not value so much their eyes as their ears.

---

[4] This consists of Rhizoma Atractylodis (*Cang Zhu*), Cortex Magnoliae Officinalis (*Hou Po*), Pericarpium Citri Reticulatae (*Chen Pi*), Radix Glycyrrhizae (*Gan Cao*), fresh Rhizoma Zingiberis (*Sheng Jiang*), and Fructus Zizyphi Jujubae (*Zao*).

Chapter Twenty

Dyspnea

(This disease) is (further) classified into shortness of breath, fire upflaming, phlegm, and upward counterflow of yin fire (types. In case of) chronic dyspnea, when dormant, it is vital to support the righteous qi; when active, attacking evil is the rule. In case of shortness of breath, supplement (qi) with Radix Panacis Ginseng (*Ren Shen*) and Radix Astragali Membranacei (*Huang Qi*). In case of fire upflaming, downbear heart fire and clear lung metal. In the presence of phlegm, it is the rule to downbear phlegm and precipitate qi. In case of upward counterflow of yin fire, supplement yin and downbear fire. There is (also) dyspnea with qi vacuity and shortness of breath and dyspnea with existence of phlegm in addition to shortness of breath as well as yin vacuity with fire ascending from the lower abdomen.

For rapid dyspneic breathing with existence of wind phlegm, the *Fu Ren Da Quan Liang Fang (Complete Collection of Fine Formulas for Women)*[1] (prescribes) *Qian Min Tang* (Thousand Strings of Coins Decoction) plus *Dao Tan Tang* (Conduct Phlegm Decoction). (While) rapid dyspneic breathing with yin vacuity embracing phlegm (requires) supplementing yin and downbearing fire with *Si Wu Tang* (Four Materials Decoction) plus Rhizoma Pinelliae Ternatae (*Ban Xia*) and Fructus Citri Seu Ponciri (*Zhi Qiao*), (and) qi vacuity (requires) honey-fried Radix Panacis Ginseng (*Ren Shen*), Cortex Phellodendri (*Huang Bai*), Tuber Ophiopogonis Japonicae (*Mai Men Dong*), Cortex Radicis Lycii (*Di Gu Pi*), etc. Generally speaking, bitter, cool medicinals are contraindicated in rapid dyspneic breathing because fire qi is

---

[1] This work was compiled by Chen Zi-ming in 1237 CE. It is first Chinese book specifically on gynecology in TCM.

exuberant.[2] (In this case,) *Dao Tan Tang* in combination with *Qian Min Tang* is miraculous.

For incessant dyspnea of various kinds, use the thwarting method, but do not use more than 1-2 doses. (This method) is seldom applied in persons with qi vacuity. After the thwarting settles it, (one should) treat phlegm if it is due to phlegm or fire if it is due to fire. Grind Semen Zanthoxyli Bungeani (*Jiao Mu*) very finely and take 2 *qian* brewed with fresh Rhizoma Zingiberis (*Sheng Jiang*) soup to check (dyspnea). This can be used either in the shape of powder or pills. Another (thwarting) method (is to use) steamed Semen Raphani Sativi (*Luo Bo Zi*) as the sovereign (with) ash-burned and powdered Fructus Gleditschiae Sinensis (*Zao Jiao*). Make with Succus Zingiberis (*Jiang Zhi*) and honey into pills the size of small Chinese parasol tree seeds; 50-70 pills per dose, melted in the mouth to check (dyspnea).

Dyspnea due to vacuity of original qi or dyspnea with shortness of breath (requires) *Sheng Mai San* (Generate the Pulse Powder). Qi ascension dyspnea with agitation which is ascribed to lung distention threatens to develop into wind water.[3] Diaphoresis can overcome this. (However,) between autumn and winter, dyspnea started by wind phlegm (should be treated by) *Sou Feng Hua Tan Wan* (Track Wind & Transform Phlegm Pills). (While) for dyspnea started by lung dampness, grind finely Semen Descurainiae Sophiae (*Tian Ting Li*), make into pills with Fructus Zizyphi Jujubae (*Zao*), and take.

When a patient lies down, qi is liable to float in the lungs. For any case of ascending qi, the commonly used (medicinals) are Rhizoma Cyperi Rotundi (*Xiang Fu*), Rhizoma Coptidis Chinensis (*Huang Lian*), Radix Scutellariae Baicalensis (*Huang Qin*), Fructus Gardeniae Jasminoidis

---

[2] As the author explains, when fire is raging, there must be water transformation involved. Therefore, no bitter, cool medicinals should be employed recklessly at first.

[3] Wind water is a kind of water swelling characterized by fever, aversion to wind, swelling starting from the head and face, pain in the joints, and a floating pulse.

(*Shan Zhi*), and Pericarpium Viridis Citri Reticulatae (*Qing Pi*) which can downbear (qi).

Dai comments: There are phlegm dyspnea, qi urgency dyspnea, stomach vacuity dyspnea, and fire upflaming dyspnea. Phlegm dyspnea is a dyspnea that advances and retreats (*i.e.,* comes and goes) irregularly and is always accompanied by a phlegm rale. Qi urgency dyspnea is rapid distressed breathing with no phlegm rale. Fire upflaming dyspnea is a dyspnea that advances and retreats irregularly, getting better when food is taken but recurring after eating. (In this case,) there most probably is repletion fire in the stomach and sticky phlegm above the diaphragm. As food is going down the throat, the sticky phlegm is brought down and dyspnea comes to a pause. A little while after, when the food has entered the stomach, the fire phlegm is, on the other (hand), helped to ascend again, and dyspnea attacks all the more fiercely. The vulgar (person) has no knowledge of this and treats it as stomach vacuity with dry, hot medicinals, (but this) only helps fire with fire. Governor Ye once suffered from (dyspnea) of this kind. The many (attending) physicians treated it as stomach vacuity and achieved no cure. Later he was administered *Dao Shui Wan* (Conduct Water Pills)[4] to disinhibit (water), and 5-7 times sent him to recovery. In addition, there is (also) stomach vacuity dyspnea which is a kind of incessant dyspnea with the shoulders raised and belly bulging.

To treat qi counterflow, qi dyspnea, and qi ascension, *Zi Jin Dan* (Purple Gold Elixir) can be used but not till (the condition has lasted) more than 3 years. Pork and wine are prohibited (when taking this medicine).

A two year old child suffered from phlegm dyspnea. Seeing that his essence spirit was clouded and fatigued and that the disease qi had penetrated deeply, this was definitely not an external contraction but a fetal toxin. This was impugned to his mother who, during pregnan-

---

[4]   This consists of Radix Et Rhizoma Rhei (*Da Huang*), Radix Scutellariae Baicalensis (*Huang Qin*), Talcum (*Hua Shi*), and Semen Pharbitidis (*Qian Niu*).

cy, used to like acrid, pungent, hot foods. (In this case,) no resolving or disinhibiting medicinals should be administered. Therefore, (I) prescribed Radix Panacis Ginseng (*Ren Shen*), Fructus Forsythiae Suspensae (*Lian Qiao*), Rhizoma Ligustici Wallichii (*Xiong*), Rhizoma Coptidis Chinensis (*Lian*), Radix Glycyrrhizae (*Sheng Gan Cao*), Pericarpium Citri Reticulatae (*Chen Pi*), Radix Paeoniae Lactiflorae (*Shao Yao*), and Caulis Akebiae Mutong (*Mu Tong*). These were boiled and then mixed with Succus Bambusae (*Zhu Li*). Several days after, (the child) recovered.

A female suffered for 6 or 7 months from phlegm coughing and rapid dyspneic breathing with inability to lie down. (In this case,) the rule without exception is (to treat) the lungs. (I administered) Radix Bupleuri (*Bei Chai Hu*), 1 *qian*, Herba Ephedrae (*Ma Huang*), 2 *qian*, Gypsum (*Shi Gao*), 2 *qian*, Cortex Radicis Mori Albi (*Sang Bai Pi*), 1 *qian*, Radix Glycyrrhizae (*Gan Cao*), one half *qian*, and Radix Scutellariae Baicalensis (*Huang Qin*), 1.5 *qian*. Recovery followed sweating. Then (she) was administered Fructus Schizandrae Chinensis (*Wu Wei Zi*), Radix Glycyrrhizae (*Gan Cao*), Cortex Radicis Mori Albi (*Sang Pi*), Radix Panacis Ginseng (*Ren Shen*), and Radix Scutellariae Baicalensis (*Huang Qin*).

Chapter Twenty-one

Wheezing

For wheezing, the exclusive rule is to treat phlegm. Ejection is the appropriate method, but in the presence of vacuity, ejection may not be allowed. To treat wheezing, it is necessary to keep away (from food rich in) flavor. Because the exclusive rule is to treat phlegm, it is necessary to perform great ejection. The emetics should include vinegar in large quantities. Merely using cool medicinals is not allowed. (One should also use) those to dissipate the exterior since this is (a case of) heat wrapped up by cold. (For this use) Rhizoma Pinelliae Ternatae (*Ban Xia*), stir-fried Fructus Citri Seu Ponciri (*Zhi Qiao*), Radix Platycodi Grandiflori (*Jie Geng*), Radix Scutellariae Baicalensis (*Pian Huang Qin*), stir-fried Fructus Perillae Frutescentis (*Zi Su*), Herba Ephedrae (*Ma Huang*), Semen Pruni Armeniacae (*Xing Ren*), and Radix Glycyrrhizae (*Gan Cao*). In cold weather, add Cortex Cinnamomi (*Gui*). Another formula (consists) of taking *Xiao Wei Dan* (Minor Stomach Elixir) with decocted *Er Chen Tang* (Two Aged Decoction) with Radix Glycyrrhizae (*Gan Cao*) subtracted but Rhizoma Atractylodis (*Cang Zhu*) and Radix Scutellariae Baicalensis (*Huang Qin*) added. This medication should vary depending on vacuity and repletion.

One method to treat wheezing with accumulation is to slightly crack a hen's egg with the (inner) membranes kept intact and submerge in a urinal for 3-4 days. Then boil and take at night. (This is) effective since eggs are able to dispel wind phlegm.

Zi Jin Dan (Purple Gold Elixir) for the treatment of wheezing (is made by) cutting 30 *liang* of lean pork into cubes the size of dice. Obtain 1 *liang* of Arsenicum (*Xin*) which should be bright, grind very finely, and mix with the pork, necessarily very evenly. Divide into 6 portions, wrap with paper-cemented clay, bake dry, and then, away from people, calcine with a charcoal fire till green-blue smoke is no longer seen. To rid (this) of fire toxins, lay (the meat) on the ground for one night and then grind, make with watersoaked steamed cake into pills the size of mung beans, and take with tea water before a meal; 20 pills for adults, 10 pills for children. This dosage can vary depending on vacuity and repletion.

A person suffered from wheezing. (They were given) Rhizoma Arisaematis (*Nan Xing*), Rhizoma Pinelliae Ternatae (*Ban Xia*), Semen Pruni Armeniacae (*Xing Ren*), Semen Trichosanthis Kirlowii (*Gua Lou Ren*), Rhizoma Cyperi Rotundi (*Xiang Fu*), Pericarpium Citri Rubri (*Ju Hong*), Pulvis Indigonis (*Qing Dai*), Semen Raphani Sativi (*Lai Fu Zi*), and carbonized Fructus Gleditschiae Sinensis (*Zao Jiao Hui*). All the above were powdered, made into pills with the paste of Massa Medica Fermentata (*Shen Qu*), and taken with ginger soup.

Chapter Twenty-two

Diarrhea

(This disease) is (further) classified into dampness, qi vacuity, fire, phlegm, and accumulation (types). The vulgar (only) use astringing medicinals to treat dysentery and diarrhea. (Such treatment) may be practical if (diarrhea) has accumulated long and is accompanied by vacuity, but it never fails to add transmuted patterns to a recent (diarrhea, and this) results in no small disastrous consequence. It should be known that, because (diarrhea) is usually due to dampness, the most far-sighted policy is to separate and disinhibit small water (*i.e.*, urination). To treat dampness and dry dampness, it is appropriate to carry out percolation and drainage with *Si Ling San* (Four *Ling* Powder)[1] plus Rhizoma Atractylodis (*Cang Zhu*) and Rhizoma Atractylodis Macrocephalae (*Bai Zhu*). In severe cases, the two *Zhu*, (*i.e.*, Rhizoma Atractylodis [*Cang Zhu*] and Atractylodis Macrocephalae [*Bai Zhu*]), should be stir-fried (for use).

In case of qi vacuity, use Radix Panacis Ginseng (*Ren Shen*), Rhizoma Atractylodis Macrocephalae (*Bai Zhu*), Radix Paeoniae Lactiflorae (*Shao Yao*), and stir-fried Rhizoma Cimicifugae (*Sheng Ma*). Fire requires attacking fire and disinhibiting small water with Radix Scutellariae Baicalensis (*Huang Qin*) and Caulis Akebiae Mutong (*Mu Tong*) introduced into *Si Ling San*. Phlegm requires sweeping phlegm with Pumice (*Hai Shi*), Pulvis Indigonis (*Qing Dai*), Radix Scutellariae Baicalensis (*Huang Qin*), and Massa Medica Fermentata (*Shen Qu*) taken in the shape of pills. Or perform ejection to provoke vomiting in order to upraise the clear qi. Food accumulation requires dispersing and abducting, coursing and flushing with Massa Medica Fermentata (*Shen*

---

[1] This consists of Sclerotium Poriae Cocoris (*Fu Ling*), Sclerotium Polypori Umbellati (*Zhu Ling*), Rhizoma Alismatis (*Ze Xie*), and Rhizoma Atractylodis Macrocephalae (*Bai Zhu*).

Qu) or Radix Et Rhizoma Rhei (*Da Huang*) and the like. Diarrhea of large quantities of water makes it imperative to use *Wu Ling San* (Five *Ling* Powder).[2]

A diarrhea-checking formula (consists of) Semen Myristicae Fragrantis (*Rou Dou Kou*), 5 *liang*, and Talcum (*Hua Shi*), 1.25 *liang* in the spring and winter, 2.5 *liang* in the summer, and 2 *liang* in the autumn. Make the above into pills with the paste of Succus Zingiberis (*Jiang Zhi*) and Massa Medica Fermentata (*Shen Qu*). Another formula, *Jiang Qu Wan* (Ginger & Medicated Leaven Pills, is composed of) Rhizoma Zingiberis (*Jiang*), 2 *liang*, and old Massa Medica Fermentata (*Shen Qu*), 6 *liang*. (This should be) stir-fried and (that which is) 1-2 years old is desirable. New Massa Medica Fermentata is not usable, for it generates heat. Old Semen Tritici Aestivi (*Mai*) can be used (instead. This formula also) includes one half *liang* of Fructus Foeniculi Vulgaris (*Hui Xiang*).[3]

A formula to treat spleen diarrhea[4] (consists of) stir-fried Rhizoma Atractylodis Macrocephalae (*Bai Zhu*), stir-fried Massa Medica Fermentata (*Shen Qu*), and stir-fried Radix Paeoniae Lactiflorae (*Shao Yao*). Take in the form of decoction, powder, or pills. This is particularly effective against spleen diarrhea when it is necessary to greatly supplement the spleen qi to restore its movement and transformation to normal.

---

[2] This consists of Sclerotium Polypori Umbellati (*Zhu Ling*), Sclerotium Poriae Cocoris (*Fu Ling*), Rhizoma Atractylodis Macrocephalae (*Bai Zhu*), Rhizoma Alismatis (*Ze Xie*), and Ramulus Cinnamomi (*Gui Zhi*).

[3] It is equally possible that Semen Hordei Vulgaris (*Mai Ya*) is meant here instead of wheat. It also seems likely to the translator that this sentence should be combined with the immediately preceding to form a single sentence reading: Old Massa Medica Fermentata (*Shen Qu*) can be replaced by one half *liang* of Fructus Foeniculi Vulgaris (*Hui Xiang*).

[4] Spleen diarrhea is outpour diarrhea due to spleen vacuity with the manifestations of abdominal distention and fullness and vomiting and retching upon ingestion.

(However,) to treat an enduring illness of large intestine qi diarrhea[5], use prepared Radix Rehmanniae (*Shu Di Huang*), 5 *qian*, stir-fried Radix Albus Paeoniae Lactiflorae (*Bai Shao Yao*), and Rhizoma Anemarrhenae (*Zhi Mu*), 3 *qian* each, dry Rhizoma Zingiberis (*Gan Jiang*), 2 *qian*, and mix-fried Radix Glycyrrhizae (*Zhi Gan Cao*), 1 *qian*. Powder the above and take. (While) for diarrhea or vomiting and retching, take *Liu Yi San* (Six to One Powder) brewed with Succus Zingiberis (*Jiang Zhi*) soup. Diarrhea due to accumulated phlegm requires precipitation.

Qing Liu Wan (Green-Blue Six Pills)[6] can eliminate dampness from the triple burner. They are usually used when treating diarrhea in combination with some other kind of pills rather than used singly. If (one) wants to treat blood dysentery, postpartum abdominal pain, or loose bowels, (one should) administer these with spleensupplementing and blood-supplementing medicinals. For enduring disease with qi vacuity and incessant diarrhea, moxa *Bai Hui* (GV 20)[7] with three cones.

An old person who was over-nourished and whose spleen was damaged by food and drink suffered from frequent diarrhea. This was a case of spleen diarrhea. (The patient was given) stir-fried Rhizoma Atractylodis Macrocephalae (*Bai Zhu*), 2 *liang*, Radix Albus Paeoniae Lactiflorae (*Bai Shao Yao*), stir-fried with wine, 1 *liang*, stir-fried Massa Medica Fermentata (*Shen Qu*), 2 *liang*, Fructus Crataegi (*Shan Zha*), 1.5 *liang*, Rhizoma Pinelliae Ternatae (*Ban Xia*), 1 *liang*, soaked with boiled water, and stir-fried Radix Scutellariae Baicalensis (*Huang Qin*), one half *liang*. Powder the above and make into pills with rice cooked with green lotus leaves as a wrapping.

---

[5]   Large intestine diarrhea is manifest with rectal pressure arising immediately upon ingestion, whitish stools, lancinating abdominal pain, a deep, slow pulse, and clear urine.

[6]   This consists of Talcum (*Hua Shi*), Radix Glycyrrhizae (*Gan Cao*), and Massa Medica Fermentata Cum Semenis Oryzam Sativam (*Hong Qu*).

[7]   Meeting of Hundreds

An(other) old person, aged 70, had a white facial complexion. His pulses were bowstring and rapid except for the stomach pulse which was deep and slippery. As a result of drinking alcohol, he contracted dysentery with blood and thin pus in his stools, abdominal pain, inhibited urination, abdominal urgency, and rectal heaviness. Radix Panacis Ginseng (*Ren Shen*) and Rhizoma Atractylodis Macrocephalae (*Bai Zhu*) were used as the sovereigns with Radix Glycyrrhizae (*Gan Cao*), Talcum (*Hua Shi*), Semen Arecae Catechu (*Bing Lang*), Radix Saussureae Seu Vladimiriae (*Mu Xiang*), and Rhizoma Atractylodis (*Cang Zhu*) as the assistants. (These) were taken with 25 pills of *Bao He Wan* (Protect & Harmonize Pills).[8] The next day his signs reduced and only his urination remained inhibited. Then *Yi Yuan San* (Boost the Origin Powder)[9] alone was administered and was effective.

A male who suffered, as a result of toiling and drudgery, from fever, pain in the lower back and legs, and simultaneous vomiting and diarrhea was prescribed Rhizoma Atractylodis Macrocephalae (*Bai Zhu*), 2 *qian*, Radix Panacis Ginseng (*Ren Shen*), 1 *qian*, Talcum (*Hua Shi*), 2 *qian*, Caulis Akebiae Mutong (*Mu Tong*), 1.5 *qian*, Radix Glycyrrhizae (*Gan Cao*), one half *qian*, Pericarpium Citri Reticulatae (*Chen Pi*), 2 *qian*, and Radix Bupleuri (*Chai Hu*), 1 *qian*.

For water diarrhea in summer months (use) *Gui Ling Gan Lu Yin* (Cinnamom & Poria Sweet Dew Drink). This consists of Cortex Cinnamomi (*Guan Gui*) and Radix Panacis Ginseng (*Ren Shen*), 5 *qian* each, Radix Saussureae Seu Vladimiriae (*Mu Xiang*), 1 *fen*, Sclerotium

---

[8]   This consists of Rhizoma Anemarrhenae (*Zhi Mu*), Bulbus Fritillariae (*Bei Mu*), Tuber Asparagi Cochinensis (*Tian Men Dong*), Flos Tussilagi Farfarae (*Kuan Dong Hua*), Radix Trichosanthis Kirlowii (*Tian Hua Fen*), Semen Coicis Lachryma-jobi (*Yi Yi Ren*), Semen Pruni Armeniacae (*Xing Ren*), Fructus Schizandrae Chinensis (*Wu Wei Zi*), Radix Glycyrrhizae (*Gan Cao*), Fructus Aristolochiae (*Ma Dou Ling*), Radix Asteris Tatarici (*Zi Wan*), Bulbus Lilii (*Bai He*), Radix Platycodi Grandiflori (*Jie Geng*), Gelatinum Corii Asini (*E Jiao*), Radix Angelicae Sinensis (*Dang Gui*), Radix Rehmanniae (*Di Huang*), Fructus Perillae Frutescentis (*Zi Su*), Herba Menthae (*Bo He*), and Radix Stemonae (*Bai Bu*).

[9]   I.e., Liu Yi San; see Note 4, Ch. 18, present Bk.

Poriae Cocoris (*Fu Ling*), Rhizoma Atractylodis Macrocephalae (*Bai Zhu*), Radix Glycyrrhizae (*Gan Cao*), Rhizoma Alismatis (*Ze Xie*), Radix Puerariae Lobatae (*Ge Gen*), Gypsum (*Shi Gao*), and Calcareous Spar (*Han Shui Shi*), 1 *liang* for each of the above, and Talcum (*Hua Shi*), 2 *liang*.

For diarrhea due to disharmony of the spleen and stomach with food damage, use *Wei Ling Tang* (Stomach *Ling* Decoction).[10] For gathering and accumulation diarrhea, (use) *Sheng Hong Wan* (Conquer the Red Pills).[11] For long persisting diarrhea with rumbling intestines, (use) *He Li Le Wan* (Terminalia Pills).[12] For diarrhea due to accumulated (food) with generalized fever and watery diarrhea, (use) *Da Chai Hu Tang* (Major Bupleurum Decoction). For watery diarrhea, (use) Rhizoma Atractylodis Macrocephalae (*Bai Zhu*), Rhizoma Atractylodis (*Cang Zhu*), Cortex Magnoliae Officinalis (*Hou Po*), Pericarpium Citri Reticulatae (*Chen Pi*), stir-fried Massa Medica Fermentata (*Shen Qu*), Sclerotium Poriae Cocoris (*Fu Ling*), Sclerotium Polypori Umbellati (*Zhu Ling*), Rhizoma Alismatis (*Ze Xie*), Radix Sanguisorbae (*Di Yu*), Radix Glycyrrhizae (*Gan Cao*), and, in winter, add dry Rhizoma Zingiberis (*Gan Jiang*), all in equal amounts. (However,) to treat water diarrhea in

---

[10] This consists of Radix Glycyrrhizae (*Gan Cao*), Sclerotium Poriae Cocoris (*Fu Ling*), Rhizoma Atractylodis (*Cang Zhu*), Pericarpium Citri Reticulatae (*Chen Pi*), Rhizoma Atractylodis Macrocephalae (*Bai Zhu*), Cortex Cinnamomi (*Guan Gui*), Rhizoma Alismatis (*Ze Xie*), Sclerotium Polypori Umbellati (*Zhu Ling*), and Cortex Magnoliae Officinalis (*Hou Po*).

[11] This consists of Rhizoma Sparganii (*San Leng*), Rhizoma Curcumae Zedoariae (*Peng E Zhu*), Pericarpium Viridis Citri Reticulatae (*Qing Pi*), fresh Rhizoma Zingiberis (*Sheng Jiang*), Fructus Immaturus Citri Seu Ponciri (*Zhi Shi*), Rhizoma Atractylodis Macrocephalae (*Bai Zhu*), Semen Raphani Sativi (*Lai Fu Zi*), and Rhizoma Cyperi Rotundi (*Xiang Fu*).

[12] This consists of Pericarpium Fructi Terminaliae Chebulae (*He Zi Pi*), Rhizoma Zingiberis (*Jiang*), Fructus Schizandrae Chinensis (*Wu Wei Zi*), Cortex Cinnamomi (*Gui Zhi*), Radix Platycodi Grandiflori (*Jie Geng*), Radix Praeparatus Aconiti Carmichaeli (*Fu Zi*), Radix Saussureae Seu Vladimiriae (*Mu Xiang*), Radix Panacis Ginseng (*Ren Shen*), Lignum Aquilariae Agallochae (*Chen Xiang*), Rhizoma Atractylodis Macrocephalae (*Bai Zhu*), and Fructus Citri Seu Ponciri (*Zhi Qiao*).

old persons, (use) Rhizoma Atractylodis Macrocephalae (*Bai Zhu*), 1 *liang*, Rhizoma Atractylodis (*Cang Zhu*), 1 *liang*, Cortex Magnoliae Officinalis (*Hou Po*), one half *liang*, stir-fried Massa Medica Fermentata (*Shen Qu*), 1 *liang*, Semen Myristicae Fragrantis (*Rou Dou Kou*), 1 *liang*, Pericarpium Citri Reticulatae (*Chen Pi*), 5 *qian*, stir-fried Radix Paeoniae Lactiflorae (*Shao Yao*), 1 *liang*, stir-fried Talcum (*Hua Shi*), 1 *liang*, processed Radix Glycyrrhizae (*Gan Cao*), 3 *qian*, and stir-fried Cortex Ailanthi Altissimae (*Chu Pi*), 1 *liang*. Make the above into pills with rice; 80 pills (per dose) taken with thin gruel before a meal.

A person suffered from chest fullness and incessant diarrhea. It was necessary to disperse food and supplement the spleen. Then the diarrhea would certainly be checked. In (food) accumulation disease, there may be incessant diarrhea in spite of a strong stomach. (Therefore,) it is necessary to apply precipitation to eliminate accumulation. Then the diarrhea will be stopped.

Whenever internal or external evils bring damage to the function of engendering and transformation, yin and yang fail to keep to their constant abodes and the viscera and bowels fail to fulfill the duties in their charge. Thus, although the stomach and intestines continue to ferment and foam, the office of conveyance and transformation is out of action and there arises diarrhea nonetheless.

A person had qi desertion and vacuity. Violent diarrhea issued in loss of consciousness of people with mouth and eyes shut and extremely faint breathing (as if) on the verge of death. Moxa was performed at *Qi Hai* (CV 6)[13] without delay. (The patient was made to) drink *Ren Shen Gao* (Ginseng Paste). After more than 10 *jin* (of ginseng) was administered, (he) recovered.

In case of yin vacuity and kidneys unable to exercise their power of imposing confinement and curbing, (one should) greatly supplement the kidneys. When phlegm accumulates in the lungs and consequently makes the qi of its associate, the large intestine, insecure, if phlegm in

---

[13]   Sea of Qi

the upper burner is (helped) gush out, lung qi will descend and large intestine vacuity will naturally be overcome. If excessive worry and thought have made the spleen qi bound up, unable to uplift, and sunken in the lower burner thus resulting in diarrhea, (one should) open depression and bind and supplement the spleen and stomach so as to make the grain qi ascend and effuse.

Dai comments: All kinds of watery diarrhea without abdominal pain are (ascribed to) dampness. Food and drink not staying in the stomach after having entered it (but becoming) untransformed food in the stools is (ascribed to) qi vacuity. Rumbling intestines, watery diarrhea, and (abdominal) pain followed by diarrhea are (ascribed to) fire. Intermittent diarrhea with varying amounts of stools is (ascribed to) phlegm. Severe abdominal pain followed by diarrhea and diarrhea followed by relief of pain is (ascribed to) food accumulation.

A formula to treat watery diarrhea (consists of) dry Rhizoma Zingiberis (*Gan Jiang*), 1 *qian*, Radix Angelicae Sinensis (*Dang Gui*), 2.5 *qian*, Fructus Pruni Mume (*Wu Mei*), 3 pieces, Cortex Phellodendri (*Huang Bai*), 1 *qian*, and Rhizoma Coptidis Chinensis (*Huang Lian*), 2 *qian*, or all in equal amounts. Boil in water.

Chapter Twenty-three

Sudden Turmoil (*i.e.*, Choleralike Disease)

When there is accumulation internally and affection externally, there will appear vomiting and diarrhea. If (the discharge of accumulation) is not yet thorough, ejection should be performed nevertheless in order to upraise the qi. Ejection can be carried out with modified *Er Chen Tang* (Two Aged Decoction). Salt water, whether boiled or unboiled, can (also) provoke vomiting.

To treat sudden turmoil (use) Rhizoma Atractylodis (*Cang Zhu*), Cortex Magnoliae Officinalis (*Hou Po*), Pericarpium Citri Reticulatae (*Chen Pi*), and Radix Puerariae Lobatae (*Ge Gen*), 1.5 *qian* for each of the above, Talcum (*Hua Shi*), 3 *qian*, Rhizoma Atractylodis Macrocephalae (*Bai Zhu*), 2 *qian*, Caulis Akebiae Mutong (*Mu Tong*), 1 *qian*, and processed Radix Glycyrrhizae (*Gan Cao*). Another method (is to) take 40 pills of *Bao He Wan* (Protect & Harmonize Pills) with ginger soup.

The general method for treating dry sudden turmoil is effusion. (When doing this,) even diaphoresis (together with) ejection does no harm since the internal is damaged and the external is confined by evil qi. In some cases, ejection is used, (in which case, this) means effusion and dissipation. (However,) in other cases, warm medicinals are used for the purpose of resolution and dissipation. This method of resolving and dissipating does not allow the introduction of cool medicinals (but requires) *Er Chen Tang* plus Rhizoma Ligustici Wallichii (*Chuan Xiong*), Rhizoma Atractylodis (*Cang Zhu*), Radix Ledebouriellae Sesloidis (*Fang Feng*), Radix Angelicae (*Bai Zhi*), and other such medicinals.

In summer months, sudden turmoil of vomiting and diarrhea may give rise to a great desire to drink water, mania, and frenetic running about. (For this use) ginger-processed Cortex Magnoliae Officinalis (*Hou Po*), Cortex Cinnamomi (*Guan Gui*), dry Rhizoma Zingiberis (*Gan Jiang*), Sclerotium Poriae Cocoris (*Fu Ling*), and Rhizoma Pinelliae Ternatae (*Ban Xia*).

A formula for sudden turmoil (consists of) Herba Agastachis Seu Pogostemi (*Huo Xiang*), Rhizoma Atractylodis (*Cang Zhu*), Cortex Magnoliae Officinalis (*Hou Po*), Pericarpium Citri Reticulatae (*Chen Pi*), Fructus Amomi (*Suo Sha*), Radix Angelicae (*Bai Zhi*), Radix Glycyrrhizae (*Gan Cao*), Rhizoma Pinelliae Ternatae (*Ban Xia*), Sclerotium Poriae Cocoris (*Fu Ling*), Radix Panacis Ginseng (*Ren Shen*), and stir-fried Massa Medica Fermentata (*Shen Qu*), all in equal amounts. In cold weather, add dry Rhizoma Zingiberis (*Gan Jiang*). In case of severe cold, add Radix Praeparatus Aconiti Carmichaeli (*Fu Zi*).

For vomiting and diarrhea sudden turmoil in summer months take *Yi Yuan San* (Boost the Origin Powder) brewed in ice water with Succus

Zingiberis (*Jiang Zhi*) added. Or take *Gui Ling Gan Lu Yin* (Cinnamom & Poria Sweet Dew Drink) brewed with clear spring water or fresh water from the well since substances of consummate yin are able to engender yin within yang.[1] For sudden turmoil with slight vexation, agitation, and thirst, (use) Qian's[2] *Bai Zhu San* (Atractylodes Powder).[3] The above two formulas are both found in the *Bao Jian (Precious Mirror)*.[4] For vomiting and diarrhea in summer months, cool *Huang Lian Xiang Ru Tang* (Coptis & Elsholtzia Decoction) in a well and take.

In sudden turmoil, the pulse is often hidden or expiring. As a general method, *Li Zhong Tang* (Rectify the Center Decoction)[5] is a good formula (for this condition). If it is yang failing to ascend and yin to descend and thus overwhelming the diaphragm and giving rise to sudden turmoil, do not make (the patient) drink millet water[6] or imminent death is incurred.

---

[1] Fresh or cool water is consummate yin because water is yin nature and coolness is also yin in nature. Sudden turmoil is a disease of the spleen, a yin viscus. However, this disease is contracted in the yang season, summer.

[2] *I.e.*, Qian Yi, styled Zhong-yang (circa 1035-1117 CE), forefather of TCM pediatrics.

[3] There are at least nine different formulas bearing the same name of which the translator is aware. Here it apparently refers to the one designed by Qian Yi. This is composed of Radix Panacis Ginseng (*Ren Shen*), Sclerotium Poriae Cocoris (*Fu Ling*), Rhizoma Atractylodis Macrocephalae (*Bai Zhu*), Folium Agastachis Seu Pogostemi (*Huo Xiang Ye*), Radix Saussureae Seu Vladimiriae (*Mu Xiang*), Radix Glycyrrhizae (*Gan Cao*), and Radix Puerariae Lobatae (*Ge Gen*).

[4] *Dong Yi Bao Jian (Precious Mirror of Oriental Medicine)* in full, a comprehensive medical work by a Korean TCM scholar published in 1611 CE.

[5] This consists of Radix Panacis Ginseng (*Ren Shen*), dry Rhizoma Zingiberis (*Gan Jiang*), mix-fried Radix Glycyrrhizae (*Zhi Gan Cao*), and Rhizoma Atractylodis Macrocephalae (*Bai Zhu*).

[6] When processed in a special way, usually fermented in cold water, it is cool in nature and penetrating. This should be used in only the sudden turmoil caused by food accumulation.

In summer months, eating too much fruit, drinking too many cold beverages, and reposing in breezy (places) may cause retention of food with inability to transform it. (Then) glomus may be caused by food, forming obstruction between the above and below. Thus sudden turmoil results. Prescribe *Liu He Tang* (Six Harmonies Decoction)[7] with Herba Agastachis Seu Pogostemi (*Huo Xiang*) in double amounts.

Commotion and tumult (in the center) with inability to vomit or defecate is called dry sudden turmoil. It is most difficult to treat. It requires ejection with boiled saltwater. (But) to treat intestinestirring sand, boil powdered Lignum Cinnamomi Camphorae (*Zhang Mu*) down to a thick decoction and take one bowl sip by sip. Presently vomiting will be provoked and there will be diarrhea. Recovery will issue (after this). [A (variant) version adds, Dry sudden turmoil is also known popularly as intestinestirring sand. {later editor}] Another method (is to) prick the purple spot around *Wei Zhong* (Bl 40)[8] to let out blood, and recovery will follow. Pricking the tips of the ten fingers to let out blood is also a good method. A method to treat death from sudden turmoil with warm qi still remaining in the abdomen (is to) put salt in (the navel) and moxa at the umbilicus, 7 cones. Then go on to moxa *Qi Hai* (CV 6).[9]

---

[7] This is composed of Radix Angelicae Sinensis (*Dang Gui*), Radix Albus Paeoniae Lactiflorae (*Bai Shao Yao*), Cortex Cinnamomi (*Guan Gui*), prepared Radix Rehmanniae (*Shu Di*), Rhizoma Ligustici Wallichii (*Chuan Xiong*) and Rhizoma Curcumae Zedoariae (*Peng E Zhu*).

[8] Commission the Middle

[9] Sea of Qi

Chapter Twenty-four

Dysentery

The treatment (of this condition depends on) the differentiation of qi and blood (types). Red (dysentery) is ascribed to the blood. White (dysentery is ascribed to) the qi. (In dysentery,) there are body heat, rectal pressure, and abdominal pain. Body heat is (due to) embraced external evils which justify resolving the exterior. If there is no aversion to cold, use *Xiao Chai Hu* (Minor Bupleurum [Decoction]) with Radix Panacis Ginseng (*Ren Shen*) deleted. Rectal pressure is the result of accumulation and depressed qi sagging below. (This requires) the combination of upraising and dispersing. Abdominal pain is (caused by) the qi of lung metal being depressed in the large intestine. (This requires) bitter Radix Platycodi Grandiflori (*Jie Geng*) to effuse (the qi) and, afterwards, dysentery-curing medicinals. (In addition,) qi (problems) require qi medicinals, while blood (problems) require blood medicinals. For dysentery with abdominal pain in people with repletion, it is appropriate to precipitate by Liu's[1] method, and then treat it with certain dysentery-curing medicinals in accordance with qi and blood (conditions).

Blood in the stools is usually governed by food accumulation and heat, (thus) making it necessary to cool and quicken the blood with Radix Angelicae Sinensis (*Dang Gui*), Semen Pruni Persicae (*Tao Ren*), Radix Scutellariae Baicalensis (*Huang Qin*), and the like, and, in some cases, with (additional) slaked lime (*Po Xiao*). *Qing Liu Wan* (Green-Blue Six Pills) offer an effective treatment for blood dysentery. (These consist of) 1 packet of *Liu Yi San* (Six To One Powder) and one half *qian* of stir-fried Massa Medica Fermentata Cum Semenis Oryzam Sativam

---

[1] See Note 1, Ch. 1, Bk. 1. Liu He-jian is famous for choosing cool and acrid medicinals to treat many types of diseases. The author recommends his method here because the patient is strong with repletion.

(*Hong Qu*). This is able to quicken the blood. (This is made) into pills with steamed rice. Abdominal pain (on the other hand) requires warm, dissipating medicinals, such as Rhizoma Zingiberis (*Jiang*) and Cortex Cinnamomi (*Gui*) to harmonize (the qi). If there is heat, use medicinals such as Radix Scutellariae Baicalensis (*Huang Qin*) and Radix Paeoniae Lactiflorae (*Shao Yao*. The treatment of) those who are strong or at the initial stage entails precipitation. (While the treatment of) those who are vacuous and weak, decrepit and old entails upraising. Dysentery during its initial stage, (only) 1-2 days old, justifies disinhibition by precipitation with *Da* or *Xiao Tiao Wei Cheng Qi Tang* (Major or Minor Regulate the Stomach & Support the Qi Decoction).

Medicinals (used) should depend on the qi and blood (conditions). For a qi disease, use Radix Panacis Ginseng (*Ren Shen*) and Rhizoma Atractylodis Macrocephalae (*Bai Zhu*). For a blood disease, it is the rule to employ *Si Wu Tang* (Four Materials Decoction). If there is heat, first abate the heat. In case of rectal pressure, it is necessary to harmonize qi with Radix Saussureae Seu Vladimiriae (*Mu Xiang*), Semen Arecae Catechu (*Bing Lang*), and the like. For rectal pressure due to accumulation, *Bao He Wan* (Protect & Harmonize Pills) is the ruling (formula). Five days after (contraction of dysentery), precipitation is no longer allowed since the spleen and the stomach are vacuous (by then).

The formula of *Bao He Wan* (consists of) Fructus Crataegi (*Shan Zha Rou*), 3 *liang*, Massa Medica Fermentata (*Shen Qu*), 2 *liang*, Pericarpium Citri Reticulatae (*Chen Pi*), Rhizoma Pinelliae Ternatae (*Ban Xia*), and Sclerotium Poriae Cocoris (*Fu Ling*), 1 *liang* for each of the above, Fructus Forsythiae Suspensae (*Lian Qiao*), 5 *qian*, and Semen Raphani Sativi (*Lai Fu Zi*), 5 *qian*. Stir-fry the above seven flavors (*i.e.*, ingredients), powder, make into pills with gruel, and take with ginger soup. Two *liang* of Rhizoma Atractylodis Macrocephalae (*Bai Zhu*) can be added.

Fever at the beginning of dysentery must be treated by precipitation with *Da Cheng Qi Tang* (Major Support the Qi Decoction) and afterwards with other formulas in accordance with signs. (But) long persisting dysentery with fever is ascribed to yin vacuity and requires cool and cold medicinals necessarily in combination with upraising and warm ones. A (variant) version says, Long persistent bleeding with fever is ascribed to yin vacuity, and (for it) *Si Wu Tang* is the ruling (formula). Body heat arising with dysentery is an external contraction.

Abdominal pain at the beginning of dysentery contraindicates Radix Panacis Ginseng (*Ren Shen*) and Rhizoma Atractylodis Macrocephalae (*Bai Zhu*). They cannot be used even in case of qi vacuity and stomach vacuity. Blood in the stools (on the other hand) may be caused by sunken wind evils. (This condition) requires upraising. It is a result of wind damaging the liver which rules the blood. Dampness may (also) damage the blood (resulting in blood in the stools. This) requires moving the dampness and clearing heat.

Rectal pressure is caused by sagging accumulation and qi and requires harmonizing the qi by combined upraising and dispersing with Radix Saussureae Seu Vladimiriae (*Mu Xiang*), Semen Arecae Catechu (*Bing Lang*), and the like. In case of no effect, use Fructus Gleditschiae Sinensis (*Zao Jiao Zi*), roasted Radix Et Rhizoma Rhei (*Da Huang*), Radix Angelicae Sinensis (*Dang Gui*), Semen Pruni Persicae (*Tao Ren*), Rhizoma Coptidis Chinensis (*Huang Lian*), and Fructus Citri Seu Ponciri (*Zhi Qiao*), all made into pills. (In this case,) rectal pressure is caused by exuberant wind in the large intestine.

There are two (conditions) in the disease of dysentery that are half life, half death (*i.e.*, border on death). Stools like fish brains border on death, and body heat with a large pulse (also) borders on death. There are (also) five incurable patterns: Diarrhea of blood points to death. Diarrhea of dusty (*i.e.*, grimy) stools and decaying color (points) to death. Diarrhea like a leaking roof (points) to death. Dysentery with the lips red like cinnabar (points) to death. (And) dysentery like (pouring) from a bamboo tube (points) to death.

Dysentery with ability to eat indicates that the stomach is not yet diseased. If damp heat toxins of the spleen and stomach ascend, fuming and steaming the clear passageways so as to shut and block the openings of the stomach, then the pattern of inability to eat develops. A formula that treats dysentery with inability to eat (is)

Xiang Lian Wan (Saussureae & Coptis Pills)[2] and Semen Nelumbinis Nuciferae (*Lian Rou*), half to half in amount. Grind and take with half soup.[3] To treat dysentery with inability to eat, (one may also) cover the umbilicus with a river snail (*Tian Luo*) with a small amount of Secretio Moschi Moschiferi (*She Xiang*) put inside. Pound together (these two) to conduct heat downward. When heat is removed, desire for food returns.

A dysentery-treating formula (consists of) Rhizoma Atractylodis (*Cang Zhu*), Rhizoma Atractylodis Macrocephalae (*Bai Zhu*), Radix Scutellariae Baicalensis (*Tiao Qin*), Radix Angelicae Sinensis (*Dang Gui*), Radix Albus Paeoniae Lactiflorae (*Bai Shao Yao*), Radix Rehmanniae (*Sheng Di*), Pericarpium Viridis Citri Reticulatae (*Qing Pi*), Rhizoma Coptidis Chinensis (*Huang Lian*), Talcum (*Hua Shi*), and Radix Glycyrrhizae (*Gan Cao*). Boil in water and (take) all in one dose.

In case of abdominal urgency and rectal pressure, (use) Rhizoma Coptidis Chinensis (*Huang Lian*) and Talcum (*Hua Shi*) plus Semen Pruni Persicae (*Tao Ren*) and Semen Arecae Catechu (*Bing Liang*). For severe cases, add Radix Et Rhizoma Rhei (*Da Huang*) In case of vomiting, add Rhizoma Pinelliae Ternatae (*Ban Xia*). Boil with ginger. Another formula (consists of) dry Rhizoma Zingiberis (*Gan Jiang*), 1 *qian*, Radix Angelicae Sinensis (*Dang Gui*), 2.5 *qian*, Fructus Pruni Mume (*Wu Mei*), 3 pieces, Cortex Phellodendri (*Huang Bai*), 1.5 *qian*, Rhizoma Coptidis Chinensis (*Huang Lian*), 2 *qian*, all the above as one dose; boil in water.

A physician, Sun, who suffered from inflating fullness of the abdomen and dysentery of white stools as a result of taking too much food and drink was prescribed Rhizoma Atractylodis (*Cang Zhu*), Rhizoma Atractylodis Macrocephalae (*Bai Zhu*), Cortex Magnoliae Officinalis

---

[2]   This is composed of Kaolin (*Bai Shi Zhi*), Os Draconis (*Long Gu*), blast-fried Rhizoma Zingiberis (*Pao Jiang*), Rhizoma Coptidis Chinensis (*Huang Lian*), and Alumen (*Ku Fan*).

[3]   Millet may be read for half. In Chinese, these two words are similar in strokes.

(*Hou Po*), Radix Glycyrrhizae (*Gan Cao*), Sclerotium Poriae Cocoris (*Fu Ling*), and Talcum (*Hua Shi*). These were boiled and taken with 30 pills of *Bao He Wan* (Protect & Harmonize Pills). Another formula contains stir-fried Massa Medica Fermentata (*Shen Qu*, in addition).

If the feet are becoming weak and gradually thin with dysentery, (use) Rhizoma Atractylodis (*Cang Zhu*), 2 *liang*, wine-processed Radix Paeoniae Lactiflorae (*Shao Yao*), 2.5 *liang*, Plastrum Testudinis (*Gui Ban*), 3 *liang*, and wine-processed Cortex Phellodendri (*Huang Bai*), one half *liang*. Powder the above, make into pills with gruel, and swallow with decocted *Si Wu Tang* (Four Materials Decoction) plus Pericarpium Citri Reticulatae (*Chen Pi*) and Radix Glycyrrhizae (*Gan Cao*. However,) if there arise lumbago and weak feet with dysentery, (use) Pericarpium Citri Reticulatae (*Chen Pi*), Rhizoma Pinelliae Ternatae (*Ban Xia*), and Radix Albus Paeoniae Lactiflorae (*Bai Shao Yao*), 1 *qian* for each of the above, Sclerotium Poriae Cocoris (*Fu Ling*), Rhizoma Atractylodis (*Cang Zhu*), Radix Angelicae Sinensis (*Dang Gui*), and wine-processed Radix Scutellariae Baicalensis (*Huang Qin*), one half *qian* for each of the above, Rhizoma Atractylodis Macrocephalae (*Bai Zhu*), 1 *qian*, and Radix Glycyrrhizae (*Gan Cao*), 2 *qian*, all the above as one dose. Boil with 3 slices of ginger and take before a meal.

A person suffered from diarrhea and (as a result of) toiling and taxation, (developed) dysentery with white accumulated (substance in stools. They were prescribed) powdered, stir-fried Talcum (*Hua Shi*), Pericarpium Citri Reticulatae (*Chen Pi*), Radix Paeoniae Lactiflorae (*Shao Yao*), Rhizoma Atractylodis Macrocephalae (*Bai Zhu*), Sclerotium Poriae Cocoris (*Fu Ling*), and Radix Glycyrrhizae (*Gan Cao*). The above were boiled and taken before a meal.

A female who suffered from scant blood and stomachache with dysentery was prescribed Rhizoma Ligustici Wallichii (*Chuan Xiong*), Radix Angelicae Sinensis (*Dang Gui*), Pericarpium Citri Reticulatae (*Chen Pi*), and Radix Paeoniae Lactiflorae (*Shao Yao*). The above were boiled and taken with brewed *Liu Yi San* (Six To One Powder).

A formula to treat chronic dysentery (consists of) Pericarpium Papaveris Somniferi (*Ying Su Ke*), one half *liang*, Cortex Ailanthi

Altissimae (*Chu Bai Pi*), 1 *qian*, and Semen Glycineae Max (*Hei Dou*), 21 pieces. Boil the above together and take before a meal. For dysentery with seasonal qi (*i.e.*, epidemic) fever, (use) Rhizoma Atractylodis (*Cang Zhu*), Cortex Magnoliae Officinalis (*Hou Po*), Radix Rubrus Paeoniae Lactiflorae (*Chi Shao Yao*), Radix Angelicae Sinensis (*Dang Gui*), Radix Scutellariae Baicalensis (*Huang Qin*), Cortex Phellodendri (*Huang Bai*), Radix Sanguisorbae (*Di Yu*), Pericarpium Papaveris Somniferi (*Su Ke*), Fructus Citri Seu Ponciri (*Zhi Qiao*), Semen Arecae Catechu (*Bing Lang*), Radix Saussureae Seu Vladimiriae (*Mu Xiang*), Radix Glycyrrhizae (*Gan Cao*), and dry Rhizoma Zingiberis (*Gan Jiang*). For dysentery with fresh blood (in the stool), add Rhizoma Coptidis Chinensis (*Huang Lian*). In case of urinary stoppage, add Talcum (*Hua Shi*) and Semen Plantaginis (*Che Qian Zi*. And) what about dysentery with blood and water (in the stools)? Add Gelatinum Corii Asini (*E Jiao*).

Pills to treat dysentery (consist of) Cacumen Biotae Orientalis (*Ce Bai Ye*), Rhizoma Coptidis Chinensis (*Huang Lian*), Cortex Phellodendri (*Huang Bai*), Radix Scutellariae Baicalensis (*Huang Qin*), Radix Angelicae Sinensis (*Dang Gui*), Radix Paeoniae Lactiflorae (*Shao Yao*), Pericarpium Papaveris Somniferi (*Su Ke*), Radix Rehmanniae (*Sheng Di Huang*), Radix Sanguisorbae (*Di Yu*), Fructus Citri Seu Ponciri (*Zhi Qiao*), Rhizoma Cyperi Rotundi (*Xiang Fu*), Radix Saussureae Seu Vladimiriae (*Mu Xiang*), and Semen Arecae Catechu (*Bing Lang*). Make into pills with thick rice gruel and take 70-80 pills. If there is food and accumulation and abdominal pain, add Rhizoma Curcumae Zedoariae (*E Zhu*), Rhizoma Sparganii (*San Leng*), and Fructus Amomi (*Suo Sha*).

Visceral toxins in alcoholics resembling blood dysentery is a disease that should be impugned to drinking in the past. It requires abandoning wine before the (following) medicinals can offer a cure: Rhizoma Atractylodis (*Cang Zhu*), 1 *qian*, Radix Rubrus Paeoniae Lactiflorae (*Chi Shao Yao*), 2 *qian*, stir-fried Flos Immaturus Sophorae Japonicae (*Huai Hua*), 1.5 *qian*, Radix Sanguisorbae (*Di Yu*), 2 *qian*, Fructus Citri Seu Ponciri (*Zhi Qiao*), 1 *qian*, mix-fried Radix Glycyrrhizae (*Zhi Gan Cao*), 3 *fen*, stir-fried Rhizoma Coptidis Chinensis (*Huang Lian*), 5 *fen*, dry Radix Puerariae Lobatae (*Gan Ge*), 2 *qian*, and Radix Angelicae Sinensis (*Dang Gui*), 5 *fen*. (Take) all the above as one dose. Boil in water, take before a meal, and recovery will follow. Another formula (consists of)

Cortex Ailanthi Altissimae (*Chu Pi*), 2 *liang*, stir-fried Massa Medica Fermentata (*Shen Qu*), 5 *qian*, Radix Albus Paeoniae Lactiflorae (*Bai Shao Yao*), 1 *liang*, stir-fried Talcum (*Hua Shi*), 1 *liang*, and Fructus Citri Seu Ponciri (*Zhi Qiao*), 5 *qian*. Powder the above, make into pills the size of Chinese parasol tree seeds with well-cooked rice, and take 70 pills with thin millet gruel.

For several months long enduring dysentery with inability to rise up, inability to take in food and drink, and extreme fatigue (administer) Radix Panacis Ginseng (*Ren Shen*), 5 *fen*, Rhizoma Atractylodis Macrocephalae (*Bai Zhu*), 1 *qian*, Radix Astragali Membranacei (*Huang Qi*), 5 *fen*, Radix Angelicae Sinensis (*Dang Gui*), 6 *fen*, Radix Paeoniae Lactiflorae (*Shao Yao*), 1 *qian*, mix-fried Radix Glycyrrhizae (*Zhi Gan Cao*), 3 *fen*, Pericarpium Papaveris Somniferi (*Su Ke*), 3 *qian*, Radix Sanguisorbae (*Di Yu*), 5 *fen*, Radix Saussureae Seu Vladimiriae (*Mu Xiang*), 3 *fen*, Fructus Amomi (*Suo Sha*), 5 *fen*, Pericarpium Citri Reticulatae (*Chen Pi*), 1 *qian*, Rhizoma Cimicifugae (*Sheng Ma*), 3 *fen*, Fructus Cardamomi (*Bai Dou Kou Ren*), 3 *fen*, and Rhizoma Alismatis (*Ze Xie*), 5 *fen*, all the above as one dose. If there is heat, add Radix Scutellariae Baicalensis (*Huang Qin*). In case of a thin pulse and aversion of the limbs to cold, add dry Rhizoma Zingiberis (*Gan Jiang*) or roasted Semen Myristicae Fragrantis (*Rou Dou Kou*) plus several slices of Radix Praeparatus Aconiti Carmichaeli (*Chuan Fu Zi*). Several doses will make food intake increase gradually.

For damp heat dysentery with inhibited voiding of scant urine, distressed thirst, ability to eat, a surging, large, and retarded pulse, abdominal pain, rectal pressure, and frequent evacuation in the night, take 30 pills of *Bao He Wan* with *Gui Ling Gan Lu Yin* (Cinnamom & Poria Sweet Dew Drink). A (variant) version recommends taking (these pills) with *Wei Ling Tang* (Stomach *Ling* Decoction). If there is more dampness than heat, disharmony of the spleen and the stomach, low food intake, abdominal pain, rectal pressure, and frequent evacuation in the night, take 30 pills of *Bao He Wan* with *Wei Ling Tang*. A (variant) version recommends taking (the pills) with *Gui Ling Gan Lu Yin*. People whose qi is vacuous and have a yellowish white facial complexion or those with fatigued limbs and with frequent (diarrhea with abdominal) pain, rectal pressure, inability to eat, and a thin, weak pulse or sweating should swallow 30 pills of *Bao He Wan* with *Huang Qi Jian Zhong Tang* (Astragalus Build the Center Decoction).[4] In case of damp heat with absence of thirst, take *Bao He Wan* with (*Huang Qi*) *Jian Zhong Tang* plus [like instead of plus in the original text, the correction made by the tr.] Rhizoma Atractylodis (*Cang Zhu*) and Sclerotium Poriae Cocoris (*Fu Ling*).

For disharmony of the spleen and stomach with low food intake, abdominal distention and pain, dysentery with rectal pressure, and a bowstring, tight pulse, take *Ping Wei San* (Level the Stomach Powder) plus Radix Paeoniae Lactiflorae (*Shao Yao*), Cortex Cinnamomi (*Guan Gui*), and Radix Puerariae Lobatae (*Ge Gen*), or take *Bao He Wan* with *Bai Zhu Fu Ling Tang* (Atractylodes & Poria Decoction).[5] (However, for) dysentery with white accumulated (substance in the stool, use) *Huang Qin Shao Yao Tang* (Scutellaria & Peony Decoction)[6] plus Rhizoma Atractylodis Macrocephalae (*Bai Zhu*), Pericarpium Citri Reticulatae (*Chen Pi*), Radix Glycyrrhizae (*Gan Cao*), Talcum (*Hua Shi*), and Semen Pruni Persicae (*Tao Ren*. But) for dysentery with red accumulated (substance in the stools) and body heat, take *Bao He Wan* with decocted *Yi Yuan San* (Boost the Origin Powder) plus Caulis Akebiae Mutong (*Mu Tong*), stir-fried Radix Paeoniae Lactiflorae (*Shao Yao*), stir-fried Pericarpium Citri Reticulatae (*Chen Pi*), and Rhizoma Atractylodis Macrocephalae (*Bai Zhu*).

As a result of drinking alcohol, an old person contracted dysentery with thin (stools) of blood, water, and pus, abdominal pain, urinary stoppage, abdominal urgency, and rectal pressure. (They were prescribed) Radix Panacis Ginseng (*Ren Shen*), Rhizoma Atractylodis Macrocephalae (*Bai Zhu*), Talcum (*Hua Shi*), Rhizoma Atractylodis

---

[4]   This consists of Radix Astragali Membranacei (*Huang Qi*), Ramulus Cinnamomi (*Gui Zhi*), Radix Glycyrrhizae (*Gan Cao*), fresh Rhizoma Zingiberis (*Sheng Jiang*), Radix Paeoniae Lactiflorae (*Shao Yao*), Maltose (*Yi Tang*), and Fructus Zizyphi Jujubae (*Zao*).

[5]   This consists of Rhizoma Atractylodis Macrocephalae (*Bai Zhu*) and Sclerotium Poriae Cocoris (*Fu Ling*) in equal amounts.

[6]   This consists of Radix Scutellariae Baicalensis (*Huang Qin*), Radix Paeoniae Lactiflorae (*Shao Yao*), and Radix Glycyrrhizae (*Gan Cao*).

(*Cang Zhu*), Semen Arecae Catechu (*Bing Lang*), Radix Saussureae Seu Vladimiriae (*Mu Xiang*), and Radix Glycyrrhizae (*Gan Cao*). The above were boiled and taken with 30 pills of *Bao He Wan*. The next day all the above signs were improved except inhibited urination. (Then) *Yi Yuan San* was used.

To treat dysentery, the formula (Zhang) Zhong-jing used whenever he spoke about precipitation being indicated was *Cheng Qi Tang* (Support the Qi Decoction). Radix Et Rhizoma Rhei (*Da Huang*), which is cold, is good by nature at penetrating and, with the help of the warmth of Cortex Magnoliae Officinalis (*Hou Po*), is good at moving stagnant qi. Moderated by the sweetness of Radix Glycyrrhizae (*Gan Cao*) and drunk in the form of a decoction, (this formula) pours into the stomach and intestines, flushing and moistening (them), expediting (the qi), and allowing no stagnated and obstructed (substances) to be left behind. Thus accumulation is moved and (dysentery) stopped. Liu He-jian (also) shed light on the pattern of stasis in the lower. (His exposition) is particularly important and pertinent. It is stated that once blood is moved, defecation will be restored to normal by itself, and once qi is regulated, rectal pressure will disappear by itself. This is the sun and the moon to the blind or the thunder to the deaf.

A person suffered from dysentery with inability to take in food. (They were given) *Si Jun Zi Tang* (Four Gentlemen Decoction) plus Rhizoma Ligustici Wallichii (*Chuan Xiong*), Radix Angelicae Sinensis (*Dang Gui*), Radix Paeoniae Lactiflorae (*Shao Yao*), Pericarpium Citri Reticulatae (*Chen Pi*), stir-fried Massa Medica Fermentata (*Shen Qu*), Rhizoma Coptidis Chinensis (*Huang Lian*), Fructus Amomi (*Sha Ren*), and Rhizoma Pinelliae Ternatae (*Ban Xia*. These) were boiled with fresh Rhizoma Zingiberis (*Sheng Jiang*) and taken.

A friend named Hu of Dong Yi, aged above 40, had suffered from dysentery for over 100 days and showed no improvement after being treated by a hundred (different) prescriptions. It was early in the ninth month. His six pulses were urgent and skipping, deep and wiry, thin and weak, and particularly so on the left hand. He had dozens of movements in a day and night but evacuated only a little static substance, almost entirely clear stagnated (food) with purplish black blood threads. (He) had had nothing to eat at all. This was not dysentery and should be treated as static blood. It may be asked what is the cause of this static blood? Rapid running after eating till full, shouting and quarrelling at the top of the voice, beating and wrestling, the infliction of a great deal of pain, unappeased anger, excessive supplementation and filling, fire (-natured) wine and fire (-natured) meat, all this, for example, is capable of causing (static blood). It turned out that this person had been wronged and caned (in court) the previous year. He had been involved in a suit for the past two years and consequently contracted blood stasis. After taking an (appropriate) formula, if (he evacuated) static blood, he would survive. Accordingly, Gummum Olibani (*Ru Xiang*), Myrrha (*Mo Yao*), Semen Pruni Persicae (*Tao Ren*), and Talcum (*Hua Shi*) together with Radix Saussureae Seu Vladimiriae (*Mu Xiang*) and Semen Arecae Catechu (*Bing Lang*) as the assistants were made into pills with the paste of Massa Medica Fermentata (*Shen Qu*). A little more than 100 pills were administered with thin gruel. Towards midnight, (static blood) still refused to be stirred. Then 200 more pills of the above formula were administered. Towards daybreak, (he) evacuated a great quantity of foul substance like putrid fish intestines, as much as 1-2 *sheng*. Drowsiness and fatigue lasted for a whole day. Then he was given some gruel, little by little, and (he) recovered.

A person suffered from dysentery with extreme rectal pressure. A person suffered from dysentery but with large food intake and rapid hungering. (They) are seen (*i.e.*, discussed) in the *Yi Yao (Essentials of Medicine)*. The vulgar use only astringing medicinals to treat dysentery and diarrhea. (Such treatment) may be practical if (diarrhea) has accumulated long and (is accompanied) by vacuity, but it never fails to add transmuted patterns to recent (diarrhea), resulting in no small disastrous consequence. It should be known that because (dysentery) is usually due to dampness, the most long-sighted policy is to separate and disinhibit the small water (*i.e.*, urination). However, it is stated in the *Nei Jing (Inner Classic)*, "If the lower body is hot, death follows, (but) if it is cold, (there will be) survival. This is a (only) a rough statement (of principle) and a careful study of other signs must be made before (a prognosis) is certain. Now, are there not deaths from absence of body heat with presence of cold? A deep, small, and interrupted or faint pulse (suggests) easy treatment. (Whereas) a floating, surging, large, and rapid pulse (suggests) difficult treatment. It is desirable (in this disease) for the pulse to be slippery and large. It is undesirable that it be bowstring and urgent.

To treat dysentery, (Zhang) Zhong-jing enumerated five (conditions) indicating warming methods and ten (conditions) indicating precipitation methods. He (also) prescribed exteriorresolving or urination-disinhibiting (depending on the patient's diagnosis) or let (the condition) develop itself to become easy or difficult to treat. His (explanations) are quite exquisite. (He) treated (dysentery), however, in the same way as diarrhea and failed to classify prescriptions in light of (pattern) identification. Students should be aware of this. Great extensive (abdominal) pain, (for instance,) was said to be treated by warming or by clearing. It should be noted that enduring disease with a cold body, spontaneous sweating, and a deep, small pulse indicates warming, while sudden disease or hot body with a floating, surging pulse indicates clearing. Body cold with spontaneous sweating (requires) using warm medicinals. Some (cases) can be treated by ejection; some by diaphoresis; some by precipitation. At the outset, the original qi has not yet become vacuous and it is necessary to apply pushing and flushing. This is a common method applied for (diseases of) a common cause. Shortly after, if qi has become vacuous, (this treatment) becomes invalid.

Red dysentery comes from the small intestine; white dysentery from the large intestine. In both of them, damp heat is the root. Red and white vaginal discharges have this in common with red and white turbidity. (However,) watery diarrhea followed by pus and blood is due to transmission from the spleen to the kidneys. (This kind of) bandit evil is difficult to cure. Diarrhea of pus and blood followed by water is due to transmission from the kidney channel to the spleen. This is said to be a mild evil and easy to cure. Stool like bean juice[7] is

---

[7] This is a very common food in north China. It is made from soaked soybeans which are then ground, pressing out the juice which is then filtered.

due to dampness. The spleen and stomach are the sea of water and grains, receiving whatever comes in. They often involve the other four viscera. Therefore, (they act) like [two characters missing] mutually infecting. It is necessary first to apply flow-freeing and disinhibition. This means advancing to confront and snatch [two characters missing]. In case of vacuity, (however,) a careful study is necessary. (Dysentery) caused by heat contraindicates such medicinals as Semen Crotonis (*Ba Dou*). In case of damage by cold substance, they may possibly be brought into use. This calls for caution. Moreover, dysentery may be epidemic. In a neighborhood or in a family, the infected bear similar (signs). This requires application in treatment (of the law) of the conquering and subordination of the movements and qi.

Dysentery with inability to eat may be (due to) heat binding the openings of the stomach. Obtain Rhizoma Coptidis Chinensis (*Huang Lian*) plus a large amount of Radix Panacis Ginseng (*Ren Shen*). Boil in water, take sip by sip, and continue sipping (even) after vomiting is provoked. To downbear (heat), it is necessary to open (the bind). Many people are ignorant of this and usually use warm medicinals of sweet flavor only to assist fire with fire and to stagnate what is stagnated. There have been cases where, after warm medicinals were taken by mistake, the toxic qi attacked the stomach. (In that case,) it is necessary to identify these toxins and dispel them accordingly.

Chapter Twenty-five

Retching, Vomiting, & Belching

These are treated in accordance with the quantities of qi and blood. In the stomach, there may exist heat and phlegm. For heat existing in the stomach and phlegm existing above the diaphragm, use *Er Chen Tang* (Two Aged Decoction) plus Fructus Gardeniae Jasminoidis (*Shan Zhi*), stir-fried with Succus Zingiberis (*Jiang Zhi*), and Rhizoma Coptidis

Chinensis (*Huang Lian*). Boil with fresh Rhizoma Zingiberis (*Sheng Jiang*) and take.

Chronic retching and vomiting disease is (due to) the stomach (being) too vacuous to receive grains. (For this, administer) fresh Rhizoma Zingiberis (*Sheng Jiang*), Radix Panacis Ginseng (*Ren Shen*), Radix Astragali Membranacei (*Huang Qi*), Rhizoma Atractylodis Macrocephalae (*Bai Zhu*), and Rhizoma Cyperi Rotundi (*Xiang Fu*). Retching and vomiting on board a boat with burning thirst may end in death once water is drunk. Child's urine is good (in this case). For retching and vomiting in people with vacuity detriment of the spleen and stomach or seen in other than the summer months, administer *Li Zhong Tang* (Rectify the Center Decoction). This should not be administered unless severe vacuity is demonstrated, and, what's more, it should be drunk when cool to conform to the nature (of the formula).

Phlegm and rheum may make the troubles of retching or vomiting with nausea, a spinning head, discomfort in the middle venter, (alternating) cold and heat, or eating raw and cold substances with disharmony of the spleen and stomach. (In this case, use) *Er Chen Tang* plus Flos Caryophylli (*Ding Xiang*), Fructus Pruni Mume (*Wu Mei*), and 7 slices of fresh Rhizoma Zingiberis (*Sheng Jiang*). In case of glomus pain, add Semen Alpiniae Katsumadai (*Cao Dou Kou*). For stomach qi vacuity weakness with inability to take in food and drink and retching and vomiting, (use) *Huo Xiang An Wei San* (Agastaches Calm the Stomach Powder): Herba Agastachis Seu Pogostemi (*Huo Xiang*), Flos Caryophylli (*Ding Xiang*), Radix Panacis Ginseng (*Ren Shen*), and Pericarpium Citri Reticulatae (*Chen Pi*). Boil together with fresh Rhizoma Zingiberis (*Sheng Jiang*). For liver fire penetrating through the stomach giving rise to upward counterflow retching and vomiting, (use) *Yi Qing Wan* (Suppress the Green-Blue Pills).[1] (But for) phlegm heat retching and vomiting, if the qi is exuberant, (use) *Dao Tan Tang* (Conduct Phlegm Decoction) plus Fructus Amomi (*Suo Sha*), ginger-processed Rhizoma Coptidis Chinensis (*Huang*

---

[1] This consists of Rhizoma Coptidis Chinensis (*Huang Lian*) and Fructus Evodiae Rutecarpae (*Wu Zhu Yu*). First boil these and then remove Fructus Evodiae Rutecarpae. Bake Rhizoma Coptidis Chinensis dry and make into pills.

Lian), and Caulis Bambusae In Taeniis (*Zhu Ru*). For incessant retching and vomiting of phlegm, (use) Pericarpium Citri Reticulatae (*Chen Pi*), Rhizoma Pinelliae Ternatae (*Ban Xia*), and Succus Zingiberis (*Jiang Zhi*. However, for) incessant retching and vomiting in summer months, (administer) *Wu Ling San* (Five *Ling* Powder) plus Succus Zingiberis (*Jiang Zhi*).

In decoctions for retching and vomiting, it is prohibited to include Fructus Trichosanthis Kirlowii (*Gua Lou Ren*), Semen Pruni Armeniacae (*Xing Ren*), Semen Pruni Persicae (*Tao Ren*), Semen Raphani Sativi (*Lai Fu Zi*), and Fructus Gardeniae Jasminoidis (*Shan Zhi*), all of which provoke vomiting. If a formula contains aromatic medicinals in order to move and disperse (phlegm), this presents no problem. For diarrhea possibly with retching and vomiting (use) *Yi Yuan San* (Boost the Origin Powder) brewed with Succus Zingiberis (*Jiang Zhi*) soup.

A person who retched out wine in the morning was prescribed Fructus Trichosanthis Kirlowii (*Gua Lou*), Bulbus Fritillariae (*Bei Mu*), stir-fried Fructus Gardeniae Jasminoidis (*Shan Zhi*), calcined Gypsum (*Shi Gao*), Rhizoma Cyperi Rotundi (*Xiang Fu*), Rhizoma Arisaematis (*Nan Xing*), ginger-processed Massa Medica Fermentata (*Shen Qu*), and stir-fried Fructus Crataegi (*Shan Zha*), 1 *liang* for each of the above, stir-fried Fructus Immaturus Citri Seu Ponciri (*Zhi Shi*), Rhizoma Curcumae (*Jiang Huang*), steamed Semen Raphani Sativi (*Lai Fu Zi*), Fructus Forsythiae Suspensae (*Lian Qiao*), and Alkaloid (*Shi Jian*), one half *liang* for each of the above, and Rhizoma Cimicifugae (*Sheng Ma*), 2.5 *qian*. The above were powdered and made into pills with Succus Zingiberis (*Jiang Zhi*) cake.

As a result of hunger and surfeit, taxation and toiling, a person suffered from a disease of retching and vomiting which was intermittent. He vomited clear water and had constipation at one time and diarrhea at another, abdominal pain attacking upward to the cardiac region and the upper back, and a bowstring pulse. (He was given) Rhizoma Atractylodis Macrocephalae (*Bai Zhu*), 1.5 *liang*, Fructus Gardeniae Jasminoidis (*Shan Zhi*), 1 *liang*, stir-fried with 2 *qian* of Fructus Evodiae Rutecarpae (*Zhu Yu*) which was removed afterwards, Rhizoma Coptidis Chinensis (*Huang Lian*), 1 *liang*, stir-fried with 2 *qian* of Fructus Evodiae Rutecarpae which was removed afterwards, Massa Medica Fermentata (*Shen Qu*), Fructus Germinatus Hordei Vulgaris

(*Mai Ya*), and Semen Pruni Persicae (*Tao Ren*), skinned and stir-fried with 20 pieces of Semen Crotonis (*Ba Dou*) which were removed afterward, 1 *liang* for each of the above, Rhizoma Curcumae (*Jiang Huang*), Semen Pruni Armeniacae (*Xing Ren*), skinned and stir-fried with 20 pieces of Semen Crotonis which were removed afterward, each 1 *liang*, Rhizoma Curcumae Zedoariae (*Peng Zhu*), 1 *liang*, stir-fried with 20 pieces of Semen Crotonis which were removed afterward, Rhizoma Cyperi Rotundi (*Xiang Fu*), 1 *liang*, Rhizoma Sparganii (*San Leng*), 1 *liang*, stir-fried with 20 pieces of Semen Crotonis which were removed afterward, Fructus Cardamomi (*Bai Dou Kou*), Fructus Amomi (*Sha Ren*), Radix Saussureae Seu Vladimiriae (*Mu Xiang*), Semen Raphani Sativi (*Lai Fu Zi*), and Pericarpium Citri Reticulatae (*Chen Pi*), 5 *qian* for each of the above, Rhizoma Arisaematis (*Nan Xing*), 1 *liang*, processed with ginger, Fructus Crataegi (*Shan Zha*), 1 *liang*, Radix Et Rhizoma Rhei (*Da Huang*), 1 *liang*, steamed, and Pericarpium Viridis Citri Reticulatae (*Qing Pi*), 5 *qian*. All the above were powdered and made into pills with Succus Zingiberis (*Jiang Zhi*) cake; 20-30 pills per dose.

Master of Ceremonies Zhu[2] prescribed Rhizoma Pinelliae Ternatae (*Ban Xia*), Pericarpium Citri Reticulatae (*Ju Pi*), and fresh Rhizoma Zingiberis (*Sheng Jiang*) as the ruling (ingredients). The Immortal Sun[3] mistook retching for counterflow hiccough. In any case, if the patient is inclined to vomit, it is absolutely not allowed to apply precipitation of counterflow.

When Liu He-jian ascribed retching to fire qi upflaming, this is but one particular (condition). It may be due to phlegm obstructing the middle burner and disabling food from descending, to qi counterflow, to cold qi depressed in the stomach, or to food stagnated somewhere near the heart and lungs and having to reflux because of inability to descend. In most

---

[2] A.k.a. Zhu Hong of the Northern Song Dynasty who specialized in the study of the *Shang Han Lun (Treatise on Damage by Cold)*.

[3] A.k.a. Sun Si-miao. Because he lived more than one hundred years, he is sometimes called an Immortal. Emperor Tai Zong of the Tang Dynasty proclaimed Sun "one who has truly attained the Dao."

cases, however, phlegm and fire existing in the stomach are the cause of retching and vomiting. Besides, chronic retching disease is due to the stomach too vacuous to receive grains, (requiring) Rhizoma Zingiberis (*Jiang*), Radix Panacis Ginseng (*Ren Shen*), Radix Astragali Membranacei (*Huang Qi*), Rhizoma Atractylodis Macrocephalae (*Bai Zhu*), Rhizoma Cyperi Rotundi (*Xiang Fu*), and so on.

Chapter Twenty-six

Heart-turning (*i.e.*, Nausea)

This is classified into phlegm, heat, and vacuity (types). Fresh Rhizoma Zingiberis (*Sheng Jiang*) is used in all (these categories) and other medicinals should be chosen in accordance with signs. If phlegm and rheum are the trouble makers, retching and vomiting with heart-turning (indicate) *Er Chen Tang* (Two Aged Decoction) plus Flos Caryophylli (*Ding Xiang*) and Fructus Pruni Mume (*Wu Mei*). Boil with 7 slices of fresh Rhizoma Zingiberis (*Sheng Jiang*) and take.

Dai comments: Heart-turning, making no noise and discharging no substance, is just a desire below the heart yet inability to vomit and retch. Although it is called heart-turning, it is not a disease of the heart but entirely involves the openings of the stomach. Rhizoma Zingiberis (*Jiang*) is necessarily used because it is able to open the stomach and sweep (away) phlegm.

Book Three

Chapter Twenty-seven

Stomach Reflux

Stomach reflux is also known as esophageal constriction, (and conversely,) esophageal constriction is (the result of) gradual development of stomach reflux. In detail, there are four (categories of this condition), blood vacuity, qi vacuity, heat, and phlegm. In addition, there may be complications. In the case of blood vacuity, the pulse is invariably rapid yet weak. In the case of qi vacuity, it is invariably moderate and weak. In the case of vacuity of both blood and qi, there is frequently foaming at the mouth. If this foaming is seen to be profuse, death is doomed. In the presence of heat, the pulse is rapid and strong. In the presence of phlegm, it is slippery and rapid. The (last) two are curable. It is also said that the stomach reflux pulse is weak on the left hand in case of blood vacuity; weak on the right hand in case of qi vacuity; and deep or hidden and large in the *cun* and *guan* sections if there is phlegm.

For blood vacuity, *Si Wu* (Four Materials [Decoction]) is the ruling (formula). For qi vacuity, *Si Jun Zi* (Four Gentlemen [Decoction]) is the ruling (formula). For heat, toxin-resolving (medicinals) are the ruling (ingredients), (and) for phlegm, *Er Chen* (Two Chen [Decoction]) is the ruling (formula). In any case, it is necessary to introduce child's urine, Succus Zingiberis (*Jiang Zhi*), Succus Bambusae (*Zhu Li*), Succus Allii Tuberosi (*Jiu Zhi*), and cow or sheep's milk. If the stools look like sheep droppings, there is no cure. For those in advanced age, though incurable, it is necessary to use Radix Panacis Ginseng (*Ren Shen*) and Rhizoma Atractylodis Macrocephalae (*Bai Zhu*) to attend to and prevent qi vacuity and stomach vacuity.

Stomach reflux may (also) be caused by yin fire upflaming, and this should be treated as yin fire. It may be caused by bound qi, (in which case) its pulse is deep and choppy in the *cun* and *guan* sections. This requires stagnation-opening and qi-conducting medicinals. It may (also) be caused by accumulated blood internally, and (in this case) it is necessary to disperse in order to drive this out. In case of bound stools, it is difficult to treat. If (one) often eats rabbit meat, defecation will be disinhibited.

The disease of stomach reflux in people with phlegm repletion and exuberant fire can be treated first with *Gua Di San* (Melon Pedicle Powder) to provoke vomiting and then with Radix Et Rhizoma Rhei (*Da Huang*), Fructus Gleditschiae Sinensis (*Zao Jiao*), Semen Pharbitidis (*Hei Qian Niu*), and slaked lime (*Po Xiao*). Powder, make into pills with paste, and take 15 pills with ginger soup. (While) a formula that treats stomach reflux with accumulated rheum uses *Yi Yuan San* (Boost the Origin Powder) as the basis. Make into pills with juice extracted from ginger after being allowed to settle and take at short intervals. Another formula consists of Rhizoma Coptidis Chinensis (*Huang Lian*), Fructus Evodiae Rutecarpae (*Zhu Yu*), stir-fried Bulbus Fritillariae (*Bei Mu*), Fructus Trichosanthis Kirlowii (*Gua Lou*), Pericarpium Citri Reticulatae (*Chen Pi*), Rhizoma Atractylodis Macrocephalae (*Bai Zhu*), Fructus Immaturus Citri Seu Ponciri (*Zhi Shi*), and Herba Eleusineae Indicae (*Niu Zhuan Cao*).

Once obstruction and congestion in swallowing arise with inability to turn the nape of the neck and the back or to stretch (the body), a seeming pattern of esophageal constriction with inability of food and drink to descend, with heart pain succeeded by generalized yellowing, (one) should first administer Rhizoma Ligustici Wallichii (*Chuan Xiong*), Radix Platycodi Grandiflori (*Jie Geng*), Fructus Gardeniae Jasminoidis (*Shan Zhi*), powdered Folium Camelliae Sinensis (*Xi Cha*), fresh Rhizoma Zingiberis (*Sheng Jiang*), and pickle. (Then) after 2 bowlfuls of phlegm are vomited, administer *Dao Tan Tang* (Conduct Phlegm Decoction) plus Radix Et Rhizoma Notopterygii (*Qiang Huo*), Radix Scutellariae Baicalensis (*Huang Qin*), and Flos Carthami Tinctorii (*Hong Hua*). This method is (only) applicable in strong persons.

An old person suffered from stomach reflux. (Therefore, they were given) Fructus Trichosanthis Kirlowii (*Gua Lou*), Bulbus Fritillariae (*Bei Mu*), Rhizoma Atractylodis Macrocephalae (*Bai Zhu*), Pericarpium Citri Reticulatae (*Chen Pi*), Fructus Evodiae Rutecarpae (*Wu Zhu Yu*), Rhizoma Coptidis Chinensis (*Huang Lian*), Radix Glycyrrhizae (*Sheng Gan Cao*), Radix Panacis Ginseng (*Ren Shen*), Sclerotium Poriae Cocoris (*Fu Ling*), and Fructus Immaturus Citri Seu Ponciri (*Zhi Shi*. However,) those who are young should be treated with *Si Wu Tang* to clear the venter. When dry, blood fails to moisten the stool and hence gives rise to bound stools. The *Ge Zhi Yu Lun (Extra Treatises Based on Investigation & Inquiry)*[1] gives a very detailed discussion about this.

Bing Lian Wan (Areca & Coptis Pills) treat stomach reflux (characterized by) food taken in the morning being turned back out in the evening, vomiting upon swallowing, pain in the venter, by relief not being experienced till all (food) is vomited, or by vomiting at the sight of any food. (They are composed of) Rhizoma Atractylodis Macrocephalae (*Bai Zhu*), Rhizoma Coptidis Chinensis (*Huang Lian*), Fructus Amomi (*Sha Ren*), Pericarpium Citri Reticulatae (*Chen Pi*), Pinellia-processed Massa Medica Fermentata (*Ban Xia Qu*), Massa Medica Fermentata (*Shen Qu*), and Rhizoma Curcumae Zedoariae (*Peng Zhu*), 1 *liang* for each of the above, Herba Agastachis Seu Pogostemi (*Huo Xiang*), Semen Arecae Catechu (*Bing Lang*), Pericarpium Viridis Citri Reticulatae (*Qing Pi*), Flos Caryophylli (*Ding Xiang*), Fructus Germinatus Hordei Vulgaris (*Mai Ya*), Rhizoma Sparganii (*San Leng*), Rhizoma Curcumae (*Jiang Huang*), Rhizoma Alpiniae Officinari (*Liang Jiang*), Fructus Cardamomi (*Bai Dou Kou*), Sclerotium Poriae Cocoris (*Fu Ling*), Flos Osmanthi Fragrantis (*Gui Hua*), Fructus Forsythiae Suspensae (*Lian Qiao*), and Fructus Crataegi (*Shan Zha*), 5 *qian* for each of the above, Radix Praeparatus Aconiti Carmichaeli (*Chuan Fu*), one half piece, and Fructus Evodiae Rutecarpae (*Wu Zhu Yu*), 2 *qian*. Powder the above medicinals and make into pills with ginger paste; 70-80 pills per dose taken with ginger soup or boiled water 3 times per day.

A person in the prime of his life suffered from (stomach) reflux. (He was given) *Yi Yuan San* plus Pericarpium Citri Reticulatae (*Chen Pi*) and Rhizoma Pinelliae Ternatae (*Ban Xia*. All the ingredients) were soaked in undiluted Succus Zingiberis (*Jiang Zhi*), dried in the sun, powdered, and taken brewed with Succus Bambusae (*Zhu Li*) and Succus Sacchari Sinensis (*Gan Zhe Zhi*).

---

[1] This is another of Zhu Dan-xi's important medical works completed in 1347 CE. It is a collection of essays expounding his new approaches to many theoretical problems. It will be issued as a companion volume to the present book as part of Blue Poppy's Great Masters Series.

An(other) person was able to eat nothing but a spoonful of gruel. If by chance he took (even) a (single) leaf of vegetable mixed in the gruel, it would be held up at the diaphragm and then even the gruel would also be unable to descend. He could swallow neither meat nor fish but thin gruel. However, he was normal in doing his daily life activities. (He was) administered *Liang Ge San* (Cool the Diaphragm Powder) plus Radix Platycodi Grandiflori (*Jie Geng*). If (in such cases) the face often feels hot with bound stools, this is due to throat constriction imposed by dried phlegm. (In that case,) drink (the above powder) with white honey. This is a treatment for stomach reflux with the venter not yet dried and desiccated.

A male in the prime of his life never ate but he had to vomit several mouthfuls. Yet he never (vomited) all that was taken in. Frequently there was a noise above the diaphragm. His facial complexion, however, was like that of a normal person. (In this case,) the trouble must exist at the diaphragm rather than in the spleen and stomach. When asked about the cause of (his) disease, (he said that he) contracted this pattern after he had eaten wheat flour food before an enraging anger was appeased. With violent anger, blood is depressed above and accumulates at the diaphragm, impeding qi from either ascending or descending. As a result, fluids gather to turn into phlegm and rheum which come into conflict with the blood, (thus) becoming stirred. Hence a noise is made. (He) was given *Er Chen Tang* plus Rhizoma Cyperi Rotundi (*Xiang Fu*), Radix Raphani Sativi (*Lai Fu*), and Succus Allii Tuberosi (*Jiu Zhi*) for one day and then *Gua Di San* and fermented millet water (*Suan Jiang*) to induce vomiting the next day. The third day, ejection was administered again. One cupful of blood was seen in the phlegm vomited. The next day, ejection continued. Another cupful of blood was observed (in the vomit) and this was followed by recuperation.

A middle-aged person suffered from a pain in the middle venter and vomiting immediately upon eating with a purplish, chilly facial complexion and a quite choppy pulse in the *guan* section. This was a blood disease. The pain in the middle venter occurred immediately after a fall. (He was) prescribed a formula to engender new and dispel old blood. He vomited about a bowlful of flaky blood and then recovered.

As a result of the seven affects, a female felt something like a kernel stuck in (her) throat which refused to be either spit out or swallowed down. In addition, there was pain in the flanks and the cardiac region with low food intake. She had been pregnant for 3 months. (I) prescribed Rhizoma Cyperi Rotundi (*Xiang Fu*), Fructus Amomi (*Sha Ren*), Sclerotium Poriae Cocoris (*Fu Ling*), and Pericarpium Citri Reticulatae (*Chen Pi*), 2 *qian* for each of the above, Tuber Ophiopogonis Japonicae (*Mai Dong*), Cortex Magnoliae Officinalis (*Hou Po*), Rhizoma Atractylodis Macrocephalae (*Bai Zhu*), Radix Panacis Ginseng (*Ren Shen*), and Radix Glycyrrhizae (*Gan Cao*), 5 *fen* for each of the above, Fructus Citri Seu Ponciri (*Zhi Qiao*), Radix Paeoniae Lactiflorae (*Shao Yao*), and Fructus Cardamomi (*Bai Dou Kou*), 8 *fen* for each of the above, and Caulis Bambusae In Taeniis (*Zhu Ru*), 2 *qian*. (These) were boiled with 5 slices of ginger and taken. If there is constant heart pain, add Semen Alpiniae Katsumadai (*Cao Dou Kou*).

A person who had suffered from esophageal constriction in the past had a bad relapse of the disease and acid regurgitation after eating mutton. They were was prescribed *Er Chen Tang* plus Rhizoma Atractylodis (*Cang Zhu*), Rhizoma Atractylodis Macrocephalae (*Bai Zhu*), Rhizoma Cyperi Rotundi (*Xiang Fu*), Fructus Amomi (*Sha Ren*), Fructus Citri Seu Ponciri (*Zhi Qiao*), Fructus Evodiae Rutecarpae (*Wu Zhu*), Rhizoma Coptidis Chinensis (*Huang Lian*), and Massa Medica Fermentata (*Shen Qu*. These) were boiled with ginger and taken. Later, because there arose abdominal urgency and rectal pressure, Radix Saussureae Seu Vladimiriae (*Mu Xiang*) and Semen Arecae Catechu (*Bing Lang*) were added.

A tubercle of bound phlegm qi in the throat that cannot either be spit or hacked out is the result of the seven affects. For this and phlegm fire upflaming with congestion in the chest and diaphragm, add Rhizoma Cyperi Rotundi (*Xiang Fu*), Fructus Amomi (*Sha Ren*), Fructus Trichosanthis Kirlowii (*Gua Lou*), Rhizoma Atractylodis Macrocephalae (*Bai Zhu*), Cortex Magnoliae Officinalis (*Hou Po*), Fructus Perillae Frutescentis (*Su Zi*), Rhizoma Coptidis Chinensis (*Huang Lian*), Fructus Evodiae Rutecarpae (*Wu Zhu Yu*), and Fructus Citri Seu Ponciri (*Zhi Qiao*) to *Er Chen Tang*. Boil with fresh Rhizoma Zingiberis (*Sheng Jiang*) and take. In case of spinning head, add Radix Peucedani (*Qian Hu*).

If the blocked qi is a result of excessive desire for food, it should be treated as dead blood. (In that case,) add Radix Angelicae Sinensis (*Dang Gui*), Semen Pruni Persicae (*Tao Ren*), Rhizoma Cyperi Rotundi (*Xiang Fu*), Fructus Amomi (*Sha Ren*), Rhizoma Atractylodis Macrocephalae (*Bai Zhu*), Fructus Immaturus Citri Seu Ponciri (*Zhi Shi*), Herba Agastachis Seu Pogostemi (*Huo Xiang*), and ginger-processed Rhizoma Coptidis Chinensis (*Huang Lian*) to *Er Chen Tang*. In case of incessant vomiting, add Flos Caryophylli (*Ding Xiang*). Boil (and take). Before taking, add small amounts of Succus Allii Tuberosi (*Jiu Zhi*), Succus Zingiberis (*Jiang Zhi*), and Succus Bambusae (*Zhu Li*), but it is still better to add cow's milk.

A person suffered from phlegm fire esophageal constriction with congestion in the chest and diaphragm. (They were given) *Er Chen Tang* plus Fructus Perillae Frutescentis (*Zi Su*), Cortex Magnoliae Officinalis (*Hou Po*), Rhizoma Cyperi Rotundi (*Xiang Fu*), Fructus Amomi (*Sha Ren*), ginger-processed Rhizoma Coptidis Chinensis (*Huang Lian*), Radix Saussureae Seu Vladimiriae (*Mu Xiang*), Semen Arecae Catechu (*Bing Lang*), Fructus Cardamomi (*Bai Dou Kou*), and Fructus Evodiae Rutecarpae (*Wu Zhu Yu*. These) were boiled with fresh Rhizoma Zingiberis (*Sheng Jiang*) and taken.

For retching and vomiting with pain in the chest and diaphragm, (use) *Er Chen Tang* plus Rhizoma Curcumae (*Jiang Huang*), Rhizoma Cyperi Rotundi (*Xiang Fu*), Fructus Amomi (*Sha Ren*), Flos Caryophylli (*Ding Xiang*), Herba Agastachis Seu Pogostemi (*Huo Xiang*), Rhizoma Atractylodis Macrocephalae (*Bai Zhu*), Fructus Cardamomi (*Bai Dou Kou*), Fructus Citri Seu Ponciri (*Zhi Qiao*), and ginger-processed Rhizoma Coptidis Chinensis (*Huang Lian*). In case of cardiac and abdominal pain with acid regurgitation, delete Fructus Citri Seu Ponciri and add Fructus Evodiae Rutecarpae (*Wu Zhu Yu*). In case of fever, delete Fructus Citri Seu Ponciri and Fructus Evodiae Rutecarpae and add dry Radix Puerariae Lobatae (*Gan Ge*), Caulis Bambusae In Taeniis (*Zhu Ru*), and Folium Eriobotryae Japonicae (*Pi Ba Ye*), (all of which) are stir-fried with Succus Zingiberis (*Jiang Zhi*). In case of severe heat, add Semen Forsythiae Suspensae (*Lian Qiao Ren*). Boil (all these ingredients) with ginger and take.

Chapter Twenty-eight

Jaundice

It is not necessary to divide (this condition) into five categories since all of them have damp heat in common like covered dough. (If accompanied by) thirst, it is difficult to treat. Without thirst, it is easy to treat. A floating pulse warrants ejection. A deep pulse warrants precipitation. For a moderate (condition use) *Xiao Wen Zhong Wan* (Minor Warm the Center Pills). For a severe (condition use) *Da Wen Zhong Wan* (Major Warm the Center Pills). In case of spleen vacuity, administer (*Wen Zhong Wan*) with Rhizoma Atractylodis Macrocephalae (*Bai Zhu*) soup and the like. For disharmonious spleen and stomach jaundice with fatigue and low food intake, (use) *Wei Ling Tang* (Stomach *Ling* Decoction). In case of dark colored urine, add Talcum (*Hua Shi*).

For damp heat jaundice with inhibited voiding of dark colored urine, (use) *Yin Chen Wu Ling San* (Artemisia Capillaris Five *Ling* Powder).[1] (However, for) damp cold jaundice with disharmony of the spleen and stomach, inability to eat, a deep, thin pulse, and uninhibited voiding of clear urine, (use) *Li Zhong Tang* (Rectify the Center Decoction). For a severe case, add Radix Praeparatus Aconiti Carmichaeli (*Fu Zi*). This is so-called yin jaundice. For accumulated spleen dampness jaundice with cardiac and abdominal pain, (use) *Wei Ling Tang*. (But for) damp heat developing into diarrhea as a result of administering medicinals which have emptied the stomach qi, (use) Radix Panacis Ginseng (*Ren Shen*), Rhizoma Atractylodis Macrocephalae (*Bai Zhu*), and the like plus Herba Artemisiae Capillaris (*Yin Chen*), Fructus Gardeniae Jasminoidis (*Shan Zhi*), and Radix Glycyrrhizae (*Gan Cao*). For abundant heat, (use) *Wen Zhong Wan* plus Rhizoma Coptidis Chinensis (*Huang Lian*. For) abundant dampness, (use) *Yin Chen Wu Ling San* plus food accumulation (dispersing) medicinals. A yellow facial

---

[1]   This consists of *Wu Ling San* (Note 10, Ch. 5, Bk. 1) plus Herba Artemisiae Capillaris (*Yin Chen*).

complexion, fatigued limbs, and uninhibited voiding of clear urine are said to be the result of wood overwhelming in the center and earth escaping to the external. (In this case, use) *Huang Qi Jian Zhong Tang* (Astragalus Build the Center Decoction).

An overdose of Herba Artemisiae Capillaris (*Yin Chen*) may result in a yin pattern of yellowing of the body, including the eyes, cold skin, pain below the heart, dry eyes with inability to open (them), and loose bowels. (For this, use) *Yin Chen Fu Zi Gan Jiang Tang* (Artemisia, Aconite & Dried Ginger Decoction. But) grain jaundice is a disease of (alternating) cold and heat, inability to eat, spinning head arising upon eating, restlessness in the heart and chest, and, over time, yellowing. (For this) prescribe Herba Artemisiae Capillaris (*Yin Chen*), Fructus Gardeniae Jasminoidis (*Zhi Zi*), and Radix Et Rhizoma Rhei (*Da Huang*). These can also treat yellowing in cold damage.

Persons with qi repletion and cardiac pain with yellowing should be treated by ejection with *Fu Xiong San* (Ligusticum Powder).[2] (But for) jaundice with (alternating) cold and heat, retching and vomiting, thirst with desire for cold drinks, yellowing of the body, including the face and eyes, inhibited urination, no desire at all for food, and sleeplessness at night, (use) *Fu Ling Shen Shi Tang* (Poria Percolate Dampness Decoction which is) composed of *Yin Chen Si Ling San* (Artemisia Four *Ling* Powder)[3] plus Radix Scutellariae Baicalensis (*Huang Qin*), Rhizoma Coptidis Chinensis (*Huang Lian*), Fructus Gardeniae Jasminoidis (*Zhi Zi*), Radix Stephaniae Tetrandrae (*Fang Ji*), Rhizoma Atractylodis (*Cang Zhu*), Pericarpium Viridis Citri Reticulatae (*Qing Pi*), and Pericarpium Citri Reticulatae (*Chen Pi*). A (variant) formula (also) includes Fructus Immaturus Citri Seu Ponciri (*Zhi Shi*). Boil in river water and take.

---

[2]   This consists of Rhizoma Ligustici Wallichii (*Chuan Xiong*), Rhizoma Atractylodis Macrocephalae (*Bai Zhu*), Pericarpium Citri Rubri (*Ju Hong*), and Radix Glycyrrhizae (*Gan Cao*).

[3]   *Si Ling San* (Note 1, Ch. 22, Bk. 2) plus Herba Artemisiae Capillaris (*Yin Chen*).

A formula for jaundice (consists of) stir-fried Rhizoma Coptidis Chinensis (*Huang Lian*), stir-fried Radix Scutellariae Baicalensis (*Huang Qin*), stir-fried Gardeniae Jasminoidis (*Shan Zhi*), Sclerotium Polypori Umbellati (*Zhu Ling*), Rhizoma Alismatis (*Ze Xie*), Rhizoma Atractylodis (*Cang Zhu*), Herba Artemisiae Capillaris (*Yin Chen*), Pericarpium Viridis Citri Reticulatae (*Qing Pi*), and Radix Gentianae Scabrae (*Long Dan Cao*), 1 *qian* for each of the above. For taxation and dietary jaundice, add Rhizoma Sparganii (*San Leng*) and Rhizoma Curcumae Zedoariae (*Peng E Zhu*), 1 *qian* each, and Fructus Amomi (*Sha Ren*), Pericarpium Citri Reticulatae (*Chen Pi*), and Massa Medica Fermentata (*Shen Qu*), 5 *fen* for each of the above.

Yin Chen Fu Zi Gan Jiang Tang (consists of) blast-fried Radix Praeparatus Aconiti Carmichaeli (*Fu Zi*), blast-fried dry Rhizoma Zingiberis (*Pao Gan Jiang*), Herba Artemisiae Capillaris (*Yin Chen*), Sclerotium Album Poriae Cocoris (*Bai Fu Ling*), Semen Alpiniae Katsumadai (*Cao Dou Kou*), Fructus Immaturus Citri Seu Ponciri (*Zhi Shi*), Rhizoma Pinelliae Ternatae (*Ban Xia*), Rhizoma Alismatis (*Ze Xie*), Rhizoma Atractylodis Macrocephalae (*Bai Zhu*), and Pericarpium Citri Reticulatae (*Chen Pi*). Boil the above with ginger and take when cooled.

Xiao Wen Zhong Wan (Minor Warm the Center Pills) treat jaundice and food accumulation. They consist of stir-fried Rhizoma Atractylodis (*Cang Zhu*), stir-fried Massa Medica Fermentata (*Shen Qu*), iron dust (*Zhen Sha*), calcined with vinegar, and Rhizoma Pinelliae Ternatae (*Ban Xia*), 2 *liang* for each of the above, Rhizoma Ligustici Wallichii (*Chuan Xiong*) and Fructus Gardeniae Jasminoidis (*Zhi Zi*), 1 *liang* each, and Rhizoma Cyperi Rotundi (*Xiang Fu*), 4 *liang*. Add more Rhizoma Ligustici Wallichii (*Chuan Xiong*) in the spring, Radix Sophorae Flavescentis (*Ku Shen*) or Rhizoma Coptidis Chinensis (*Huang Lian*) in the summer, and Fructus Evodiae Rutecarpae (*Wu Zhu Yu*) or dry Rhizoma Zingiberis (*Gan Jiang*) in the winter. Powder the above and make into pills with vinegar paste.

Da Wen Zhong Wan (Major Warm the Center Pills), also known as *Nuan Zhong Wan* (Heat the Center Pills), treat food accumulation jaundice with swelling and also can be borrowed to restrain the liver and to dry the spleen. They consist of Pericarpium Citri Reticulatae (*Chen Pi*), Rhizoma Atractylodis (*Cang Zhu*), soaked with rice water and stir-fried, Cortex Magnoliae Officinalis (*Hou Po*), ginger-processed, Rhizoma Sparganii (*San*

Leng), stir-fried with vinegar, Rhizoma Curcumae Zedoariae (*Peng Zhu*), stir-fried with vinegar, and Pericarpium Viridis Citri Reticulatae (*Qing Pi*), 5 *liang* for each of the above, Radix Glycyrrhizae (*Gan Cao*), 2 *liang*, Rhizoma Cyperi Rotundi (*Xiang Fu*), 1 *jin*, stir-fried with vinegar, and iron dust (*Zhen Sha*), calcined with vinegar, 10 *liang*. Powder the above, make into pills with vinegar paste, and take on an empty stomach with ginger soup (or) with wine before lunch and supper. In case of spleen vacuity, take with a decoction of Rhizoma Atractylodis Macrocephalae (*Bai Zhu*), Radix Panacis Ginseng (*Ren Shen*), Radix Paeoniae Lactiflorae (*Shao Yao*), Pericarpium Citri Reticulatae (*Chen Pi*), and Radix Glycyrrhizae (*Gan Cao*). Fat meat, fruits, and vegetables are prohibited.

A (variant) formula for *Xiao Wen Zhong Wan* treats dampness retained in the spleen and stomach with stools of mixed water and (untransformed) grain and a withered yellowish facial complexion. (It consists of) iron dust (*Zhen Sha*), stir-fried with vinegar, 8 *liang*, Rhizoma Cyperi Rotundi (*Xiang Fu*) [no quantity given {tr.}], stir-fried Massa Medica Fermentata (*Shen Qu*), 8 *liang*, stir-fried Rhizoma Atractylodis Macrocephalae (*Bai Zhu*), 5 *liang*, washed Rhizoma Pinelliae Ternatae (*Ban Xia*), 5 *liang*, Radix Glycyrrhizae (*Gan Cao*), 2 *liang*, Pericarpium Citri Reticulatae (*Chen Pi*), 5 *liang*, with it's inner white skin preserved, Rhizoma Coptidis Chinensis (*Huang Lian*), 2 *liang*, and Radix Sophorae Flavescentis (*Ku Shen*), 3 *liang*. Powder the above, make into pills with vinegar paste; 50 pills per dose taken with a decoction of Rhizoma Atractylodis Macrocephalae (*Bai Zhu*) and Pericarpium Citri Reticulatae (*Chen Pi*). In winter, delete Rhizoma Coptidis Chinensis and add Cortex Magnoliae Officinalis (*Hou Po*).

Chapter Twenty-nine

Wasting Thirst

The pattern of wasting thirst is a disease involving the triple burner. (Li) Dong-yuan devised a method of treating it (based on categorizing it according to) the upper, middle, and lower (burners). Upper burner wasting thirst is (a condition involving) the lungs (whose symptoms include) drinking quantities of water, low food intake, and normal defecation and urination or, in other words, uninhibited voiding of clear urine. (In this case,) dryness resides in the upper burner. The appropriate treatment is to flow dampness to moisten this dryness. Middle burner wasting thirst is (a condition involving) the stomach (whose symptoms include) thirst and drinking quantities of water with reddish yellow urine. To cure it, precipitation should go on till (excessive) drinking of water is discontinued. Lower burner wasting thirst is (a condition involving) the kidneys (whose symptoms include) dribbling of turbid, grease-like urine. (In this case,) it is appropriate to nurture the blood and depurate (heat). When the clear is separated from the turbid, recovery ensues naturally.

The great method is to nurture the lungs, downbear fire, and engender blood as the ruling (measures). For wasting thirst with diarrhea, first stir-fry, powder, and take Rhizoma Atractylodis Macrocephalae (*Bai Zhu*) and Radix Albus Paeoniae Lactiflorae (*Bai Shao Yao*). Then take *Bai Lian Ou Zhi Gao* (Lotusroot Juice Paste). Following relief of internal damage, unresolved dryness and thirst are (symptoms of) heat remaining in the lungs. Boil Radix Panacis Ginseng (*Ren Shen*), Radix Scutellariae Baicalensis (*Huang Qin*), and a small amount of Radix Glycyrrhizae (*Gan Cao*), put in Succus Zingiberis (*Jiang Zhi*), and take when cooled or take (while hot) little by little with a spoon. In case of vacuity, (one) can take *Du Shen Tang* (Solitary Ginseng Decoction). Wasting thirst with frequent urination requires the fluid-engendering *Gan Lu Yin* (Sweet Dew Drink).[1] *Qiong Yu Gao* (Fine Jade Paste) is also remarkable. (However, for) dry mouth and

---

[1] This consists of Folium Eriobotryae Japonicae (*Pi Ba Ye*), prepared Radix Rehmanniae (*Shu Di*), Tuber Asparagi Cochinensis (*Tian Men Dong*), stir-fried Fructus Citri Seu Ponciri (*Zhi Qiao*), Herba Artemisiae Capillaris (*Yin Chen*), Radix Rehmanniae (*Sheng Di*), Tuber Ophiopogonis Japonicae (*Mai Men Dong*), Herba Dendrobii (*Shi Hu*), mix-fried Radix Glycyrrhizae (*Zhi Gan Cao*), and Radix Scutellariae Baicalensis (*Huang Qin*), all in equal amounts.

tongue, frequent voiding of reddish urine, and a red, cracked tongue surface, (use) *Di Huang Yin Zi* (Rehmannia Drink).[2]

A pregnant woman who had thirst and an (excessive) desire for water in the middle of summer was prescribed *Si Wu Tang* (Four Materials Decoction) plus Radix Scutellariae Baicalensis (*Huang Qin*), Pericarpium Citri Reticulatae (*Chen Pi*), Radix Glycyrrhizae (*Sheng Gan Cao*), and Caulis Akebiae Mutong (*Mu Tong*). Several doses sent her to recovery.

Bai Ou Zhi Gao (Lotusroot Juice Paste, consists of) powdered Rhizoma Coptidis Chinensis (*Huang Lian*), Succus Radicis Rehmanniae (*Sheng Di Zhi*), cow's milk, and Succus Rhizomatis Nelumbinis Nuciferae (*Bai Lian Ou Zhi*), 1 *jin* each. Simmer the above liquids over a small fire down to a paste. Then put in the powdered Rhizoma Coptidis Chinensis and make into pills; 20-30 pills per dose taken with warm water several times a day.

Sao Si Tang (Silk Reeling Decoction) consists of Radix Trichosanthis zKirlowii (*Tian Hua Fen*), Succus Rhizomatis Phragmitis Communis (*Lu Gen Zhi*), Caulis Bambusae In Taeniis (*Dan Zhu Ru*), Tuber Ophiopogonis Japonicae (*Mai Men Dong*), Rhizoma Anemarrhenae (*Zhi Mu*), and cow's milk. All these ingredients are important medicinals for wasting thirst.

Chapter Thirty

Water Swelling

When the spleen is too vacuous to move turbid qi, the qi gathers into water which floods, running recklessly. (In this case,) it is necessary to

---

[2] This consists of prepared Radix Rehmanniae (*Shu Di*), Radix Morindae Officinalis (*Ba Ji Tian*), Fructus Corni Officinalis (*Shan Zhu Yu*), Herba Dendrobii (*Shi Hu*), Herba Cistanchis (*Rou Cong Rong*), blast-fried Radix Praeparatus Aconiti Carmichaeli (*Fu Zi*), Fructus Schizandrae Chinensis (*Wu Wei Zi*), Cortex Cinnamomi (*Guan Gui*), Sclerotium Poriae Cocoris (*Fu Ling*), Tuber Ophiopogonis Japonicae (*Mai Men Dong*), Rhizoma Acori Graminei (*Shi Chang Pu*), and Radix Polygalae Tenuifoliae (*Yuan Zhi*).

supplement the spleen with Radix Panacis Ginseng (*Ren Shen*) and Rhizoma Atractylodis Macrocephalae (*Bai Zhu*) so as to solidify the spleen qi. Then (the spleen qi) will easily become strong enough to move and transform, to uplift and downbear, and to move the pivots and mechanisms up and down. (Thus) water will be able to move by itself. This is not a case calling for *Wu Ling* (Five *Ling* [Powder]) or *Shen You* (God Bless [Pills]) to move water. Generally speaking, (in this case) it is necessary to supplement the center, move dampness, and disinhibit urination. It is absolutely not allowed to apply precipitation unwarrantedly. Add to *Er Chen Tang* (Two Aged Decoction) Radix Panacis Ginseng (*Ren Shen*), Rhizoma Atractylodis (*Cang Zhu*), and Rhizoma Atractylodis Macrocephalae (*Bai Zhu*) as the ruling (ingredients) with Radix Scutellariae Baicalensis (*Huang Qin*), Tuber Ophiopogonis Japonicae (*Mai Dong*), and Fructus Gardeniae Jasminoidis (*Zhi Zi*) as the assistants to restrain liver wood. (Thus) earth qi is leveled to restrain water. In case of abdominal distention, add a small amount of Cortex Magnoliae Officinalis (*Hou Po*) as an assistant. In case of qi failing to circulate, add Radix Saussureae Seu Vladimiriae (*Mu Xiang*) and Caulis Akebiae Mutong (*Mu Tong*), (and) in case of qi sinking, add Radix Bupleuri (*Chai Hu*) and Rhizoma Cimicifugae (*Sheng Ma*. Therefore,) it is all right only to add and subtract (from this formula) in accordance with the signs.

The classic[1] says: The various kinds of qi gathering and depression are all ascribed to the lungs. The various kinds of dampness, swelling, and fullness are all ascribed to the spleen. (And) the various kinds of abdominal distention and enlargement are all ascribed to heat. Dampness is the qi of earth, while earth is the child of fire. Therefore, more often than not, damp disease is generated by heat. (However,) heat qi cannot become damp by itself. But the qi of the child can affect the mother. (Thus) there is a transmutation from dampness. To treat the disease of swelling, the treatment of dampness should always be the rule. Nonetheless, since there may be various complications, the (particular) treatment methods (also) vary.

---

[1]   This statement is found in Ch. 74, *Su Wen* (*Simple Questions*).

In the treatment of swelling, some (practitioners) hue to a theory of treating water (exclusively) by conducting the kidneys to drain (water). This is by no means a reasonable view. Because of the seven affects internally and the six qi[2] externally, spleen earth may become decrepit and weak so as to lose its function of conveyance and transformation. (Consequently,) the clear and turbid, (now) mixed and confused together, become depressed (and transform) into water which infiltrates and penetrates into the channels and connecting vessels, pouring into the ravines and valleys. In this case, the turbid, putrid qi, retarding and obstructing fluids and humor, pours into the tunnels for a long time, (thus) also turning blood into water. (Therefore,) it is desirable that (this situation) be brought under control by the strength of that which lies above the spleen. It should be understood that when earth is diseased, metal qi becomes decrepit, and wood, now in awe of nothing, comes and bullies earth.[3] (Thus) the spleen, though desirous of escaping, has no means to escape from disease.

(In this case,) the appropriate treatment method is to clear the fire of the heart channel and to supplement and nurture spleen earth. When the function of conveyance and transformation is renewed, lung qi will descend and the infiltrated passageways will become open and free. (In addition,) the comparatively clear will restore the turbid vanquished qi to qi, blood, and fluids and humor. The most vanquished and turbid part will become sweat if it is located above and urine if it is located below. (Thus it is) gradually separated and dispersed.

It is also said: Open the ghost gates and purge the clean mansion. The ghost gates are the interstices of the skin which are ascribed to the lungs, while the clean mansion is the urinary bladder which is ascribed to the kidneys. (But I) have never heard of the kidney-conducting theory. (Zhang) Zhong-jing says, Dampness should be treated through disinhibiting urination. This is what is meant in the classic by the statement of

---

[2]   These are wind, cold, summer heat, dampness, dryness, and fire.

[3]   That which is above spleen earth is heart fire, and metal is the phase which restrains wood. When metal is insufficient or impaired, wood will run wild.

138

purging the clean mansion. Qian Zhong-yang[4] says, In relationship to the kidneys, there are no draining methods. Please look from their points of view and see, is conduction appropriate for the kidneys?

Practically (speaking), water swelling arises (mostly) from the center palace, while (people of) various schools know nothing but the theory of treating dampness through disinhibiting urination with, as a rule, water-removing medicinals. This is the way to hasten death. When the spleen is extremely vacuous, so much so that it is vanquished, the more precipitation (is carried out), the more vacuous (it becomes). Even though a thwarting effect may be achieved for the time being, an insidious detriment has been caused to the righteous qi. How can (a more serious) disease not follow upon the heels (of such a treatment)? The appropriate treatment is to greatly supplement the center palace as the ruling (method), and additions and subtractions should be made in accordance with the complications (of the case at hand). Otherwise, death follows.

A pulse coming on deep and slow, usually a green-blue, whitish complexion, absence of vexation and thirst, inhibited voiding of scant yet clear urine, and frequent diarrhea, these are (indications of) yin water. The appropriate treatment is (to use) warming formulas. (However,) a pulse coming on deep and rapid, usually a yellowish red complexion, vexation or thirst, inhibited voiding of scant reddish urine, and frequent constipation, these are (indications of) yang water. The appropriate treatment is to (use) clearing and leveling formulas.

In enduring disease of qi vacuity and floating, there may arise swollen hands and feet. This is (due to) frenetic movement of vacuous qi. (Whereas) the disease of swelling arising postpartum or with excessive menstrual flow is (due to) blood vacuity.

Swelling above the waist requires diaphoresis. Swelling below the waist requires disinhibition of urination. This is (Zhang) Zhong-jing's method. Radix Stephaniae Tetrandrae (*Fang Ji*) treats damp heat swelling below the waist, but it cannot be used in case of internal damage with a weak stomach. Water swelling in pregnant women is

---

[4]   A.k.a Qian Yi. See Note 2, Ch. 23, Bk. 2.

called swelling (with) child. For water swelling arising with dysentery, take internally *Yi Shen San* (Boost the Kidneys Powder)[5] and externally shower and wash with Radix Glycyrrhizae (*Gan Cao*) soup. Postpartum water swelling must necessarily be treated with blood and qi-supplementing (medicinals) as the ruling ones.

(In terms of) water swelling, five (types) are incurable. This is because none of the five viscera remain unimpaired. Discharging of bloody water is incurable. (But) for puffy swelling with diarrhea in persons of vacuity weakness, add Pericarpium Citri Reticulatae (*Chen Pi*), Radix Glycyrrhizae (*Gan Cao*), Radix Albus Paeoniae Lactiflorae (*Bai Shao Yao*), Rhizoma Cimicifugae (*Sheng Ma*), stir-fried Massa Medica Fermentata (*Shen Qu*), Rhizoma Alismatis (*Ze Xie*), Caulis Akebiae Mutong (*Mu Tong*), Fructus Amomi (*Sha Ren*), and Rhizoma Zingiberis (*Jiang*) to *Si Jun Zi Tang* (Four Gentlemen Decoction. Boil and take.

For females suffering from generalized water swelling, nausea, congealed and stagnated malign blood, and abdominal pain as a result of menopause, use Radix Angelicae Sinensis (*Dang Gui*), Radix Rubrus Paeoniae Lactiflorae (*Chi Shao*), Pericarpium Viridis Citri Reticulatae (*Qing Pi*), Caulis Akebiae Mutong (*Mu Tong*), Cortex Radicis Moutan (*Mu Dan Pi*), Rhizoma Corydalis Yanhusuo (*Xuan Hu Suo*), Talcum (*Hua Shi*), Myrrha (*Mo Yao*), and Sanguis Draconis (*Xue Jie*).

For a puffy face due to decrepit and scant original qi, weakness, and vacuous spleen, use Radix Angelicae Sinensis (*Dang Gui*), Rhizoma Atractylodis Macrocephalae (*Bai Zhu*), Caulis Akebiae Mutong (*Mu Tong*), Rhizoma Atractylodis (*Cang Zhu*), and dry Radix Puerariae Lobatae (*Gan Ge*), 1 *qian* for each of the above, Radix Panacis Ginseng (*Ren Shen*), Radix Astragali Membranacei (*Huang Qi*), and Radix Albus Paeoniae Lactiflorae (*Bai Shao*), 5 *fen* for each of the above, and Radix Bupleuri (*Chai Hu*), 4 *fen*, (while for) overwhelming dampness resulting

---

[5] This consists of Magnetitum (*Ling Ci Shi*), Radix Morindae Officinalis (*Ba Ji*), Fructus Zanthoxyli Bungeani (*Hua Jiao*), Rhizoma Acori Graminei (*Shi Chang Pu*), and Lignum Aquilariae Agallochae (*Chen Xiang*), 2 *qian* per dose. Obtain one pig's kidney, cut finely, mix with salt and Bulbus Allii Fistulosi (*Cong Bai*) together with the above ingredients, wrap with wet paper, and roast. Chew well before swallowing.

in swelling or diarrhea with low food intake, (use) *Wei Ling Tang* (Stomach *Ling* Decoction) plus Caulis Akebiae Mutong (*Mu Tong*) and Tuber Ophiopogonis Japonicae (*Mai Men Dong*. And) for puffy swelling of the face and eyes or all over the body, add Fructus Perillae Frutescentis (*Zi Su*), Herba Ephedrae (*Ma Huang*), and Radix Platycodi Grandiflori (*Jie Geng*) to *Wu Jia Pi San* (Acanthopanax Powder).[6]

To treat damp swelling, use Rhizoma Atractylodis (*Cang Zhu*), Cortex Magnoliae Officinalis (*Hou Po*), Pericarpium Citri Reticulatae (*Chen Pi*), Semen Raphani Sativi (*Lai Fu Zi*), Sclerotium Polypori Umbellati (*Zhu Ling*), Rhizoma Alismatis (*Ze Xie*), Semen Plantaginis (*Che Qian*), Talcum (*Hua Shi*), Sclerotium Poriae Cocoris (*Fu Ling*), Fructus Citri Seu Ponciri (*Zhi Qiao*), Caulis Akebiae Mutong (*Mu Tong*), Pericarpium Arecae (*Da Fu Pi*), and Semen Arecae Catechu (*Bing Lang*). Boil the above and take. In case of distressed rapid breathing, add Semen Lepidii Apetali (*Ku Ting Li*). In case of inhibited urination, add Semen Pharbitidis (*Qian Niu*). For severe cases, add *Jun Chuan San* (Dredge the River Powder)[7] and damp toxins will disperse by themselves.

For puffy swelling after malaria, (use) *Si Ling San* (Four *Ling* Powder) plus Pericarpium Viridis Citri Reticulatae (*Qing Pi*), Caulis Akebiae Mutong (*Mu Tong*), Pericarpium Arecae (*Fu Pi*), Radix Saussureae Seu Vladimiriae (*Mu Xiang*), and Semen Arecae Catechu (*Bing Lang*). For puffy swelling of the backs of the feet with coughing of red phlegm, (use) *Er Chen (Tang)* plus Caulis Akebiae Mutong (*Mu Tong*), Rhizoma Alismatis (*Ze Xie*), Radix Scutellariae Baicalensis (*Huang Qin*), Rhizoma Atractylodis Macrocephalae (*Bai Zhu*), Cortex Radicis Mori Albi (*Sang Pi*), Bulbus Fritillariae (*Bei Mu*), Tuber Ophiopogonis Japonicae (*Mai*

---

[6] This consists of Cortex Eucommiae Ulmoidis (*Du Zhong*), Radix Acanthopanacis (*Wu Jia Pi*), Gelatinum Corii Asini (*E Jiao*), Radix Ledebouriellae Sesloidis (*Fang Feng*), Semen Cibotii Barometsis (*Gou Ji*), Rhizoma Ligustici Wallichii (*Chuan Xiong*), Radix Albus Paeoniae Lactiflorae (*Bai Shao Yao*), Herba Cum Radice Asari Sieboldi (*Xi Xin*), Rhizoma Dioscoreae Hypoglaucae (*Bei Xie*), and Semen Pruni Armeniacae (*Xing Ren*). Boil and put in Gelatinum Corii Asini (*E Jiao*).

[7] This consists of Radix Et Rhizoma Rhei (*Da Huang*), Semen Pharbitidis (*Qian Niu*), Semen Pruni (*Yu Li Ren*), Mirabilitum (*Mang Xiao*), Radix Euphorbiae Kansui (*Gan Sui*), and Radix Saussureae Seu Vladimiriae (*Mu Xiang*).

Dong), Fructus Schizandrae Chinensis (*Wu Wei*), and Fructus Perillae Frutescentis (*Su Zi*).

A formula that treats water swelling (consists of) Fructus Gardeniae Jasminoidis (*Shan Zhi Ren*), stir-fried (and) powdered. Take about a soup-spoonful with thin gruel. A (variant) version says, For heat disease in the venter that is located in the upper, use Fructus Gardeniae Jasminoidis with the peel preserved. Another formula (consists of) Fructus Gardeniae Jasminoidis (*Shan Zhi*), 5 *qian*, Radix Saussureae Seu Vladimiriae (*Mu Xiang*), 1 *qian*, and Rhizoma Atractylodis Macrocephalae (*Bai Zhu*), 2.5 *qian*. Boil with water from rapids and take. (While) a thwarting formula against water swelling (is made by) powdering Herba Cirsii Japonici (*Da Ji*) and making this into pills with Fructus Zizyphi Jujubae (*Zao Rou*). Take 11 pills. These can thwart qi repletion, but they are not applicable in vacuity cases.

Chapter Thirty-one

Drum Distention

(This) is classified into repletion and vacuity (types). Repletion distention is hard and gives pain when pressed. Vacuity distention is not hard and gives no pain when pressed. Repletion requires precipitation and whittling and afterwards supplementation, while vacuity requires warming and upbearing, supplementation being the key. Loosening (*i.e.*, relaxing) in the morning and tightening in the evening indicates blood vacuity, (while) loosening in the evening and tightening in the morning indicates qi vacuity. Tautness by day and night indicates vacuity of both qi and blood. Drum distention is also known as *gu*.[1] It is, in fact, so-called simple abdominal distention.[2] Details about it can be found in the *Ge Zhi Yu Lun (Extra Treatises Based on Investigation & Inquiry)*. The treatment method is to greatly supplement center qi and move dampness as the rule. Since this is (a disease of) extremely vacuous spleen, it is necessary to keep away from music and refrain from (food of) thick flavors.[3]

If there is qi vacuity, (use) large doses of Radix Panacis Ginseng (*Ren Shen*) and Rhizoma Atractylodis Macrocephalae (*Bai Zhu*) with the assistance of Pericarpium Citri Reticulatae (*Chen Pi*), Sclerotium Poriae Cocoris (*Fu Ling*), Radix Scutellariae Baicalensis (*Huang Qin*), and Rhizoma Atractylodis (*Cang Zhu*). If there is blood vacuity, (use) *Si Wu* (Four Materials [Decoction]) as the ruling (formula) with additions and subtractions in accordance with the signs. Attacking medicinals are only allowed in (the treatment of) strong and sturdy persons with repletion. Afterwards wind up with Rhizoma Atractylodis Macrocephalae (*Bai Zhu*) as the ruling (medicinal).

For center fullness with qi vacuity (use) *Si Jun Zi* (Four Gentleman [Decoction]) plus Rhizoma Ligustici Wallichii (*Chuan Xiong*), Radix Angelicae Sinensis (*Dang Gui*), Radix Paeoniae Lactiflorae (*Shao Yao*), Rhizoma Coptidis Chinensis (*Huang Lian*), Pericarpium Citri Reticulatae (*Chen Pi*), Cortex Magnoliae Officinalis (*Hou Po*), and Radix Glycyrrhizae (*Sheng Gan Cao*. But for) abdominal distention with stomach vacuity, (use) *Tiao Zhong Tang* (Regulate the Center Decoction, which consists of) Radix Panacis Ginseng (*Ren Shen*), Rhizoma Atractylodis Macrocephalae (*Bai Zhu*),

---

[1]   This was traditionally believed to be a kind of poisonous worm which could enter the abdomen and cause a disease characterized by abdominal distention.

[2]   *I.e.*, swelling or distention limited to the abdomen. Sometimes, however, even when the limbs or the head and face are swollen, the abdominal distention or swelling can be also called simple one if it does not advance into a generalized one.

[3]   This refers to music made by bamboo or wooden instruments. Since the spleen corresponds to earth and is restrained by wood, music made by wooden instruments is contraindicated in spleen vacuity. In addition, thick flavors may cause stagnation in the center and, therefore, should be prohibited in spleen disease.

Pericarpium Citri Reticulatae (*Chen Pi*), Radix Glycyrrhizae (*Gan Cao*), Rhizoma Pinelliae Ternatae (*Ban Xia*), Cortex Magnoliae Officinalis (*Hou Po*), and fresh Rhizoma Zingiberis (*Sheng Jiang*). Abdominal distention complicated by vacuity should be treated with *Fen Xiao Wan* (Separate & Disperse Pills).[4] Cold and abdominal distention complicated by vacuity should be treated with *Fen Xiao Tang* (Separate & Disperse Decoction).[5] Cold distention should be treated with *Chen Xiang Zun Zhong Wan* (Aquilaria Respectable Pills).[6] For abdominal distention complicated by a vacuity pattern of internal damage, (use) *Mu Xiang Shun Qi Tang* (Saussurea Normalize the Qi Decoction)[7] and *Chen Xiang Jiao Tai Wan* (Aquilaria Crossing Prosperity Pills).[8]

---

[4] This consists of Radix Et Rhizoma Notopterygii (*Qiang Huo*), Radix Angelicae (*Bai Zhi*), Radix Bupleuri (*Chai Hu*), Rhizoma Ligustici Wallichii (*Chuan Xiong*), Fructus Citri Seu Ponciri (*Zhi Qiao*), Fructus Crataegi (*Shan Zha*), Pericarpium Citri Reticulatae (*Chen Pi*), Sclerotium Polypori Umbellati (*Zhu Ling*), and Rhizoma Alismatis (*Ze Xie*).

[5] The ingredients in this formula are the same as in the preceding formula but prepared in the form of a decoction.

[6] This consists of Lignum Aquilariae Agallochae (*Chen Xiang*), Radix Praeparatus Aconiti Carmichaeli (*Fu Zi*), Radix Aconiti (*Wu Tou*), dry Rhizoma Zingiberis (*Gan Jiang*), Rhizoma Alpiniae Officinari (*Gao Liang Jiang*), Fructus Foeniculi Vulgaris (*Hui Xiang*), Cortex Cinnamomi (*Guan Gui*), and Fructus Evodiae Rutecarpae (*Wu Zhu Yu*).

[7] This consists of Radix Saussureae Seu Vladimiriae (*Mu Xiang*), Rhizoma Atractylodis (*Cang Zhu*), Semen Alpiniae Katsumadai (*Cao Dou Kou*), Cortex Magnoliae Officinalis (*Hou Po*), Pericarpium Viridis Citri Reticulatae (*Qing Pi*), Pericarpium Citri Reticulatae (*Chen Pi*), Fructus Alpiniae Oxyphyllae (*Yi Zhi Ren*), Sclerotium Poriae Cocoris (*Fu Ling*), Rhizoma Alismatis (*Ze Xie*), Rhizoma Zingiberis (*Jiang*), Rhizoma Pinelliae Ternatae (*Ban Xia*), Fructus Evodiae Rutecarpae (*Wu Zhu Yu*), Radix Angelicae Sinensis (*Dang Gui*), Rhizoma Cimicifugae (*Sheng Ma*), and Radix Bupleuri (*Chai Hu*).

[8] This consists of Rhizoma Atractylodis Macrocephalae (*Bai Zhu*), Pericarpium Citri Reticulatae (*Chen Pi*), Fructus Immaturus Citri Seu Ponciri (*Zhi Shi*), Fructus Evodiae Rutecarpae (*Wu Zhu Yu*), Sclerotium Poriae Cocoris (*Fu Ling*), Rhizoma Alismatis (*Ze Xie*), Radix Angelicae Sinensis (*Dang Gui*), Radix Saussureae Seu Vladimiriae (*Mu Xiang*), Pericarpium Viridis Citri Reticulatae (*Qing Pi*), Radix Et Rhizoma Rhei (*Da Huang*), and Cortex Magnoliae Officinalis (*Hou Po*).

For cold damage with the four signs of glomus, fullness, dryness, and repletion in strong persons or miscellaneous patterns of abdominal fullness with signs similar to these four, prescribe *Da Cheng Qi Tang* (Major Support the Qi Decoction)). For the *tai yin* disease of abdominal distention and fullness, swelling of the four limbs or all over the body, chest glomus, inability to eat, scant urine, difficult defecation or diarrhea, or spleen distention with frequent hiccough, great fullness, and generalized heaviness, administer Suo Ju's *San He Tang* (Three Harmonies Decoction). For spleen dampness with abdominal distention and fullness, a yellow facial complexion, and inhibited voiding of urine, (use) *Wei Ling Tang* (Stomach *Ling* Decoction). For vacuity below with abdominal distention and qi ascension, (use) *Si Wu (Tang)* plus Radix Panacis Ginseng (*Ren Shen*), Pericarpium Citri Reticulatae (*Chen Pi*), Caulis Akebiae Mutong (*Mu Tong*), Radix Glycyrrhizae (*Gan Cao*), and Fructus Forsythiae Suspensae (*Lian Qiao*. However,) in case of food accumulation, swallow *Bao He Wan* (Protect & Harmonize Pills). (While for) distention in alcoholics with turbid urine and swelling of the feet arising at night, (use) *Gui Ling Gan Lu Yin* (Cinnamom & Poria Sweet Dew Drink) plus Radix Panacis Ginseng (*Ren Shen*), dry Radix Puerariae Lobatae (*Gan Ge*), Herba Agastachis Seu Pogostemi (*Huo Xiang*), and Radix Saussureae Seu Vladimiriae (*Mu Xiang*).

For abdominal distention without the feeling of fullness caused by eating too much meat (use) Rhizoma Coptidis Chinensis (*Huang Lian*), 1 *liang*, powdered, and Resina Ferulae Asafoetidae (*A Wei*), one half *liang*, soaked with vinegar. Grind into a paste, make into pills, and take with *Wen Zhong Wan* (Warm the Center Pills) and Rhizoma Atractylodis Macrocephalae (*Bai Zhu*) soup. In case of eating meat often resulting in abdominal distention, prescribe the ingredients comprising *San Bu Wan* (Three Supplementation Pills) as the basis plus Rhizoma Cyperi Rotundi (*Xiang Fu*) and Plastrum Amydae (*Xia Jia, i.e.,* the ventral shell of the turtle). Make into pills with cake and take.

Cortex Magnoliae Officinalis (*Hou Po*) treats abdominal distention because its flavor is acrid. However, (in the treatment of this condition) it must be processed with Rhizoma Zingiberis (*Jiang*, before use). It is said in a (variant) edition, Distention disease necessitates the use of Radix Panacis Ginseng (*Ren Shen*), Radix Astragali Membranacei (*Huang Qi*), and Rhizoma Atractylodis Macrocephalae (*Bai Zhu*) in large doses to supplement the spleen. Then the (distending) qi will move by itself. Moreover, Rhizoma Atractylodis Macrocephalae as the sovereign ingredient needs to be combined with Cortex Magnoliae Officinalis (*Hou Po*) to loose (*i.e.*, relax) fullness.

A person who suffered from qi weakness with abdominal inflation and puffy swelling was prescribed Radix Panacis Ginseng (*Ren Shen*), Radix Angelicae Sinensis (*Dang Gui*), Sclerotium Poriae Cocoris (*Fu Ling*), Radix Paeoniae Lactiflorae (*Shao Yao*), 1 *qian* for each of the above, Rhizoma Atractylodis Macrocephalae (*Bai Zhu*), 2 *qian*, Rhizoma Ligustici Wallichii (*Chuan Xiong*), 7.5 *fen*, Pericarpium Citri Reticulatae (*Chen Pi*), Pericarpium Arecae (*Fu Pi*), Caulis Akebiae Mutong (*Mu Tong*), Cortex Magnoliae Officinalis (*Hou Po*), Spora Lygodii Japonici (*Hai Jin Sha*), 5 *fen* for each of the above, Ramulus Perillae Frutescentis (*Zi Su Geng*), and Radix Saussureae Seu Vladimiriae (*Mu Xiang*), 3 *fen* each. After several doses were taken, the puffy swelling completely disappeared except in the head and face. This (residuum) was due to *yang ming* qi vacuity and, therefore, was difficult to eliminate. Thus the use of Sclerotium Poriae Cocoris and Rhizoma Atractylodis Macroce-phalae was continued.

A female suffered from chronic abdominal vacuity distention, (*i.e.,*) simple distention, because her qi was dejected (and) unable to circulate. If, however, the face is swollen or swollen qi progresses from the hands and feet upwards and the yang phase comes to respond, (the condition) is still curable. (In this case,) Radix Panacis Ginseng (*Ren Shen*), Rhizoma Atractylodis Macrocephalae (*Bai Zhu*), Rhizoma Ligustici Wallichii (*Chuan Xiong*), and Radix Angelicae Sinensis (*Dang Gui*) are the sovereigns, assisted by Radix Albus Paeoniae Lactiflorae (*Bai Shao Yao*) to astringe distention with its sourness, Talcum (*Hua Shi*) to simultaneously dry dampness and disinhibit water, Pericarpium Arecae (*Da Fu Pi*) to astringe the qi, and Ramulus Perillae Frutescentis (*Zi Su Geng*), Semen Raphani Sativi (*Lai Fu Zi*), and Pericarpium Citri Reticulatae (*Chen Pi*) to drain fullness, Spora Lygodii Japonici (*Hai Jin Sha*) and Caulis Akebiae Mutong (*Mu Tong*) to disinhibit water, Radix Saussureae Seu Vladimiriae (*Mu Xiang*) to promote movement and transportation, and Radix Glycyrrhizae (*Sheng Gan Cao*) to co-ordinate the various medicinals.

An(other) female suffered from qi vacuity simple distention with a swollen face. (For this she was given) Radix Panacis Ginseng (*Ren Shen*), Rhizoma Atractylodis Macrocephalae (*Bai Zhu*), Sclerotium Poriae Cocoris (*Fu Ling*), Cortex Magnoliae Officinalis (*Hou Po*), Pericarpium Arecae (*Da Fu Pi*), Rhizoma Ligustici Wallichii (*Chuan Xiong*), Radix Angelicae Sinensis (*Dang Gui*), Radix Albus Paeoniae Lactiflorae (*Bai Shao*), Radix Glycyrrhizae (*Sheng Gan Cao*), and Talcum (*Hua Shi*).

A person who was addicted to wine and had suffered from malaria for half a year had distention of the abdomen with spiderweb-like (vessels visible on it). An(other) person who was addicted to wine suffered from distention following hemafecia with a black complexion and an enlarged belly like that of a ghost. [Both cases are found in the *Yi Yao* {*Essentials of Medicine*, later editor}]. Of the above two cases, one was treated by supplementation of qi and the other by supplementation of blood. The other medicinals (in their prescriptions) varied little, and both recovered.

Chapter Thirty-two

Spontaneous Sweating

(This condition) is ascribed to qi vacuity and to yang qi. [The second may be a misprint for vacuity which, in this context, makes more sense. {tr.}] The existence of phlegm may give rise to spontaneous sweating, as may dampness and so may heat. (According to) the great method, the appropriate (medicinals) are Radix Panacis Ginseng (*Ren Shen*) and Radix Astragali Membranacei (*Huang Qi*) with a small amount of Ramulus Cinnamomi (*Gui Zhi*) as an assistant. In case of yang vacuity, Radix Praeparatus Aconiti Carmichaeli (*Fu Zi*) can also be used.

For qi vacuity with spontaneous sweating, (use) *Huang Qi Jian Zhong Tang* (Astragalus Build the Center Decoction). For qi vacuity with cold and heat, spontaneous sweating, taxation fatigue, low food intake, and a weak pulse, (use) *Bu Zhong Yi Qi Tang* (Supplement the Center & Boost the Qi Decoction. But for) great vacuity (due to) taxation and toiling with a deep, thin pulse, massive sweating, moisture on the surface of the tongue, absence of vexation and agitation yet perspiration arising due to fright or a scare, (which) is similar to vacuity desertion in cold damage, (use) *Bu Zhong Yi Qi Tang* with Radix Bupleuri (*Chai Hu*) deleted but Fructus Schizandrae Chinensis (*Wu Wei Zi*) and Radix Ephedrae (*Ma Huang Gen*) added.

Upward fire qi steaming dampness in the stomach can also produce sweat. It requires *Liang Ge San* (Cool the Diaphragm Powder) as the ruling (formula). Or (use) the method of applying powder (directly on the body). For stomach repletion with copious sweating on the hands and feet as well as the axillae, and dry, bound stools, (use) *Da Cheng Qi Tang* (Major Support the Qi Decoction) as the ruling (formula. However, for) phlegm repletion obstruction and stagnation with (alternating) cold and heat, spontaneous sweating, ability to eat, dry, bound stools, and a replete pulse, (use) *Da Chai Hu Tang* (Major Bupleurum Decoction) as the ruling (formula). In general, qi heat spontaneous sweating is, in most cases, a pattern of superabundance.

If, when eating or drinking, sweat never fails to exit, the impetuous and swift qi should be suppressed and contracted with *An Wei Tang* (Calm the Stomach Decoction).[1] (Whereas) great draining of sweat is fluid desertion and requires checking without delay with Radix Panacis Ginseng (*Ren Shen*), Radix Astragali Membranacei (*Huang Qi*), Tuber Ophiopogonis Japonicae (*Mai Dong*), Fructus Schizandrae Chinensis (*Wu Wei*), stir-fried Cortex Phellodendri (*Huang Bai*), and Rhizoma Anemarrhenae (*Zhi Mu*. However,) for damp heat spontaneous sweating due to the defensive qi being too vacuous and weak to resist

---

[1]   This consists of Rhizoma Coptidis Chinensis (*Huang Lian*), Fructus Schizandrae Chinensis (*Wu Wei Zi*), Fructus Pruni Mume (*Wu Mei*), Radix Glycyrrhizae (*Sheng Gan Cao*), mix-fried Radix Glycyrrhizae (*Zhi Gan Cao*), and Rhizoma Cimicifugae (*Sheng Ma*).

wind cold, (use) *Tiao Wei Tang* (Regulate the Defensive Decoction).[2] (And for) vacuity desertion with spontaneous sweating in cold damage, (use) *Zhen Wu Tang* (Turtle & Snake Decoction).[3] Externally use the powder method.

Chapter Thirty-three

Thief Sweating (*i.e.*, Night Sweating)

This is ascribed to yin vacuity and blood vacuity. Thief sweating in infants needs no (special) treatment. It is appropriate to administer *Liang Ge San* (Cool the Diaphragm Powder). For thief sweating with fever, which is ascribed to yin vacuity, prescribe *Si Wu Tang* (Four Materials Decoction) plus Cortex Phellodendri (*Huang Bai*). In case of qi vacuity, add Radix Panacis Ginseng (*Ren Shen*), Radix Astragali Membranacei (*Huang Qi*), and Rhizoma Atractylodis Macrocephalae (*Bai Zhu*).

Sweating nowhere except on the patch (of skin over) the cardiac region which gets worse the more thoughts and worries (there are) is a disease caused by straining the heart. It is called heart's juice. It requires nurturing heart blood by taking powdered Sclerotium Poriae

---

[2] This consists of Radix Ephedrae Chinensis (*Ma Huang Gen*), Radix Astragali Membranacei (*Huang Qi*), Radix Et Rhizoma Notopterygii (*Qiang Huo*), Radix Angelicae Sinensis (*Dang Gui*), Radix Glycyrrhizae (*Sheng Gan Cao*), Radix Scutellariae Baicalensis (*Huang Qin*), Rhizoma Pinelliae Ternatae (*Ban Xia*), Tuber Ophiopogonis Japonicae (*Mai Dong*), Radix Rehmanniae (*Sheng Di Huang*), Sclerotium Polypori Umbellati (*Zhu Ling*), Lignum Sappanis (*Su Mu*), Flos Carthami Tinctorii (*Hong Hua*), and Fructus Schizandrae Chinensis (*Wu Wei Zi*).

[3] This consists of Sclerotium Poriae Cocoris (*Fu Ling*), Radix Paeoniae Lactiflorae (*Shao Yao*), fresh Rhizoma Zingiberis (*Sheng Jiang*), Rhizoma Atractylodis Macrocephalae (*Bai Zhu*), and Radix Praeparatus Aconiti Carmichaeli (*Fu Zi*).

Cocoris (*Fu Ling*) brewed with Folium Artemisiae Argyii (*Ai Ye*) soup.

Dang Gui Liu Huang Tang (*Dang Gui* Six Yellows Decoction)[1] is a divine formula for thief sweating. Radix Astragali Membranacei (*Huang Qi*) should be twice as much as the rest of the ingredients, which are (otherwise) equal in amount. Powder these ingredients; 5 *qian* per dose. For children, the dosage should be reduced by half. Another formula (consists of) adding to the above formula Rhizoma Anemarrhenae (*Zhi Mu*), Radix Panacis Ginseng (*Ren Shen*), Rhizoma Atractylodis Macrocephalae (*Bai Zhu*), Radix Glycyrrhizae (*Gan Cao*), Cortex Radicis Lycii (*Di Gu*), Fructus Levis Tritici (*Fu Mai*), and Folium Mori Albi (*Sang Ye*). In case of incessant sweating, add Concha Ostreae (*Chi Gen Mu Li*). In case of fright sleeplessness, add Radix Polygalae Tenuifoliae (*Yuan Zhi*) and administer *Zhu Sha An Shen Wan* (Cinnabar Calm the Spirit Pills)[2] between (doses of the above, while) *Si Chao Bai Zhu San* (Four [Times] Stir-fried Atractylodes Powder)[3] is a formula which treats thief sweating with extreme efficacy. [Its composition can be found in the *Yi Yao* {*Essentials of Medicine*. later editor}]

A person who was worried and depressed suffered from thief sweating and not wide (*i.e.*, constricted) chest and diaphragm. (They were given) *Dang Gui Liu Huang Tang* plus Radix Ledebouriellae Sesloidis (*Fang Feng*), Pericarpium Viridis Citri Reticulatae (*Qing Pi*), Fructus Citri Seu Ponciri (*Zhi Qiao*), Rhizoma Cyperi Rotundi (*Xiang Fu*), and Fructus Amomi (*Sha Ren*).

---

[1] This consists of Radix Angelicae Sinensis (*Dang Gui*), Radix Rehmanniae (*Sheng Di Huang*), prepared Radix Rehmanniae (*Shu Di Huang*), Rhizoma Coptidis Chinensis (*Huang Lian*), Radix Scutellariae Baicalensis (*Huang Qin*), and Cortex Phellodendri (*Huang Bai*).

[2] This consists of Cinnabar (*Zhu Sha*), Radix Glycyrrhizae (*Gan Cao*), Rhizoma Coptidis Chinensis (*Huang Lian*), Radix Angelicae Sinensis (*Dang Gui*), and Radix Rehmanniae (*Sheng Di Huang*).

[3] There are quite a number of different formulas named *Bai Zhu San*. The one the author refers to may be composed of Concha Ostreae (*Mu Li*), Rhizoma Atractylodis Macrocephalae (*Bai Zhu*), and Radix Ledebouriellae Sesloidis (*Fang Feng*).

Chapter Thirty-four

Counterflow Swallowing (*i.e.*, Hiccough)

(This disease) is (further) classified into phlegm, qi vacuity, and yin fire (types). Counterflow swallowing is counterflow hiccough. It is (caused by) qi counterflow. It is so named because the qi surges straight up from below the umbilicus and, when it exits through the mouth, it makes a noise. It should be treated in accordance with superabundance and insufficiency. [Details can be found in the *Ge Zhi Yu Lun* {*Extra Treatises Based on Investigations & Inquiry*. later editor}] In case of superabundance and phlegm, apply ejection with stem-preserved Radix Panacis Ginseng (*Ren Shen Lu*) and the like. In case of insufficiency, take *Da Bu Wan* (Great Supplement Pills)[1] with *Ren Shen Bai Zhu Tang* (Ginseng & Atractylodes Decoction).[2] If phlegm impedes qi giving rise to counterflow swallowing, this is due to dry phlegm refusing to exit. Perform mechanical emesis with honey water. Generally speaking, the existence of phlegm requires Pericarpium Citri Reticulatae (*Chen Pi*) and Rhizoma Pinelliae Ternatae (*Ban Xia*, while) qi vacuity requires Radix Panacis Ginseng (*Ren Shen*) and Rhizoma Atractylodis Macrocephalae (*Bai Zhu*). Yin fire requires Rhizoma Coptidis Chinensis (*Huang Lian*), Talcum (*Hua Shi*), and Cortex Phellodendri (*Huang Bai*). In case of abundant phlegm, administer ejection or phlegm-moving. In case of extreme vacuity, use Radix Panacis Ginseng paste (*Shen Gao*) or the like. For internal damage with counterflow swallowing which will not stop, (use) *Bu Zhong Yi Qi Tang* (Supplement the Center & Boost the Qi Decoction) plus Flos Caryo-

---

[1] This consists of stir-fried Cortex Phellodendri (*Huang Bai*), Rhizoma Anemarrhenae (*Zhi Mu*), prepared Radix Rehmanniae (*Shu Di*), Plastrum Testudinis (*Gui Ban*), and the spinal marrow of a pig.

[2] This consists of Radix Panacis Ginseng (*Ren Shen*), Rhizoma Atractylodis Macrocephalae (*Bai Zhu*), Rhizoma Arisaematis (*Tian Nan Xing*), and Rhizoma Pinelliae Ternatae (*Ban Xia*).

phylli (*Ding Xiang*. But, for) vacuity cold counterflow swallowing, (use) *Ding Xiang Shi Di Tang* (Clove & Persimmon Calyx Decoction)[3] and moxa at *Qi Men* (Liv 13).[4]

In case of qi heat and phlegm heat, boil and take 72 pieces of Ramus Indocalami Tessellati (*Qing Ruo Tou*). In the blood pattern of cold damage with incessant counterflow swallowing and a rigid and shortened (*i.e.*, contracted) tongue, (use) *Tao Ren Cheng Qi Tang* (Peach Seed Support the Qi Decoction)[5] as the ruling (formula. However, for) incessant counterflow swallowing with abundant phlegm, boil and take Rhizoma Pinelliae Ternatae (*Ban Xia*), Sclerotium Poriae Cocoris (*Fu Ling*), Pericarpium Citri Reticulatae (*Chen Pi*), Semen Pruni Persicae (*Tao Ren*), Folium Eriobotryae Japonicae (*Pi Ba Ye*), and Succus Zingiberis (*Jiang Zhi*. And for) counterflow hiccough with loose bowels (use) Radix Panacis Ginseng (*Ren Shen*), Rhizoma Atractylodis Macrocephalae (*Bai Zhu*), Radix Paeoniae Lactiflorae (*Shao Yao*), Pericarpium Citri Reticulatae (*Chen Pi*), Radix Glycyrrhizae (*Gan Cao*), Talcum (*Hua Shi*), Cortex Phellodendri (*Huang Bai*), and Succus Bambusae (*Zhu Li*).

Heart pain with counterflow swallowing arising upon drinking boiled water is due to dead blood existing in the center. It should be precipitated by *Tao Ren Cheng Qi Tang*. (But for) counterflow hiccough with absence of pulse, (use) *Er Chen Tang* plus Radix Panacis Ginseng (*Ren Shen*), Rhizoma Atractylodis Macrocephalae (*Bai Zhu*), Tuber Ophiopogonis Japonicae (*Mai Dong*), Fructus Schizandrae Chinensis (*Wu Wei*), and Caulis Bambusae In Taeniis (*Zhu Ru*) which are taken after being boiled with Rhizoma Zingiberis (*Jiang*). In severe cases, add

---

[3]   This consists of Flos Caryophylli (*Ding Xiang*), Calyx Diospyroris Kaki (*Shi Di*), Radix Panacis Ginseng (*Ren Shen*), and fresh Rhizoma Zingiberis (*Sheng Jiang*).

[4]   Gate of Qi

[5]   This consists of Semen Pruni Persicae (*Tao Ren*), stir-fried Radix Et Rhizoma Rhei (*Da Huang*), Radix Glycyrrhizae (*Gan Cao*), Cortex Cinnamomi (*Rou Gui*), and a small amount of Rhizoma Zingiberis (*Jiang*).

Calyx Diospyroris Kaki (*Shi Di*) and Flos Caryophylli (*Ding Xiang*). In case of counterflow swallowing with absence of pulse in persons of vacuity, add Cortex Phellodendri (*Huang Bai*) and Rhizoma Anemarrhenae (*Zhi Mu*. Another method for) treating counterflow swallowing is to fume with and make (the patient) swallow the smoke of burning yellow wax. In cold cases, burn and swallow the smoke of Sulphur (*Liu Huang*).

A person, aged nearly 70, contracted counterflow swallowing following dysentery. A female contracted counterflow swallowing as a result of violent anger in a summer month. A person, aged nearly 50, contracted counterflow swallowing following dysentery as a result of anger. [These treatments can all be found all in the *Yi Yao* {*Essentials of Medicine*, later editor}.]

Chapter Thirty-five

Head Wind[1]

(This disease) is (further) classified into phlegm, heat, and blood vacuity (types). People of various schools limit their discussion to hemilateral head wind alone and are ignorant of its categorization. Therefore, their treatment is often not effective.

Left-sided (pain) is ascribed to wind. (In this case, use) Herba Seu Flos Schizonepetae Tenuifoliae (*Jing Jie*) and Herba Menthae (*Bo He*. It may also be) ascribed to blood vacuity, (in which case, use) Rhizoma Ligustici Wallichii (*Chuan Xiong*), Radix Angelicae Sinensis (*Dang Gui*), and Radix Paeoniae Lactiflorae (*Shao Yao*). Right-sided (pain) is

---

[1] This is a special kind of headache characterized by sudden, violent, and persistent attacks at irregular intervals.

ascribed to phlegm. (This requires the use of) Rhizoma Atractylodis (*Cang Zhu*) and Rhizoma Pinelliae Ternatae (*Ban Xia*. It may also) be ascribed to heat, (and, in that case, use) wine-fried Radix Scutellariae Baicalensis (*Huang Qin*. Further, it may also be) ascribed to damp phlegm, (thus requiring) Rhizoma Ligustici Wallichii (*Cuan Xiong*), Rhizoma Arisaematis (*Nan Xing*), and Rhizoma Atractylodis (*Cang Zhu*).

(Another method to treat) hemilateral and ambilateral head wind (is to) sniff into the nose *Gua Di San* (Melon Pedicle Powder). A sniffing (*i.e.*, inhalant) formula for thin persons (consists of) soft Gypsum (*Ruan Shi Gao*) and slaked lime (*Po Xiao*), 5 *qian* each, Borneolum (*Nao Zi*), Cortex Santali Albi (*Tan Xiang Pi*), Herba Seu Flos Schizonepetae Tenuifoliae (*Jing Jie*), and Herba Menthae (*Bo He*), 1 *qian* for each of the above, and Radix Angelicae (*Bai Zhi*) and Herba Cum Radicis Asari Sieboldi (*Xi Xin*), 2 *qian* each.

Yi Li Jin (One Nugget of Gold)[2] treats hemilateral and ambilateral head wind. Its wonder consists of (its use of) Fructus Seu Flos Piperis Longi (*Bi Ba*) and pig's gall. *Tian Xiang San* (Celestial Fragrance Powder) treats years long head wind. [Both formulas can be found in the *Yi Yao* {*Essentials of Medicine,* later editor}] Some sniffing formulas are comprised merely of Fructus Seu Flos Piperis Longi and pig's gall.

An(other) formula for head wind (uses) wine-processed Radix Scutellariae Baicalensis (*Pian Qin*), 1 *liang*, Rhizoma Atractylodis (*Cang Zhu*), Radix Ledebouriellae Sesloidis (*Fang Feng*), Radix Et Rhizoma Notopterygii (*Qiang Huo*), 5 *qian* for each of the above, Herba Xanthii Sibirici (*Cang Er*), 3 *qian*, and Herba Cum Radicis Asari Sieboldi (*Xi Xin*), 2 *qian*. Powder the above, smash 1 slice of Rhizoma Zingiberis (*Jiang*), and pound 3 *qian* of the above powders with this smashed Rhizoma Zingiberis evenly. (Then) brew with tea water, heat to a boil, and take. In a (variant) version, (it consists of) wine-processed Radix

---

[2] This consists of Fructus Seu Flos Piperis Longi (*Bi Ba*) soaked in pig's gall, 3 *qian*, and Rhizoma Ligustici Wallichii (*Chuan Xiong*), Radix Et Rhizoma Ligustici Sinensis (*Gao Ben*), Pulvis Indigonis (*Qing Dai*), Radix Angelicae (*Bai Zhi*), and Rhizoma Corydalis Yanhusuo (*Xuan Hu Suo*), 2 *qian* for each of the above.

Scutellariae Baicalensis (*Pian Qin*), 1.5 *liang*, Radix Et Rhizoma Notopterygii (*Qiang Huo*), Rhizoma Atractylodis (*Cang Zhu*), Rhizoma Ligustici Wallichii (*Chuan Xiong*), 5 *qian* for each of the above, Herba Xanthii Sibirici (*Cang Er*), Herba Cum Radicis Asari Sieboldi (*Xi Xin*), 3 *qian* each. The processing method is the same as above.

Another formula (consists of) wine-processed Radix Scutellariae Baicalensis (*Pian Qin*), Herba Xanthii Sibirici (*Cang Er*), Radix Et Rhizoma Notopterygii (*Qiang Huo*), wine-processed Rhizoma Coptidis Chinensis (*Huang Lian*), Radix Glycyrrhizae (*Sheng Gan Cao*), 1.5 *qian* for each of the above, Rhizoma Atractylodis (*Cang Zhu*), 2.5 *qian*, stir-fried Massa Medica Fermentata Cum Pinelliam (*Ban Xia Qu*), 3.5 *qian*, and Rhizoma Ligustici Wallichii (*Chuan Xiong*), 1 *qian*. The processing method is the same as above.

A formula for damp phlegm head wind (consists of) wine-processed Radix Scutellariae Baicalensis (*Pian Qin*), 3 *qian*, Rhizoma Atractylodis (*Cang Zhu*), 1 *liang*, wine-fried Rhizoma Ligustici Wallichii (*Chuan Xiong*), Herba Cum Radicis Asari Sieboldi (*Xi Xin*), 2 *qian* each, and a small amount of Radix Glycyrrhizae (*Gan Cao*). The above are powdered and processed as above. (Yet) another formula for head wind (consists of) Herba Seu Flos Schizonepetae Tenuifoliae (*Jing Jie*), Radix Ledebouriellae Sesloidis (*Fang Feng*), Apex Radicis Aconiti (*Cao Wu Jian*), Radix Glycyrrhizae (*Gan Cao*), Rhizoma Ligustici Wallichii (*Tai Xiong*), Fructus Viticis (*Man Jing Zi*), Radix Platycodi Grandiflori (*Jie Geng*), and Herba Ephedrae (*Ma Huang*). Powder, brew with tea, and take. (And for) head itching wind with (abundant) dandruff and yellowing hair, take wine-fried, powdered Radix Et Rhizoma Rhei (*Da Huang*) brewed with tea.

A person suffered from head wind with nasal congestion and snivelling. (They were given) Rhizoma Arisaematis (*Nan Xing*), Rhizoma Atractylodis (*Cang Zhu*), wine-processed Radix Scutellariae Baicalensis (*Huang Qin*), Flos Magnoliae Liliflorae (*Xin Yi*), and Rhizoma Ligustici Wallichii (*Chuan Xiong*).

An(other) person who used to take fat meat and fine grains suffered from head wind attacks immediately giving rise to spinning head and heavy(-headedness) with ache. (They were given) *Er Chen Tang* plus Herba Seu Flos Schizonepetae Tenuifoliae (*Jing Jie*), Rhizoma Arisaematis (*Nan Xing*), wine-processed Radix Scutellariae Baicalensis (*Huang Qin*), Radix Ledebouriellae Sesloidis (*Fang Feng*), Rhizoma Atractylodis (*Cang Zhu*), Rhizoma Ligustici Wallichii (*Tai Xiong*), and Rhizoma Zingiberis (*Jiang*). These were taken after being boiled. Afterwards, (they were prescribed) wine-processed Radix Scutellariae Baicalensis (*Huang Qin*), Rhizoma Arisaematis (*Nan Xing*), Rhizoma Pinelliae Ternatae (*Ban Xia*), 1 *liang* for each of the above, carbonized Fructus Gleditschiae Sinensis (*Zao Jiao Hui*), 1 *qian*, and Fructus Pruni Mume (*Wu Mei*), 20 pieces. Fructus Pruni Mume was boiled together with 10 pieces of Semen Crotonis (*Ba Dou*) which were removed afterwards. (The Fructus Pruni Mume) was mixed with the above powdered ingredients, made into pills with ginger-processed Massa Medica Fermentata (*Jiang Qu*), and melted in the mouth.

Chapter Thirty-six

Headache

This is usually ruled by phlegm. (However,) severe ache (is due to) abundant fire. Some cases indicate ejection; some contraindicate it. Some indicate precipitation. In case of phlegm heat, it is necessary to clear phlegm and downbear fire. (But) wind cold external evils should be treated by resolving and dissipating (these through the exterior). Blood vacuity headache that attacks upwards from the fish tails[1] to the eyes and head necessitates the use of *Xiong Gui Tang* (Ligusticum

---

[1] This refers to the wrinkles at the corners of the eyes.

& *Dang Gui* Decoction).[2] (While) qi vacuity headache, phlegm inversion headache[3], or dizziness with a weak pulse and low food intake embraced by internal damage disease (require the use of) *Ban Xia Bai Zhu Tian Ma Tang* (Pinellia, Atractylodes & Gastrodia Decoction).[4] (And) a spinning head, dark eyes, and headache due to yin vacuity embracing fire (requires the use of) *An Shen Tang* (Calm the Spirit Decoction).[5]

For a splitting headache, (use) wine-processed Radix Et Rhizoma Rhei (*Da Huang*), one half *liang*, which is powdered and taken brewed with tea. Headache involving the eyes is (due to) wind heat attacking upwards, (thus) requiring Radix Angelicae (*Bai Zhi*) to open (depressed wind heat). A formula for this consists of Before the Rains tea[6], Rhizoma Ligustici Wallichii (*Chuan Xiong*), Radix Angelicae Sinensis (*Dang Gui*), Radix Ledebouriellae Sesloidis (*Fang Feng*), Radix Angelicae

---

[2]   This consists of Rhizoma Ligustici Wallichii (*Chuan Xiong*), Radix Angelicae Sinensis (*Dang Gui*), Radix Rubrus Paeoniae Lactiflorae (*Chi Shao Yao*), Radix Ledebouriellae Sesloidis (*Fang Feng*), and Radix Et Rhizoma Notopterygii (*Qiang Huo*).

[3]   *I.e.*, splitting headache due to turbid phlegm counterflowing upward with dizziness, generalized heaviness, restlessness, confused speech, oppression in the chest, nausea, vexation, foaming at the mouth, and frigidity of the limbs

[4]   This consists of Cortex Phellodendri (*Huang Bai*), Rhizoma Zingiberis (*Jiang*), Rhizoma Gastrodiae Elatae (*Tian Ma*), Rhizoma Atractylodis (*Cang Zhu*), Sclerotium Poriae Cocoris (*Fu Ling*), Radix Astragali Membranacei (*Huang Qi*), Rhizoma Alismatis (*Ze Xie*), Radix Panacis Ginseng (*Ren Shen*), Rhizoma Atractylodis Macrocephalae (*Bai Zhu*), Massa Medica Fermentata (*Shen Qu*), Rhizoma Pinelliae Ternatae (*Ban Xia*), Fructus Germinatus Hordei Vulgaris (*Mai Ya*), and Pericarpium Citri Reticulatae (*Ju Pi*).

[5]   This consists of Tuber Ophiopogonis Japonicae (*Mai Men Dong*), Radix Panacis Ginseng (*Ren Shen*), Radix Angelicae Sinensis (*Dang Gui*), Rhizoma Coptidis Chinensis (*Huang Lian*), Semen Zizyphi Spinosae (*Suan Zao Ren*), Radix Rehmanniae (*Di Huang*), and Sclerotium Pararadicis Poriae Cocoris (*Fu Shen*).

[6]   This is a special kind of tea picked before the Grain Rains, one of the 24 nodes of qi which occurs in mid-April.

(*Bai Zhi*), Radix Aconiti (*Tai Wu*), and Herba Cum Radicis Asari Sieboldi (*Xi Xin*. However,) in strong persons with severe heat (head)ache and dry, bound stools, (use) *Da Cheng Qi Tang* (Major Support the Qi Decoction). Bulbus Allii Fistulosi (*Cong Bai*, also) treats splitting headache and frees the flow of yang qi above and below. (But) a pain radiating up to the top of the head and extending down to the Clay Pellet Palace[7] is a true headache. There is no remedy available for this.

Qing Kong Gao (Clear the Sky Paste)[8] treats all categories of headache except blood vacuity headache. [The formula can be found in the *Yi Yao*, {*Essentials of Medicine*, later editor}] *Xiao Qing Kong Gao* (Minor Clear the Sky Paste) treats *shao yang* headache and also hemilateral headache or (head)ache in the *tai yang* channel. (It consists of) Radix Scutellariae Baicalensis (*Pian Qin*). Soak thoroughly in wine, dry in the sun, powder, and take with wine or tea water.

A person suffered from headache with wind phlegm and hot phlegm. (They were given) wine-processed Radix Scutellariae Baicalensis (*Huang Qin*), Fructus Forsythiae Suspensae (*Lian Qiao*), Rhizoma Arisaematis (*Nan Xing*), Rhizoma Ligustici Wallichii (*Chuan Xiong*), Herba Seu Flos Schizonepetae Tenuifoliae (*Jing Jie*), Radix Ledebouriellae Sesloidis (*Fang Feng*), and Radix Glycyrrhizae (*Gan Cao*). The reason why Rhizoma Ligustici Wallichii is used together with Radix Scutellariae Baicalensis is that the latter can effect downbearing once the former accomplishes upbearing. Without Rhizoma Ligustici Wallichii, headache cannot be solved. Herba Seu Flos Schizonepetae Tenuifoliae is a cool, clearing agent. For headache, use Rhizoma Ligustici Wallichii from Sichuan. For ache in the brains, use Rhizoma Ligustici Wallichii from the Tian Tai Mountains (in Zhejiang).

---

[7] This is a supposed special place within the brain three *cun* inward from the center of the forehead.

[8] This consists of Rhizoma Ligustici Wallichii (*Chuan Xiong*), Radix Bupleuri (*Chai Hu*), Rhizoma Coptidis Chinensis (*Huang Lian*), Radix Ledebouriellae Sesloidis (*Fang Feng*), Radix Glycyrrhizae (*Gan Cao*), Radix Et Rhizoma Notopterygii (*Qiang Huo*), Radix Scutellariae Baicalensis (*Huang Qin*), and Fructus Gardeniae Jasminoidis (*Zhi Zi*).

A person, replete yet thin in form, suffered from headache with phlegm. (They were given) Radix Scutellariae Baicalensis (*Huang Qin*), Rhizoma Coptidis Chinensis (*Huang Lian*), Fructus Gardeniae Jasminoidis (*Shan Zhi*), Bulbus Fritillariae (*Bei Mu*), Fructus Trichosanthis Kirlowii (*Gua Lou*), Rhizoma Arisaematis (*Nan Xing*), and Rhizoma Cyperi Rotundi (*Xiang Fu*).

An(other) person who had small, prominent sinews (*i.e.*, veins), was a little lanky, and who taxed himself despite a vacuous root suffered from severe headache with a bowstring, rapid pulse. He was treated with Radix Panacis Ginseng (*Ren Shen*) as the sovereign and Rhizoma Ligustici Wallichii (*Chuan Xiong*) and Pericarpium Citri Reticulatae (*Chen Pi*) as the assistants. In 6 days, no improvement was shown. (However,) recovery was expected in another 2 days. Abruptly he declared that his disease had abated. On examination, his pulse seemed a little replenished. Half a day passed and an obstruction at the diaphragm made his abdomen full. I enquired in a roundabout way and knew that his brother had added Radix Astragali Membranacei (*Huang Qi*) to 3 doses of my formula. Then (I) prescribed *Er Chen Tang* (Two Aged Decoction) plus Cortex Magnoliae Officinalis (*Hou Po*), Fructus Citri Seu Ponciri (*Zhi Qiao*), and Rhizoma Coptidis Chinensis (*Huang Lian*) to drain the defensive. Three doses affected recovery.

Chapter Thirty-seven

Spinning Head[1]

This is due to) phlegm embraced by qi vacuity and fire. (In this case,) the treatment of phlegm is the ruling (method. However,) one should also employ medicinals to supplement the qi and downbear fire at the

---

[1]   This refers to feeling faint and dizzy in the head.

same time. In most cases, this pattern is ascribed to phlegm. Without phlegm, spinning (head) can never arise. Furthermore, there are (cases of) damp phlegm and (of) abundant fire. A rapid pulse on the left hand (indicates) abundant heat, (while) a choppy pulse (on the left hand indicates) the existence of dead blood. A replete pulse on the right (indicates) phlegm accumulation, (but) a large pulse (on the right) is invariably a fire disease. In a (variant) version (it is said that) enduring disease should be read for fire disease because, when a person suffers from an enduring disease, both qi and blood are vacuous and phlegm is turbid, unable to descend. For damp phlegm, (use) *Er Chen Tang* (Two Aged Decoction). For abundant fire, (use) *Er Chen Tang* plus wine-processed Radix Scutellariae Baicalensis (*Pian Qin*). When qi vacuity and ministerial fire are embraced, the ruling (method) remains the treatment of phlegm in combination with supplementing the qi and downbearing fire with formulae such as *Ban Xia Bai Zhu Tian Ma Tang* (Pinellia, Atractylodes & Gastrodia Decoction).

An old woman who had suffered from red and white vaginal discharge for 1½ years was always feeling a spinning head. She was unable to stand or sit for long but was quiet while sleeping. The treatment focused solely on her vaginal discharge. Once the vaginal discharge disease was cured, the spinning head was overcome as well.

Chapter Thirty-eight

Dizziness

If there is phlegm above and fire below, fire may flame up and stir this phlegm, (thus causing dizziness). In case of qi vacuity embracing phlegm, (use) *Si Jun* (Four Gentlemen [Decoction]) and *Er Chen* (Two Aged [Decoction] with) Radix Astragali Membranacei (*Huang Qi*), Rhizoma Ligustici Wallichii (*Chuan Xiong*), and Herba Seu Flos

Schizonepetae Tenuifoliae (*Jing Jie*). Wind phlegm dizziness (on the other hand) is treated with *Er Chen Tang* plus Radix Scutellariae Baicalensis (*Huang Qin*), Rhizoma Atractylodis (*Cang Zhu*), Radix Ledebouriellae Sesloidis (*Fang Feng*), and Radix Et Rhizoma Notopterygii (*Qiang Huo*). In case of unbearable dizziness, soak Radix Et Rhizoma Rhei (*Da Huang*) in wine, stir-fry 3 times, powder, and take brewed with tea. People with qi repletion and having phlegm with either heavy-headedness or dizziness can be treated with this too. For strong and sturdy people with severe heat pain (in the head) and dry, bound stools, (use) *Da Cheng Qi Tang* (Major Support the Qi Decoction).

Chapter Thirty-nine

Heavy-headedness

This is (due to) damp qi existing above. Sniff into the nose *Gua Di San* (Melon Pedicle Powder). *Hong Dou San* (Ormosia Powder) treats mountainlike heavy-headedness. This is (due to) damp qi in the head. (It consists of) Herba Ephedrae (*Ma Huang*), 5 *qian*, Pediculus Melonis (*Ku Ding Xiang* [*Gua Di* may also be called *Ku Ding Xiang*. {trans.}]), 5 *fen*, Radix Et Rhizoma Notopterygii (*Qiang Huo*), 3 *fen*, Fructus Forsythiae Suspensae (*Lian Qiao*), 3 *fen*, and Semen Abri Precatorii (*Hong Dou*), 15 pieces. Powder and sniff into the nose.

Chapter Forty

Swollen Head & Face

For swelling and enlargement of the head and face with heat and a bowstring, rapid pulse, (use) *Liang Ge San* (Cool the Diaphragm

Powder) minus slaked lime (*Xiao*) and Radix Et Rhizoma Rhei (*Da Huang*) but with Radix Platycodi Grandiflori (*Jie Geng*), Fructus Citri Seu Ponciri (*Zhi Qiao*), Herba Seu Flos Schizonepetae Tenuifoliae (*Jing Jie*), and Herba Menthae (*Bo He*) added. For red swelling of the face due to qi repletion use *Wei Feng Tang* (Stomach Wind Decoction).[1] For a swollen face with sores, (use) *Tiao Wei Cheng Qi Tang* (Regulate the Stomach & Support the Qi Decoction) plus Herba Menthae (*Bo He*) and Herba Seu Flos Schizonepetae Tenuifoliae (*Jing Jie*).

Chapter Forty-one

Pain in the Supraorbital Bone

This is ascribed to wind heat and phlegm. It should be treated as wind phlegm, a quasi-pattern of painful wind[1], with Radix Angelicae (*Bai Zhi*) and wine-processed Radix Scutellariae Baicalensis (*Pian Qin*) in equal amounts. Powder; 2 qian per dose taken brewed with tea water. Another formula (consists of) domesticated Radix Aconiti (*Chuan Wu*) and wild Radix Aconiti (*Cao Wu*), 1 *qian* each, as the sovereigns, both soaked with child's urine and stir-fried to rid of toxins, Herba Cum Radicis Asari Sieboldi (*Xi Xin*), Radix Et Rhizoma Notopterygii (*Qiang Huo*), wine-processed Radix Scutellariae Baicalensis (*Huang Qin*), and Radix Glycyrrhizae (*Gan Cao*), one half *fen* for each of the above, as the assistants. Powder finely, divide into 2-3 doses, and take with tea water. In a (variant) version, Rhizoma Arisaematis (*Nan Xing*) is added and (the formula) is to be taken with ginger and tea. (Yet) another

---

[1] This consists of Rhizoma Atractylodis Macrocephalae (*Bai Zhu*), Rhizoma Ligustici Wallichii (*Chuan Xiong*), Radix Panacis Ginseng (*Ren Shen*), Radix Albus Paeoniae Lactiflorae (*Bai Shao Yao*), Radix Angelicae Sinensis (*Dang Gui*), Cortex Cinnamomi (*Rou Gui*), and Sclerotium Poriae Cocoris (*Fu Ling*).

[1] This is also known as articular wind and is characterized by reddening, swelling, and inhibited mobility of the affected parts, usually the joints.

formula, *Xuan Qi Tang* (Choose the Strange Decoction, consists of) Radix Ledebouriellae Sesloidis (*Fang Feng*), Radix Et Rhizoma Notopterygii (*Qiang Huo*), wine-processed Radix Scutellariae Baicalensis (*Huang Qin*), and Radix Glycyrrhizae (*Gan Cao*). Boil and take.

Chapter Forty-two

Heart Pain

This is pain in the venter. The treatment varies with the old and the new. If it is known to be a case of cold, it is necessary to apply warm dissipation during the initial stage. (However, if) the disease lasts long, (cold) may become depressed, and depression generates heat so as to produce fire. Therefore, Fructus Gardeniae Jasminoidis (*Shan Zhi*) should be used at that point as the sovereign and certain warm medicinals as guides. If heat exists at the opening of the stomach thus giving pain, Fructus Gardeniae Jasminoidis is indispensable and it should be used together with Succus Zingiberis (*Jiang Zhi*) as its assistant and large quantities of Rhizoma Ligustici Wallichii (*Tai Xiong*) to open (depressed heat). Or (it can be treated) with *Er Chen Tang* (Two Aged Decoction) plus Rhizoma Ligustici Wallichii (*Chuan Xiong*) and Rhizoma Atractylodis (*Cang Zhu*), and stir-fried Fructus Gardeniae Jasminoidis (*Shan Zhi*) in double the amount. In case of severe pain, add stir-fried dry Rhizoma Zingiberis (*Gan Jiang*). This is following the contrary treatment method.[1]

---

[1] Contrary treatment (*fan zhi*) implies treating like by like or, in other words, hot by hot medicinals and cold by cold medicinals. It is contrary because correct treatment (*zheng zhi*) in TCM is predicated on restoring balance through the introduction of the equal opposite. Therefore, in correct treatment, cold medicinals are used to clear heat and hot medicinals are used to warm cold. In this case, hot medicinals are used to treat a hot condition. Thus, according to the logic of TCM, this is a contrary treatment.

If habitual liking for hot food results in retention of dead blood at the opening of the stomach thus giving pain, prescribe *Tao Ren Cheng Qi Tang* (Persica Support the Qi Decoction) to precipitate (the retained blood). If it is a mild case, (one) should use Succus Allii Tuberosi (*Jiu Zhi*) and Radix Platycodi Grandiflori (*Jie Geng*) in combination with qi and blood opening and upraising medicinals. (However,) pain relieved by pressing the painful place with something is embraced vacuity. (For this) use *Er Chen Tang* plus stir-fried dry Rhizoma Zingiberis (*Gan Jiang*) for harmonization.

Pain due to worms is (manifest by) white spots on the face, red lips, and ability to eat. (For this) prescribe (medicinals) such as Cortex Radicis Meliae (*Ku Lian Gen*) and carbonate of lead (*Hei Xi Hui*, i.e., *Qian Hui*, the black substance left on an iron pot when lead is heated). This pain is followed by ability to eat and is intermittent. In the first half of the month, worms have their heads upward, and are (therefore) easy to treat. In the second half, they have their heads downward and are (thus) difficult to treat. First eat some meat broth or honey to coax the worms into moving up. Then administer the medicinals. An(other) worm-killing formula (consists of) Cortex Radicis Meliae (*Lian Gen*), Semen Arecae Catechu (*Bing Lang*), and Fructus Carpesii Abrotanoidis (*He Shi*). In summer, procure and take the juice from these. In winter, it is best to boil them into a thick decoction and take with *Wang Ling Wan* (Panacea Pills).[2]

(If there is) a replete pulse and constipation or if the pain becomes more severe after precipitation, the pulse must be deep. The appropriate medicinals (in this case) are warm ones such as Radix Praeparatus Aconiti Carmichaeli (*Fu Zi*). Do not use Radix Panacis Ginseng (*Ren Shen*) or Rhizoma Atractylodis Macrocephalae (*Bai Zhu*) since various types of pain contraindicate (the use of) supplementing the qi. (However,) for qi vacuity entering the venter thus giving pain (use)

---

[2] This consists of Semen Arecae Catechu (*Bing Lang*), Radix Et Rhizoma Rhei (*Da Huang*), Semen Pharbitidis (*Hei Qian Niu*), Fructus Gleditschiae Sinensis (*Zao Jiao*), Cortex Radicis Meliae (*Ku Lian Gen Pi*), Lignum Aquilariae Agallochae (*Chen Xiang*), Radix Saussureae Seu Vladimiriae (*Mu Xiang*), and Fructificatio Polypori Mylittae (*Lei Wan*).

Cao Dou Kou Wan (Alpinia Katsumadai Pills). For *shan*[3] pain in the cardiac region, stomach, abdomen, and hypochondrium, *Er Chen Tang* plus Radix Panacis Ginseng (*Ren Shen*) and Rhizoma Atractylodis Macrocephalae (*Bai Zhu*) as well as various aromatic medicinals offer an effective treatment.

For cardiac and hypochondriac pain, (use) slightly stir-fried dry Rhizoma Zingiberis (*Gan Jiang*) and vinegar-fried Flos Daphnis Genkwae (*Yuan Hua*) in equal amounts. Make into pills with honey; several pills per dose. For heat rheum pain, (use) Rhizoma Coptidis Chinensis (*Huang Lian*) and Radix Euphorbiae Kansui (*Gan Sui*) taken in the shape of pills. For retained rheum heart/stomach pain or cold (heart/stomach) pain in winter, (use) *Gui Huang Wan* (Cinnamom & Rhubarb Pills).[4] (To treat) extremely severe heart pain, an ancient formula in which Succus Radicis Rehmanniae (*Sheng Di Huang Zhi*) is mixed with flour, proves, when boiled and taken, very effective in killing and precipitating worms. Stomach vacuity and contraction of cold with severe cardiac and abdominal pain in those of qi weakness (should be treated with) *Li Zhong Tang* (Rectify the Center Decoction. While) stomach vacuity ache with internal damage due to fever and inability to take in food (requires) *Bu Zhong Yi Qi Tang* (Supplement the Center & Boost the Qi Decoction) plus Semen Alpiniae Katsumadai (*Cao Dou Kou*).

For heart qi pain, (use) *Tian Xiang San* (Celestial Fragrance Powder). Its formula (is composed of) Radix Angelicae (*Bai Zhi*), Radix Aconiti (*Chuan Wu*), Rhizoma Arisaematis (*Nan Xing*), and Rhizoma Pinelliae Ternatae (*Ban Xia*. However), for old people with great cardiac and abdominal pain, a surging, large, but vacuous pulse, clouding inversion, and inability to eat who cannot stand a single attacking medicinal, (use) *Si Jun Zi Tang* (Four Gentlemen Decoction) plus Radix

---

[3]   This term includes all kinds of hernias as categorized by modern Western medicine as well as dragging pain in the lower abdomen.

[4]   This consists of Ramulus Cinnamomi (*Gui Zhi*), Radix Albus Paeoniae Lactiflorae (*Bai Shao*), Radix Glycyrrhizae (*Gan Cao*), and Radix Et Rhizoma Rhei (*Da Huang*).

Angelicae Sinensis (*Dang Gui*), Herba Ephedrae (*Ma Huang*), and Lignum Aquilariae Agallochae (*Chen Xiang*). Great cardiac and diaphragmatic pain travelling and attacking the upper and lower backs and inducing inversion with inability to receive any food and medicinals (should be treated) by mechanical emesis together with administration of emetics. When about a bowlful of accumulated phlegm is discharged, the pain will stop by itself. For fat persons with venter pain right opposite to the heart or glomus qi in the middle venter which refuses to dissipate, (use) *Cao Dou Kou Wan* (Alpinia Katsumadai Pills): Fructus Cardamomi (*Bai Dou Kou*), 3 *qian*, Rhizoma Atractylodis Macrocephalae (*Bai Zhu*), Rhizoma Sparganii (*San Leng*), Semen Alpiniae Katsumadai (*Cao Dou Kou*), Rhizoma Pinelliae Ternatae (*Ban Xia*), 1 *liang* for each of the above, Fructus Amomi (*Sha Ren*), Rhizoma Curcumae (*Pian Jiang Huang*), Fructus Immaturus Citri Seu Ponciri (*Zhi Shi*), Pericarpium Viridis Citri Reticulatae (*Qing Pi*), Rhizoma Alpiniae Officinari (*Liang Jiang*) [A {variant} version gives Rhizoma Zingiberis {*Jiang*} instead. {later editor}], Pericarpium Citri Reticulatae (*Chen Pi*), Cortex Cinnamomi (*Gui Pi*), Flos Caryophylli (*Ding Xiang*), Rhizoma Curcumae Zedoariae (*Peng Zhu*), Radix Saussureae Seu Vladimiriae (*Mu Xiang*), Herba Agastachis Seu Pogostemi (*Huo Xiang*), and Herba Polygalae Tenuifoliae (*Xiao Cao*), 5 *qian* for each of the above. Make into pills with steamed ginger cake; 60-70 pills per dose taken with boiled water.

Hei Wan Zhi (Black Pills) treat venter pain. (They consist of) pitted Fructus Pruni Mume (*Wu Mei*), Fructus Pruni Armeniacae (*Xing Ren*), skinned and tip-nipped, Semen Crotonis (*Ba Dou*), stripped of skin, membrane, core, and oil, Fructus Amomi (*Sha Ren*), 14 pieces for each of the above, Pulvis Fumi Carbonisati (*Bai Cao Shuang*), 2 *qian*, and Rhizoma Pinelliae Ternatae (*Ban Xia*), 21 pieces. Pound the above and make into pills; about a dozen of pills per dose.

Bei Ji Wan (Emergency Pills) treat cardiac and abdominal inversion pain with food stuffing the chest and diaphragm. (They consist of) Radix Et Rhizoma Rhei (*Da Huang*), 1 *qian*, de-oiled Semen Crotonis (*Ba Dou*), 5 *fen*, and dry Rhizoma Zingiberis (*Gan Jiang*), 5 *fen*. Make the above into pills with honey; 3-5 pills per dose.

Heart pain arising soon after medicinals are swallowed down the throat and retching arising after soup or water is drunk (is due to) dead blood existing in the center. This should be precipitated with *Tao Ren Cheng Qi Tang* (Persica Support the Qi Decoction). A rapid pulse on the left hand (indicates) abundant heat, (but) a choppy pulse (indicates) dead blood. A replete pulse on the left hand (indicates) phlegm accumulation, (but) a large pulse invariably (indicates) an enduring disease.

A formula for cardiac pain (consists of) Fructus Evodiae Rutecarpae (*Zhu Yu*), washed with boiled water, stir-fried and husked Fructus Gardeniae Jasminoidis (*Shan Zhi*), stir-fried Rhizoma Coptidis Chinensis (*Huang Lian*), and Talcum (*Hua Shi*), 5 *qian* for each of the above, and Semen Litchii Chinensis (*Li He*), burnt (but with its) nature preserved, 3 *qian*. Powder the above, make into pills with steamed cake of Succus Zingiberis (*Jiang Zhi*), and take. Another formula (consists of) stir-fried Fructus Gardeniae Jasminoidis (*Shan Zhi Ren*). Powder and take with ginger soup or in the shape of pills. In case of cold pain, add Semen Alpiniae Katsumadai (*Cao Dou Kou*). Stir-fry (all the ingredients), powder, make into pills, and take. (Yet) another formula (is composed of) Rhizoma Atractylodis Macrocephalae (*Bai Zhu*), 5 *qian*, Radix Albus Paeoniae Lactiflorae (*Bai Shao Yao*), Fructus Amomi (*Sha Ren*), Rhizoma Pinelliae Ternatae (*Ban Xia*), soaked in boiled water, Radix Angelicae Sinensis (*Dang Gui*), 3 *qian* for each of the above, Semen Pruni Persicae (*Tao Ren*), Rhizoma Coptidis Chinensis (*Huang Lian*), stripped of hair, stir-fried Massa Medica Fermentata (*Shen Qu*), Pericarpium Citri Reticulatae (*Chen Pi*), 2 *qian* for each of the above, Fructus Evodiae Rutecarpae (*Wu Zhu Yu*), 1.5 *qian*, stir-fried Bombyx Batryticatus (*Jiang Can*), Fructus Corni Officinalis (*Zhu Yu*), 1 *qian* (each), and Fructus Gardeniae Jasminoidis (*Shan Zhi*), husked and char-fried, 6 *qian*. Powder the above and make into pills the size of Fructus Zanthoxyli Bungeani (*Chuan Jiao*) with cake. Boil wine-washed Radix Rehmanniae (*Sheng Di*) together with Rhizoma Zingiberis (*Jiang*) and take 20 pills with this decoction. In addition, powder one half *liang* of Flos Piperis Longi (*Bi Ba*), mix with vinegar, roll into pellets, and swallow.

Another formula (consists of) Ramulus Cinnamomi (*Gui Zhi*), Herba Ephedrae (*Ma Huang*), and Alkaloid (*Shi Jian*), in equal amounts. Powder, soak with Succus Zingiberis (*Jiang Zhi*), and make into pills with cake. Take 15 pills with hot, pungent, ginger soup. This is usually used to treat cake pain.[5] (Again) another formula (is composed of) Fructus Viticis Negundi (*Huang Jing Zi*). Char-fry, powder, and take with thin gruel. (Still) another formula (is made from) Concha Mactrae Quadrangularis (*He Fen*) and powdered Rhizoma Cyperi Rotundi (*Xiang Fu*). Boil these with Rhizoma Ligustici Wallichii (*Chuan Xiong*) and Fructus Gardeniae Jasminoidis (*Shan Zhi*), put in and mix with Succus Zingiberis (*Jiang Zhi*), and take while hot and pungent. (And finally,) another formula (consists of) sliced Rhizoma Pinelliae Ternatae (*Ban Xia*), stir-fried with sesame oil. Powder, make into pills with cake of Succus Zingiberis (*Jiang Zhi*), and take 20 pills with ginger soup. This also treats roaring asthma. To treat qi pain, (which is) a pain in all the cavities of the body, a small amount of Radix Saussureae Seu Vladimiriae (*Mu Xiang*) is always introduced in formulas. Only thus can (the cavities) be opened and freed.

Cao Dou Kou Wan is appropriate for intruding cold inflicting stomach-ache and is also able to appease heat. One can take 1-2 doses. (They consist of) Semen Alpiniae Katsumadai (*Cao Dou Kou*), roasted wrapped in dough, 1.4 *qian*, Fructus Evodiae Rutecarpae (*Wu Zhu Yu*), washed and baked, Fructus Alpiniae Oxyphyllae (*Yi Zhi Ren*), Radix Panacis Ginseng (*Ren Shen*), Radix Astragali Membranacei (*Huang Qi*), Bombyx Batryticatus (*Bai Jiang Can*), and Pericarpium Citri Reticulatae (*Ju Pi*), 8 *fen* for each of the above, Radix Glycyrrhizae (*Sheng Gan Cao*), mix-fried Radix Glycyrrhizae (*Zhi Gan Cao*), Radix Angelicae Sinensis (*Dang Gui Shen*), and Pericarpium Viridis Citri Reticulatae (*Qing Pi*), 6 *fen* for each of the above, Rhizoma Curcumae (*Pian Jiang Huang*), stir-fried Massa Medica Fermentata (*Shen Qu*), and Radix Bupleuri (*Chai Hu*), 4 *fen* for each of the above, Rhizoma Pinelliae Ternatae (*Ban Xia*) soaked in boiled water, and Rhizoma Alismatis (*Ze Xie*), 1 *qian* each, stir-fried Fructus Germinatus Hordei Vulgaris (*Mai Ya*), 1.5 *qian*, and Semen Pruni Persicae (*Tao Ren*), 7 pieces, soaked in boiled water, skinned, and tip-nipped. Except for Semen Pruni Persicae which should be ground separately into a paste, powder all the above finely,

---

[5]   The translator has been unable to identify what cake pain is. It may refer to pain in the cardiac and abdominal regions.

mix together well, and with steamed cake soaked in boiled water make into pills the size of Chinese parasol tree seeds; 50-70 per dose taken between meals with boiled water. (This prescription) should vary in accordance with the condition of the disease. In case of copious urine, reduce Rhizoma Alismatis by half. The amount of Radix Bupleuri depends on flank pain. *Cao Dou Kou Wan* offers a remarkable treatment for heart pain in persons of dwindled and weakened qi.

Pulvis Indigonis (*Qing Dai*) treats heat heart pain and worm pain. Take it with Succus Zingiberis (*Jiang Zhi*) brewed in boiled water, or extract the juice from Folium Isatidis Daqingye (*Lan Ye*) and take it with Succus Zingiberis (*Jiang Zhi*). In case this medicinal is not available, put some water in a small jar, place some salt on the edge of a knife, heat the knife (till) hot-red, and quench it in the water. (Then) make the patient drink (this water) while hot. Heart pain can also be treated with Fructus Gardeniae Jasminoidis (*Shan Zhi*) together with (some) thwarting medicinals. In case of relapse after relief, this formula is surely ineffective. (Then) take Sodium Sulfate (*Xuan Ming Fen*). One dose offers instant relief. (In addition,) Ovum Notarchi Leachi Freeri (*Hai Fen*) plus powdered Rhizoma Cyperi Rotundi (*Xiang Fu*) taken with Succus Zingiberis (*Jiang Zhi*) are able to treat heart pain, but they should not be taken in the shape of decoction.

For internal damage with fever, inability to eat, and pain in the stomach opening[6], (use) *Bu Zhong Yi Qi* (Supplement the Center & Boost the Qi [Decoction]) plus Semen Alpiniae Katsumadai (*Cao Dou Kou*). In case of heat pain, add Fructus Gardeniae Jasminoidis (*Zhi Zi*). For heart pain with qi repletion, one can (also) use one single ingredient, Concha Ostreae (*Mu Li*). Powder this by calcination and take 2 *qian* brewed with wine. (However,) pain due to the stomach opening damaged by food requires dispersion and abduction (of food). For pain caused by stagnated blood retained in the stomach opening, prescribe blood-breaking medicinals. For heart pain possibly with phlegm, dissolve Alumen (*Ming Fan*) and prepare it with (*Bu Zhong Yi*

---

[6] Chinese often use the stomach opening to refer to the cardiac region or the venter rather than the actual opening of the stomach.

Qi Tang) in the form of pills the size of Fructus Euryalis Ferocis (*Qian Shi*), Swallow one pill with heated Succus Zingiberis (*Jiang Zhi*).

A person whose pulse was choppy suffered from constant heart and spleen pain. (They were given) Rhizoma Atractylodis Macrocephalae (*Bai Zhu*), Rhizoma Pinelliae Ternatae (*Ban Xia*), Rhizoma Atractylodis (*Cang Zhu*), Fructus Immaturus Citri Seu Ponciri (*Zhi Shi*), Massa Medica Fermentata (*Shen Qu*), Rhizoma Cyperi Rotundi (*Xiang Fu*), Sclerotium Poriae Cocoris (*Fu Ling*), and Rhizoma Ligustici Wallichii (*Tai Xiong*). Powder the above, make into pills with Massa Medica Fermentata (*Shen Qu*) paste, and take.

An(other) person suffered from heart pain and *shan* pain. (They were given) stir-fried Fructus Gardeniae Jasminoidis (*Shan Zhi*), and Rhizoma Cyperi Rotundi (*Xiang Fu*), 1 *liang* each, Rhizoma Atractylodis (*Cang Zhu*), Massa Medica Fermentata (*Shen Qu*), and Fructus Germinatus Hordei Vulgaris (*Mai Ya*), 5 *qian* for each of the above, Rhizoma Pinelliae Ternatae (*Ban Xia*), 7 *qian*, Fructus Pruni Mume (*Wu Mei*) and Alkaloid (*Shi Jian*), 3 *qian* each, and Ramulus Cinnamomi (*Gui Zhi*), 1.5 *qian*. Powder the above, make into pills with Succus Zingiberis (*Jiang Zhi*) cake; 100 pills per dose taken with ginger soup. Delete Cortex Cinnamomi in winter.

A person suffered from obstruction and congestion with pain in the chest as a result of taking hot wine and food. This was ascribed to the existence of dead blood. They were prescribed Rhizoma Atractylodis Macrocephalae (*Bai Zhu*), Bulbus Fritillariae (*Bei Mu*), Fructus Germinatus Hordei Vulgaris (*Mai Ya*), Rhizoma Cyperi Rotundi (*Xiang Fu*), Fructus Trichosanthis Kirlowii (*Gua Lou*), Semen Pruni Persicae (*Tao Ren*), Semen Pruni Armeniacae (*Xing Ren*), Cortex Radicis Moutan (*Mu Dan Pi*), Radix Glycyrrhizae (*Sheng Gan Cao*), Radix Puerariae Lobatae (*Ge Gen*), Fructus Gardeniae Jasminoidis (*Shan Zhi*), Radix Scutellariae Baicalensis (*Huang Qin*), Flos Carthami Tinctorii (*Hong Hua*), and Fructus Piperis Cubebae (*Bi Cheng Qie*). Powder the above and take either in the shape of pills or powder, whichever one prefers.

For details about other (relevant) treatment methods, refer to the *Yi Yao (Essentials of Medicine)*.

Chapter Forty-three

Low Back Pain

(This condition is further categorized into) kidney vacuity, blood stasis, damp heat, accumulated phlegm, and wrenching and contusion (types). The pulse in low back pain is invariably wiry and deep. A wiry pulse (indicates) vacuity, while a deep pulse, stagnation. When the pulse is large, the kidney is vacuous. A choppy (pulse) suggests blood stasis. A moderate (*i.e.*, a slightly retarded pulse) suggests dampness. (And) a slippery and hidden one suggests phlegm.

In case of kidney vacuity, use Cortex Eucommiae Ulmoidis (*Du Zhong*), Plastrum Testudinis (*Gui Ban*), Cortex Phellodendri (*Huang Bai*), Rhizoma Anemarrhenae (*Zhi Mu*), Fructus Lycii Chinensis (*Gou Qi*), and Fructus Schizandrae Chinensis (*Wu Wei*). One (variant formula) adds Fructus Psoraleae Corylifoliae (*Bu Gu Zhi*) and the spinal marrow of a pig. Take in the shape of pills. In case of blood stasis causing ache, the appropriate (formula) is the blood-moving and qi-rectifying *Bu Yin Wan* (Supplement Yin Pills)[1] plus Semen Pruni Persicae (*Tao Ren*), Flos Carthami Tinctorii (*Hong Hua*), and the like. Besides, prick *Wei Zhong* (BL 40) to let blood out since the blood is retarded below. (While) in case of damp heat causing the ache, it is appropriate to dry dampness and move the qi with Rhizoma Atractylodis (*Cang Zhu*), Cortex Eucommiae Ulmoidis (*Du Zhong*), Rhizoma Ligustici Wallichii (*Chuan Xiong*), Cortex Phellodendri (*Huang Bai*), etc. (Also) appropriate is

---

[1] This formula consists of wine-fried Cortex Phellodendri (*Huang Bai*), one half *liang*, wine-soaked, stir-fried Rhizoma Anemarrhenae (*Zhi Mu*) and prepared Radix Rehmanniae (*Shu Di*), 3 *liang* each, wine-soaked, fried Plastrum Testudinis (*Gui Ban*), 4 *liang*, stir-fried Radix Albus Paeoniae Lactiflorae (*Bai Shao Yao*), Pericarpium Citri Reticulatae (*Chen Pi*), and Radix Achyranthis Bidentatae (*Niu Xi*), 2 *liang* for each of the above, Herba Cynomorii Songarici (*Suo Yang*) and Radix Angelicae Sinensis (*Dang Gui*), 1.5 *liang* each, and wine-soaked, crisp-fried Os Tigridis (*Hu Gu*), 1 *liang*. Powder the above and make into pills with wine-cooked mutton.

(Zhang) Zi-he's *Wei Shen San* (Roasted Kidney Powder).[2] For phlegm causing the ache, (use) *Er Chen Tang* (Two Aged Decoction) plus Rhizoma Arisaematis (*Nan Xing*) with certain qi-quickening medicinals added as assistants to make phlegm move with the qi. In case of various (types) of repletion lumbago due to wrenching and contusion, *Dang Gui Cheng Qi Tang* (*Dang Gui* Support the Qi Decoction)[3] is used to precipitate (the malign blood).

Kidney fixity is a disease (characterized by) the lower back (feeling) cold like (being immersed in) water with generalized heaviness, absence of thirst, uninhibited urination, normal food intake, and a heavy abdomen as if there were some weights in the lower back. The appropriate treatment is to drain dampness and, at the same time, to use warming medicinals to disperse (wind cold). Cold dampness causing low back pain is treated with *Mo Yao Gao* (Rub the Low Back Paste). If the lumbus is too painful (for one) to stand, needle *Ren Zhong* (CV 26). Chronic lumbago necessarily requires Cortex Cinnamomi (*Guan Gui*) to open (cold block), and such a formula may (also) check thigh pain. It can also be used for flank pain. (However, in the treatment of) the various kinds of low back pain, do not use Radix Panacis Ginseng (*Ren Shen*) to supplement the qi. (In that case,) the qi will remain blocked and the ache will become all the more serious. (Likewise, although) various kinds of pain are all ascribed to fire, one should not over-use cold and cool medicinals. (Even in such cases,) it is proper to apply warm (medicinals) to disperse.

---

[2]   This formula consists of wine-soaked Radix Achyranthis Bidentatae (*Niu Xi*), Rhizoma Dioscoreae Hypoglaucae (*Bei Xie*), Cortex Eucommiae Ulmoidis (*Du Zhong*), Herba Cistanchis (*Rou Cong Rong*), Semen Cuscutae (*Tu Si Zi*), Radix Ledebouriellae Sesloidis (*Fang Feng*), Semen Astragali Complanati (*Bai Ji Li*), Semen Trigonellae Foeni-graeci (*Hu Luo Ba*), and Fructus Psoraleae Corylifoliae (*Bu Gu Zhi*), all in equal amounts, and half the amount of Cortex Cinnamomi (*Rou Gui*). Powder the above, cook (some) pig's kidneys well, and make all into pills.

[3]   This formula consists of Radix Angelicae Sinensis (*Dang Gui*) and Radix Et Rhizoma Rhei (*Da Huang*), 1 *liang* each, Radix Glycyrrhizae (*Gan Cao*), one half *liang*, and Mirabilitum (*Mang Xiao*), 9 *qian*. (Take) 2 *liang* per dose. Boil with 5 slices of ginger and 10 dates.

For low back pain with damp phlegm causing diarrhea, (use) mix-fried Plastrum Testudinis (*Gui Ban*), 1 *liang*, stir-fried Cortex Ailanthi Altissimae (*Chu Pi*), Rhizoma Atractylodis (*Cang Zhu*), and Talcum (*Hua Shi*), 5 *qian* for each of the above, and stir-fried Radix Paeoniae Lactiflorae (*Shao Yao*) and Rhizoma Cyperi Rotundi (*Xiang Fu*), 4 *qian* each. Make the above into pills with gruel. In case of internal damage, take these with Rhizoma Atractylodis Macrocephalae (*Bai Zhu*) soup and Fructus Crataegi (*Shan Zha*).

For damp ache of the low back and leg, (use) wine-fried Plastrum Testudinis (*Gui Ban*) and wine-fried Cortex Phellodendri (*Huang Bai*), 5 *qian* each, Pericarpium Viridis Citri Reticulatae (*Qing Pi*), 3 *qian*, and Radix Glycyrrhizae (*Sheng Gan Cao*), 1.5 *qian*. Powder the above. Pound 1 piece of Rhizoma Zingiberis (*Jiang*), put in 2 *qian* of the powdered medicinals, grind finely, brew with Succus Xanthii Sibirici (*Cang Er Zhi*), heat to a boil, and take. (But for) damp ache of the low back and foot, (use) powdered, wine-fried Plastrum Testudinis (*Gui Ban*), 2 *liang*, wine-fried Cortex Phellodendri (*Huang Bai*), Herba Xanthii Sibirici (*Cang Er*), Rhizoma Atractylodis (*Cang Zhu*), and wine-washed Radix Clematidis Chinensis (*Wei Ling Xian*), 1 *liang* for each of the above, and Cacumen Biotae Orientalis (*Bian Bai*), one half *liang*. Powder the above. Boil *Si Wu Tang* (Four Materials Decoction) in black soybean juice together with Pericarpium Citri Reticulatae (*Chen Pi*), Radix Glycyrrhizae (*Gan Cao*), and fresh Rhizoma Zingiberis (*Sheng Jiang*). After removing the dregs, brew with 2 *qian* of the above powdered medicinals and take.

Mo Yao Gao treats low back pain in old people, people with vacuity, and also (in those with) white vaginal discharge. (It consists of) Radix Aconiti (*Wu Tou*), Radix Praeparatus Aconiti Carmichaeli (*Fu Zi*), and Rhizoma Arisaematis (*Nan Xing*), 2.5 *qian* for each of the above, Realgar (*Xiong Huang*) and Cinnabar (*Zhu Sha*), 1 *qian* each, Camphora (*Zhang Nao*), Flos Caryophylli (*Ding Xiang*), dry Rhizoma Zingiberis (*Gan Jiang*), and Fructus Evodiae Rutecarpae (*Wu Zhu Yu*), 1.5 *qian* for each of the above, and Secretio Moschi Moschiferi (*She Xiang*), 5 pieces. Powder the above and make into pills the size of longans with honey. Dissolve 1 pill in Succus Zingiberis (*Jiang Zhi*) and make into a gruel-like (paste). After heating over a fire, put it onto the palm and rub the lower back (with the palm) till all the paste has adhered to the low back. Heat cotton-padded clothes, (put on, and) bind them, and the lumbus will feel fire-like hot. Apply 1 pill every other day.

To treat damp heat ache and pain in the low back and leg with spasms and hypertonicity of the flanks (due to) lying in the open on damp ground, and inability to turn over (the body, use) *Cang Zhu Tang* (Atractylodes Decoction): Rhizoma Atractylodis (*Cang Zhu*), Cortex Phellodendri (*Huang Bai*), Radix Bupleuri (*Chai Hu*), Radix Ledebouriellae Sesloidis (*Fang Feng*), Radix Praeparatus Aconiti Carmichaeli (*Fu Zi*), Cortex Eucommiae Ulmoidis (*Du Zhong*), Rhizoma Ligustici Wallichii (*Chuan Xiong*), and Cortex Cinnamomi (*Rou Gui*). Prepare these in decoction and take. In case of cold damp qi intruding the body (giving rise to) generalized heaviness, swelling, and pain with a withered yellow facial complexion, add Herba Ephedrae (*Ma Huang*).

A person, aged 60, suffered from unbearable low back pain as a result of falling from horseback. His six pulses[4] were large and scattered, but wiry, small, and long as well as slightly hard when pressure was applied. This showed the existence of malign blood. (However,) this did not allow for expelling. Supplementation and recruiting (*i.e.,* replenishing) should be used first (due to age. Therefore,) Lignum Sappanis (*Su Mu*) was boiled together with Radix Panacis Ginseng (*Ren Shen*), Radix Angelicae Sinensis (*Dang Gui*), Rhizoma Ligustici Wallichii (*Chuan Xiong*), Pericarpium Citri Reticulatae (*Chen Pi*), and Radix Glycyrrhizae (*Gan Cao*) and then taken. In half a month, the pulse gradually became astringed, and food intake gradually increased. Then the above medicinals were administered brewed with Pyritum (*Zi Ran Tong*), etc. One day later, recovery ensued.

To treat low back pain as well as cold pain in the sinews and bones, (use) Radix Angelicae Sinensis (*Dang Gui*), Radix Rubrus Paeoniae Lactiflorae (*Chi Shao Yao*), Radix Et Rhizoma Notopterygii (*Qiang Huo*), wine-fried Cortex Phellodendri (*Huang Bai*), and wine-fried Cortex

---

[4]   This refers to the superficial and deep pulses in the three sections at the radial artery, *i.e.,* the *cun* or inch, *guan* or bar, and *chi* or foot positions.

Eucommiae Ulmoidis (*Du Zhong*), 1 *qian* for each of the above, Rhizoma Atractylodis Macrocephalae (*Bai Zhu*), Rhizoma Ligustici Wallichii (*Chuan Xiong*), Radix Saussureae Seu Vladimiriae (*Mu Xiang*), Semen Arecae Catechu (*Bing Lang*), Radix Ledebouriellae Sesloidis (*Fang Feng*), Radix Angelicae (*Bai Zhi*), Rhizoma Atractylodis (*Cang Zhu*), and Fructus Illicii Veri (*Ba Jiao Hui Xiang*), one half *qian* for each of the above, and Radix Glycyrrhizae (*Gan Cao*), 3 *fen*. Prepare by decoction, brewing with 1 *qian* of Gummum Olibani (*Ru Xiang*), and take before a meal. *Mo Yao Gao* used externally is also good.

Book Four

Chapter Forty-four

Flank Pain

(This is due to either) exuberant liver fire[1], wood qi repletion[2], the existence of streaming phlegm, or the existence of dead blood. In case of a tense liver with wood qi repletion, use Rhizoma Ligustici Wallichii (*Chuan Xiong*), Rhizoma Atractylodis (*Cang Zhu*), and Pericarpium Viridis Citri Reticulatae (*Qing Pi*). Boil in water and take with *Long Hui Wan* (Gentiana & Aloe Pills). In case of exuberant liver fire, administer *Dang Gui Long Hui Wan* (*Dang Gui*, Gentiana & Aloe Pills) with Succus Zingiberis (*Sheng Jiang Zhi*). This is a very important formula for draining fire. This *Dang Gui Long Hui Wan* treats flank pain and moves phlegm (when administered) in the form of honey pills but downbears liver fire, expedites retardation, and treats various miscellaneous patterns (when administered) in the form of pills (made from) Massa Medica Fermentata (*Shen Qu*). It includes Radix Angelicae Sinensis (*Dang Gui*), Radix Gentianae Scabrae (*Long Dan Cao*), Fructus Gardeniae Jasminoidis (*Shan Zhi Ren*), Cortex Phellodendri (*Huang Bai*), Radix Scutellariae Baicalensis (*Huang Qin*), and Rhizoma Coptidis Chinensis (*Huang Lian*), 1 *liang* for each of the above, Radix Et Rhizoma Rhei (*Da Huang*) and Resina Alois (*Lu Hui*), one half *liang* each, Radix Saussureae Seu Vladimiriae (*Mu Xiang*), 1.5 *qian*, and Secretio Moschi Moschiferi (*She Xiang*), 5 *fen*. One (variant formula adds) Radix Bupleuri (*Chai Hu*) and Pericarpium Viridis Citri Reticulatae (*Qing Pi*), one half *liang* each. Another (variant) formula (adds) Pulvis Indigonis (*Qing Dai*). This also treats damp heat flank pain on both sides with remarkable efficacy.

---

[1] Liver fire is, in most cases, impugned to emotional factors, such as anger and frustration. It is manifest by red, swollen eyes, a bitter taste in the mouth, dry throat, hot face, distended head, and irritability.

[2] Wood or liver repletion is similar to liver fire but different in that it manifests distended and painful flanks, oppression in the chest, dyspepsia, and menstrual irregularity with fewer or no signs of heat, such as red, painful eyes.

First stick *Hu Po Gao* (Succinum Paste)[3] to the painful place and then take the pills with Succus Zingiberis (*Jiang Zhi*). In case of severe pain, stir-fry the pills till hot before taking. Another (variant) formula (also) includes Pulvis Indigonis (*Qing Dai*). Take 30 pills per dose with ginger soup. (Yet) another formula (is called) *Xiao Long Hui Wan* (Minor Gentiana & Aloe Pills. It consists of) Radix Angelicae Sinensis (*Dang Gui*), Radix Gentianae Scabrae (*Long Dan Cao*), Fructus Gardeniae Jasminoidis (*Shan Zhi*), Rhizoma Coptidis Chinensis (*Huang Lian*), Radix Scutellariae Baicalensis (*Huang Qin*), Radix Bupleuri (*Chai Hu*), and Rhizoma Ligustici Wallichii (*Chuan Xiong*), one half *liang* for each of the above, and Resina Alois (*Lu Hui*), 3 *qian*.

For dead blood, use Semen Pruni Persicae (*Tao Ren*), Flos Carthami Tinctorii (*Hong Hua*), and Rhizoma Ligustici Wallichii (*Chuan Xiong*). For streaming phlegm, use *Er Chen Tang* (Two Aged Decoction) plus Rhizoma Arisaematis (*Nan Xing*), Rhizoma Ligustici Wallichii (*Chuan Xiong*), and Rhizoma Atractylodis (*Cang Zhu*). In case of (phlegm) repletion, use *Kong Xian Dan* (Control Drool Elixir)[4] to downbear phlegm. (But,) when the liver is tormented by tenseness, [which has already been discussed in the *Yi Yao* {*Essentials of Medicine*, later editor}], promptly take acrid (medicinals in order to) disperse, such as Rhizoma Ligustici Wallichii (*Chuan Xiong*) and Rhizoma Atractylodis (*Cang Zhu*). In case of severe flank pain, take *Long Hui Wan* with Succus Zingiberis (*Sheng Jiang Zhi*) because, (in this case,) liver fire is exuberant, (while) for flank pain with coughing, [which has already been discussed in the *Yi Yao* {*Essentials of Medicine*, later editor}], (use) *Er Chen Tang* plus Rhizoma Arisaematis (*Nan Xing*), Rhizoma Cyperi

---

[3] This paste consists of Succinum (*Hu Po*), 1 *liang*, Caulis Akebiae Mutong (*Mu Tong*), Cortex Cinnamomi (*Gui Xin*), Radix Angelicae Sinensis (*Dang Gui*), Radix Angelicae (*Bai Zhi*), Radix Ledebouriellae Sesloidis (*Fang Feng*), Resina Pini (*Song Zhi*), Cinnabar (*Zhu Sha*), and Semen Momordicae Cochinensis (*Mu Bie Zi*), one half *liang* for each of the above, Flos Caryophylli (*Ding Xiang*) and Radix Saussureae Seu Vladimiriae (*Mu Xiang*), 3 *fen* each, and sesame oil (*Ma You*), 2 *jin*.

[4] This formula consists of Radix Euphorbiae Kansui (*Gan Sui*), Herba Cirsii Japonici (*Da Ji*), and Semen Sinapis Albae (*Bai Jie Zi*), all in equal amounts.

Rotundi (*Xiang Fu*), Pericarpium Viridis Citri Reticulatae (*Qing Pi*), Pulvis Indigonis (*Qing Dai*), and Succus Zingiberis (*Jiang Zhi*).

Zuo Jin Wan (Left Gold Pills) treat liver fire. (They are composed of) Radix Scutellariae Baicalensis (*Huang Qin*), 6 *liang*, and Fructus Evodiae Rutecarpae (*Zhu Yu*), 5 *qian*. Another formula (called) *Tui Qi San* (Push the Qi Powder) treats unbearable pain in the left lateral costal region. (It consists of) Rhizoma Curcumae (*Pian Jiang Huang*), stir-fried Fructus Citri Seu Ponciri (*Zhi Qiao*) and stir-fried Cortex Cinnamomi (*Gui Xin*), one half *liang* for each of the above, and mix-fried Radix Glycyrrhizae (*Zhi Gan Cao*), 3 *qian*. Powder the above (and) take 2 *qian* per dose with wine. *Kong Xian Dan* (on the other hand) treats qi pain all over the body and migratory pain in the flanks. In case of phlegm embracing dead blood, add Semen Pruni Persicae (*Tao Ren*) paste and make into pills. (And) to treat pain in the cardiac and lateral costal regions, (use) equal amounts of slightly stir-fried dry Rhizoma Zingiberis (*Gan Jiang*) and vinegar-fried Flos Daphnis Genkwae (*Yuan Hua*). Make into pills with honey; 12 pills per dose. This is greatly effective!

In persons with weak qi, pain in the lateral costal regions with a thin, taut, or wiry pulse is usually a result of taxation and toiling and angry qi. *Ba Wu Tang* (Eight Materials Decoction, treats this and consists of) Radix Panacis Ginseng (*Ren Shen*), Rhizoma Atractylodis Macrocephalae (*Bai Zhu*), Sclerotium Poriae Cocoris (*Bai Fu Ling*), Radix Glycyrrhizae (*Gan Cao*), Radix Angelicae Sinensis (*Dang Gui*), prepared Radix Rehmanniae (*Shu Di Huang*), Rhizoma Ligustici Wallichii (*Chuan Xiong*), and Radix Albus Paeoniae Lactiflorae (*Bai Shao Yao*) plus Radix Saussureae Seu Vladimiriae (*Mu Xiang*), Cortex Cinnamomi (*Guan Gui*), and Pericarpium Viridis Citri Reticulatae (*Qing Pi*).

For flank pain with constipation and a replete pulse, (use) *Mu Xiang Bing Lang Wan* (Saussurea & Areca Pills): Radix Saussureae Seu Vladimiriae (*Mu Xiang*), 5 *qian*, Pericarpium Viridis Citri Reticulatae (*Qing Pi*), 2 *qian*, Pericarpium Citri Reticulatae (*Chen Pi*), 2 *qian*, Fructus Citri Seu Ponciri (*Zhi Qiao*), 1 *qian*, Semen Arecae Catechu (*Bing Lang*), 2 *qian*, Rhizoma Coptidis Chinensis (*Chuan Lian*), 2 *qian*, Cortex Phellodendri (*Huang Bai*), 4 *qian*, Radix Et Rhizoma Rhei (*Da Huang*), 4 *qian*, Rhizoma Cyperi Rotundi (*Xiang Fu*), 1 *qian*, and Semen

Pharbitidis (*Qian Niu*), powdered and sifted, 8 *qian*. Powder the above and make into pills the size of Chinese parasol tree seeds by dripping water; 60-70 pills per dose taken on an empty stomach with ginger soup.

For damp heat ache and pain in the low back and leg with spasms and hypertonicity of the flanks due to lying in the open on damp ground and inability to turn over, (use) *Cang Zhu Tang* (Atractylodes Decoction) [whose formula can be found in the chapter on low back pain {later editor}].

A person who suffered from pain due to the attack of phlegm qi in the flanks was prescribed *Kong Xian Dan*. The phlegm precipitated was like (sticky) dough. Semen Sinapis Albae (*Bai Jie Zi*) precipitates phlegm and its acridity is able to disperse pain. An(other) person suffered from stabbing pain somewhere in the chest a little to the right with a sensation of internal heat attacking outward and incessant drooling at the mouth. They had contracted lung *yong* as a result of long brewing (of this heat. For this they were prescribed) Bulbus Fritillariae (*Bei Mu*), Fructus Trichosanthis Kirlowii (*Gua Lou*), and Rhizoma Arisaematis (*Nan Xing*) to rid the drool, Ramulus Perillae Frutescentis (*Zi Su Geng*) to drain lung qi, Radix Scutellariae Baicalensis (*Huang Qin*), ginger-fried Rhizoma Coptidis Chinensis (*Huang Lian*), Pericarpium Citri Reticulatae (*Chen Pi*), and Sclerotium Poriae Cocoris (*Fu Ling*) to lead downwards, Rhizoma Cyperi Rotundi (*Xiang Fu*) and Fructus Citri Seu Ponciri (*Zhi Qiao*) to loosen the diaphragm and remove its pain, Spina Gleditschiae Sinensis (*Zao Jiao Ci*) to resolve bind pain, and Radix Platycodi Grandiflori (*Jie Geng*) to upfloat. In case of inability to eat, add Rhizoma Atractylodis Macrocephalae (*Bai Zhu*). In case of vomiting of water rheum, do not use Fructus Trichosanthis Kirlowii (*Gua Lou*) in any case. Mostly medicinals such as Rhizoma Atractylodis (*Cang Zhu*) should be used instead.

A person suffered from qi pain in the left flank with a corresponding pain in the (same side of) the chest. (They were prescribed) Fructus Trichosanthis Kirlowii (*Gua Lou*), 1 *liang*, Bulbus Fritillariae (*Bei Mu*), 1 *liang*, Rhizoma Arisaematis (*Nan Xing*), 1 *liang*, Radix Angelicae Sinensis (*Dang Gui*), 5 *qian*, Semen Pruni Persicae (*Tao Ren*), 5 *qian*, Rhizoma

Ligustici Wallichii (*Chuan Xiong*), 5 *qian*, Radix Bupleuri (*Chai Hu*), 5 *qian*, stir-fried Rhizoma Coptidis Chinensis (*Huang Lian*), 5 *qian*, stir-fried Radix Scutellariae Baicalensis (*Huang Qin*), 5 *qian*, stir-fried Fructus Gardeniae Jasminoidis (*Shan Zhi*), 5 *qian*, stir-fried Rhizoma Cyperi Rotundi (*Xiang Fu*), 5 *qian*, stir-fried Rhizoma Curcumae (*Jiang Huang*), 5 *qian*, Resina Alois (*Lu Hui*), 3 *qian*, Pericarpium Viridis Citri Reticulatae (*Qing Pi*), 3 *qian*, Pericarpium Citri Reticulatae (*Chen Pi*), 3 *qian*, Pulvis Indigonis (*Qing Dai*), 1.5 *qian*, and stir-fried Radix Gentianae Scabrae (*Long Dan Cao*), 5 *qian*.

For ache and pain in the cardiac, thoracic, abdominal, and lateral costal regions, *Er Chen Tang* plus Radix Panacis Ginseng (*Ren Shen*), Rhizoma Atractylodis Macrocephalae (*Bai Zhu*), and various aromatic medicinals offer an effective treatment. In the presence of blood stasis, it is necessary to use blood-breaking and qi-moving medicinals such as tip-preserved Semen Pruni Persicae (*Tao Ren*) and Rhizoma Cyperi Rotundi (*Xiang Fu*). In case of exuberant fire, it is necessary to fell the liver. If the liver is tormented by tenseness, it is appropriate to take acrid (medicinals) to disperse it. *Xiao Chai Hu Tang* (Minor Bupleurum Decoction) can also treat this.

Wood penetrating earth with flank pain and vomiting means that wind evils are trapped between the spleen and stomach. (In that case,) use *Er Chen Tang* plus Rhizoma Gastrodiae Elatae (*Tian Ma*), Radix Albus Paeoniae Lactiflorae (*Bai Shao Yao*), stir-fried Massa Medica Fermentata (*Shen Qu*), Fructus Citri Seu Ponciri (*Zhi Qiao*), Rhizoma Cyperi Rotundi (*Xiang Fu*), Rhizoma Atractylodis Macrocephalae (*Bai Zhu*), and Fructus Amomi (*Sha Ren*). For irascible persons with frequent pain in the abdomen and flanks, (use) *Xiao Chai Hu Tang* plus Rhizoma Ligustici Wallichii (*Chuan Xiong*), Radix Paeoniae Lactiflorae (*Shao Yao*), Pericarpium Viridis Citri Reticulatae (*Qing Pi*), etc. In case of severe pain, take (the above) in the form of decoction with *Dang Gui Long Hui Wan*. This offers very rapid effect.

A person suffered from an aching spleen and flank pain with a slightly dry mouth. Inquiry revealed that (the disease) was already years old. Autumn heat was still prevailing at the time. (For this,) *Er Chen Tang* plus dry Radix Puerariae Lobatae (*Gan Ge*), Rhizoma Ligustici Wallichii

(*Chuan Xiong*), Pericarpium Viridis Citri Reticulatae (*Qing Pi*), and Caulis Akebiae Mutong (*Mu Tong*) were boiled and taken with *Long Hui Wan*.

An(other) person whose original qi was vacuous and exhausted suffered from a moderate pain in the flanks. (They were given) *Bu Zhong Yi Qi Tang* (Supplement the Center & Boost the Qi Decoction) plus Radix Albus Paeoniae Lactiflorae (*Bai Shao*), Radix Gentianae Scabrae (*Long Dan*), Pericarpium Viridis Citri Reticulatae (*Qing Pi*), Fructus Citri Seu Ponciri (*Zhi Qiao*), Rhizoma Cyperi Rotundi (*Xiang Fu*), and Rhizoma Ligustici Wallichii (*Chuan Xiong*).

(Yet) an(other) person suffered from pain in the flanks with fever arising each evening. This was due to yin vacuity. *Xiao Chai Hu Tang* was combined with *Si Wu Tang* (Four Materials Decoction) plus Radix Gentianae Scabrae (*Long Dan*), Pericarpium Viridis Citri Reticulatae (*Qing Pi*), and dry Radix Puerariae Lobatae (*Gan Ge*). In case of severe yin vacuity, add Cortex Phellodendri (*Huang Bai*) and Rhizoma Anemarrhenae (*Zhi Mu*).

Chapter Forty-five

Abdominal Pain

(This condition) is (further) classified into cold, heat, dead blood, food accumulation, and damp phlegm (types). Clear phlegm often gives rise to abdominal pain. The great method is to use Rhizoma Ligustici Wallichii (*Chuan Xiong*), Rhizoma Atractylodis (*Cang Zhu*), Rhizoma Cyperi Rotundi (*Xiang Fu*), and Radix Angelicae (*Bai Zhi*). Powder and take with hot boiled water in which Succus Zingiberis (*Jiang Zhi*) is added. Due to qi stagnation, phlegm may obstruct the passageways. The qi is not free flowing and, therefore, there is pain. (For this) it is appropriate to conduct the phlegm and resolve (the qi) depression. For qi (pain), use qi(-moving) medicinals like Radix Saussureae Seu Vladimiriae

(*Mu Xiang*), Semen Arecae Catechu (*Bing Lang*), Fructus Citri Seu Ponciri (*Zhi Qiao*), and Rhizoma Cyperi Rotundi (*Xiang Fu*). For blood (pain), use blood(-breaking) medicinals like Rhizoma Ligustici Wallichii (*Chuan Xiong*), Radix Angelicae Sinensis (*Dang Gui*), Flos Carthami Tinctorii (*Hong Hua*), and Semen Pruni Persicae (*Tao Ren*).

(Pain) in the upper (abdomen) is usually ascribed to food. (For this,) warming and dispersing with medicinals like dry Rhizoma Zingiberis (*Gan Jiang*), Rhizoma Atractylodis (*Cang Zhu*), Rhizoma Ligustici Wallichii (*Chuan Xiong*), Radix Angelicae (*Bai Zhi*), Rhizoma Cyperi Rotundi (*Xiang Fu*), and Succus Zingiberis (*Jiang Zhi*) are appropriate. (But) for cold pain, (use) *Li Zhong Tang* (Rectify the Center Decoction) and *Jian Zhong Tang* (Build the Center Decoction). A variant edition prescribes *Xiao Jian Zhong Tang* (Minor Build the Center Decoction) plus Rhizoma Zingiberis (*Jiang*), Cortex Cinnamomi (*Gui*), Rhizoma Ligustici Wallichii (*Tai Xiong*), Rhizoma Atractylodis (*Cang Zhu*), Radix Angelicae (*Bai Zhi*), and Rhizoma Cyperi Rotundi (*Xiang Fu*). In case of vomiting, add Flos Caryophylli (*Ding Xiang*).

For heat pain, (use) *Er Chen Tang* (Two Aged Decoction) plus Radix Scutellariae Baicalensis (*Huang Qin*), Rhizoma Coptidis Chinensis (*Huang Lian*), and Fructus Gardeniae Jasminoidis (*Zhi Zi*). In serious cases, add dry Rhizoma Zingiberis (*Gan Jiang*). A (variant formula) consists of *Tiao Wei Cheng Qi Tang* (Regulate the Stomach & Support the Qi Decoction) plus Radix Saussureae Seu Vladimiriae (*Mu Xiang*) and Semen Arecae Catechu (*Bing Lang*).

For dissipation in wine, overeating, and lustfulness (causing) lower abdominal distention and pain, use Radix Angelicae Sinensis (*Dang Gui*), Radix Paeoniae Lactifloriae (*Shao Yao*), Rhizoma Ligustici Wallichii (*Chuan Xiong*), Radix Bupleuri (*Chai Hu*), Pericarpium Viridis Citri Reticulatae (*Qing Pi*), Fructus Evodiae Rutecarpae (*Wu Zhu Yu*), Radix Glycyrrhizae (*Sheng Gan Cao*), and Semen Pruni Persicae (*Tao Ren*). Boil and take. In case of chest fullness and low food intake, add Sclerotium Poriae Cocoris (*Fu Ling*), Rhizoma Pinelliae Ternatae (*Ban Xia*), and Pericarpium Citri Reticulatae (*Chen Pi*. However,) to treat wine accumulation abdominal pain, it is vital to loosen the qi with Rhizoma Sparganii (*Sn Leng*), Rhizoma Curcumae Zedoariae (*E Zhu*), Rhizoma

Cyperi Rotundi (*Xiang Fu*), Cortex Cinnamomi (*Guan Gui*), Rhizoma Atractylodis (*Cang Zhu*), Cortex Magnoliae Officinalis (*Hou Po*), Pericarpium Citri Reticulatae (*Chen Pi*), Radix Glycyrrhizae (*Gan Cao*), Sclerotium Poriae Cocoris (*Fu Ling*), Radix Saussureae Seu Vladimiriae (*Mu Xiang*), and Semen Arecae Catechu (*Bing Lang*).

For wood repletion abdominal pain (so painful) the hand cannot (even) be near (it) with the six pulses all deep and thin and severe repletion and perspiration, (use) *Da Cheng Qi Tang* (Major Support the Qi Decoction) plus Cortex Cinnamomi (*Gui*). In case of (even) more severe pain in strong and sturdy (persons), add Semen Pruni Persicae (*Tao Ren*). In case of still more severe pain, add Radix Praeparatus Aconiti Carmichaeli (*Fu Zi*).

For vacuity cold causing pain in the lower abdomen, (use) *Xiao Jian Zhong Tang*. This formula consists of Radix Paeoniae Lactiflorae (*Shao Yao*), 6 *liang*, Ramulus Cinnamomi (*Gui Zhi*), 2 *liang*, Radix Glycyrrhizae (*Gan Cao*), 2 *liang*, Fructus Zizyphii Jujubae (*Da Zao*), 7 pieces, fresh Rhizoma Zingiberis (*Sheng Jiang*), 3 *liang*, and Maltose (*Yi Tang*), 1 *sheng*. (But for) spleen dampness accumulation jaundice with aching and pain in the cardiac and abdominal regions, (use) *Wei Ling Tang* (Stomach *Ling* Decoction. And for) stomach vacuity and contraction of cold causing cold and pain in the cardiac and abdominal regions in (persons with) qi weakness, (use) *Li Zhong Tang*. For great abdominal pain with deep and replete pulses, (use) *Fu Zi Li Zhong Tang* (Aconite Rectify the Center Decoction)[1] in combination with *Da Cheng Qi Tang*. Boil and take when cooled.

An old person suffered from great cardiac and abdominal pain with a large, surging pulse. (Their) pain was vacuity pain. (They also had) clouding inversion and inability to eat, and they could not stand any

---

[1] This consists of Radix Praeparatus Aconiti Carmichaeli (*Fu Zi*), dry Rhizoma Zingiberis (*Gan Jiang*), blast-fried Fructus Evodiae Rutecarpae (*Wu Zhu Yu*), Cortex Cinnamomi (*Guan Gui*), Radix Panacis Ginseng (*Ren Shen*), Radix Angelicae Sinensis (*Dang Gui*), Pericarpium Citri Reticulatae (*Chen Pi*), Cortex Magnoliae Officinalis (*Hou Po*), Rhizoma Atractylodis Macrocephalae (*Bai Zhu*), and mix-fried Radix Glycyrrhizae (*Zhi Gan Cao*). These are boiled together with ginger and dates.

attacking (formula. Therefore, they were prescribed) *Si Jun Zi Tang* (Four Gentlemen Decoction) plus Radix Angelicae Sinensis (*Dang Gui*), Herba Ephedrae (*Ma Huang*), and Lignum Aquilariae Agallochae (*Chen Xiang*).

A woman, living in widowhood and whose menses had long been absent, suffered from abdominal fullness, low food intake, occasional lower abdominal pain, weak form and body heat. (I) prescribed (her) wine-soaked Radix Angelicae Sinensis (*Dang Gui*), 1 *qian*, ginger-fried prepared Radix Rehmanniae (*Shu Di Huang*), 1 *qian*, Rhizoma Cyperi Rotundi (*Xiang Fu*), 1 *qian*, Rhizoma Ligustici Wallichii (*Chuan Xiong*), 1.5 *qian*, Radix Albus Paeoniae Lactiflorae (*Bai Shao Yao*), 1.5 *qian*, Pericarpium Citri Reticulatae (*Chen Pi*), 1.5 *qian*, stir-fried Cortex Phellodendri (*Huang Bai*), 5 *fen*, Radix Glycyrrhizae (*Sheng Gan Cao*), 3 *qian*, stir-fried Rhizoma Anemarrhenae (Zhi Mu), 5 *fen*, ginger-processed Cortex Magnoliae Officinalis (*Hou Po*), 5 *fen*, Rhizoma Corydalis Yanhusuo (*Xuan Hu Suo*), 5 *fen*, Rhizoma Atractylodis Macrocephalae (*Bai Zhu*), 2 *qian*, Pericarpium Arecae (*Da Fu Pi*), 3 *qian*, Flos Carthami Tinctorii (*Hong Hua Tou*), 9 pieces, soaked in alcohol, and ground Semen Pruni Persicae (*Tao Ren*), 9 pieces. The above were sliced and boiled in water.

For frequent vacuity pain due to spleen and stomach dampness with the existence of cold, (use) *Li Zhong Tang*. For great cardiac and abdominal pain with (alternating) cold and heat, retching and vomiting, and a deep, wiry pulse, (use) *Da Chai Hu Tang* (Major Bupleurum Decoction). Fructus Amomi (*Suo Sha*) treats vacuity pain in the abdomen. Dai comments: Cold pain is a continuous pain which is dull and does not increase or decrease. Intermittent pain (on the other hand) is (ascribed to) heat. Dead blood pain is a pain fixed in place and never moving away. Food accumulation pain is a pain which, when serious, induces a desire to defecate and which is relieved following the movement of the bowels. Damp phlegm pain is a pain that is invariably accompanied by inhibited urination.

Pain caused by food requires warm dissipation. Do not apply great precipitation since food becomes congealed when it meets with cold but is dissolved when it meets with warmth. In addition, if (warm dissipation) is assisted by qi-moving and qi-quickening medicinals, it never fails. Some may ask how phlegm can cause pain. The answer is that phlegm may gather as a result of qi stagnation. When it gathers, it obstructs the passageways. Since qi is unable to circulate, pain is caused.

Rumbling in the abdomen is fire striking and stirring water. Water tends to flow downward, while fire tends to flame upward. (Rumbling) is explained by their conflict. There are (also) cases of rumbling due to cold viscera with existence of water. It is appropriate to treat this based on the division of the three yin regions: (*i.e.,*) the venter, *tai yin*, the periumbilical abdomen, *shao yin*, and the lower abdomen, *jue yin*.

Chapter Forty-six

Disharmony of the Spleen & Stomach

Bu Pi Wan (Supplement the Spleen Pills) are appropriate to take for those with spleen vacuity and an aversion to decocted medicinals. (They consist of) Rhizoma Atractylodis Macrocephalae (*Bai Zhu*), 8 *liang*, Rhizoma Atractylodis (*Cang Zhu*), Pericarpium Citri Reticulatae (*Chen Pi*), and Sclerotium Poriae Cocoris (*Fu Ling*), 4 *liang* for each of the above. Powder the above, make into pills with gruel, and take. In a (variant edition) there is (also) Radix Paeoniae Lactifloriae (*Shao Yao*), one half *liang*. *Bai Zhu Wan* (Atractylodes Pills) have the same indications. (They consist of) Rhizoma Atractylodis Macrocephalae (*Bai Zhu*), 8 *liang*, and Radix Paeoniae Lactiflorae (*Shao Yao*), 4 *liang*. (Also) powder the above, make into pills with gruel, and take. *Da An Wan* (Great Calming Pills) fortify the spleen and stomach and disperse drink and food. (They are composed of) Fructus Crataegi (*Shan Zha*), Rhizoma Atractylodis Macrocephalae (*Bai Zhu*), 2 *liang* each, Sclerotium Poriae Cocoris (*Fu Ling*), stir-fried Massa Medica Fermentata (*Shen Qu*), Rhizoma Pinelliae Ternatae (*Ban Xia*), 1 *liang* for each of the above, Pericarpium Citri Reticulatae (*Chen Pi*), stir-fried Semen Raphani Sativi (*Lai Fu Zi*), and Fructus Forsythiae Suspensae (*Lian Qiao*), 5 *qian* for each of the above. Powder and make into pills with cake. A (variant) formula without Rhizoma Atractylodis Macrocephalae is called *Bao He Wan* (Protect & Harmonize Pills).

Chapter Forty-seven

Pain in the Upper Back & Nape of the Neck

Great pain in the heart and diaphragm radiating to attack the upper and lower back, the pain (so) great as to give rise to inversion, make it impossible to accept any medications. In case of violent vomiting, perform mechanical emesis with a goose quill in the course of vomiting and the pain will be checked when a big bowlful of accumulated phlegm is vomited.

A male suffered from rigidity of the nape of the neck with inability to look back and moderate pain arising on turning. His pulse was found to be bowstring, rapid, and replete, particularly so on the right hand. (The case) was treated as phlegm heat intruding into the *tai yang* channel. (For this, he) was administered *Er Chen Tang* plus Radix Scutellariae Baicalensis (*Huang Qin*), Radix Et Rhizoma Notopterygii (*Qiang Huo*), and Flos Carthami Tinctorii (*Hong Hua*). Two days later, recovery ensued.

A male suddenly had a thread of pain in the medial border of his scapula which spread over the shoulder and obliquely through the chest, ending in the flank. This unbearable pain continued day and night without a break. His pulse was bowstring and rapid, but when pressure was applied, it was greatly hollow. (It was also) larger on the left hand than the right. The scapula (is associated with) the small intestine channel, while the chest and flank (are associated with) the gallbladder (channel). This (condition) must be due to the heart being injured by thought and worry. Before the heart contracts disease, the bowel (*i.e.*, the small intestine) becomes diseased. Therefore, the pain started from the scapula on the back. Furthermore, as worry had not been resolved, it went to the gallbladder.[1] Hence, the pain ascended onto the chest and ended in the flank. This was small intestinal fire overwhelming gallbladder wood, the child overwhelming the mother, a repletion evil. After inquiry, it proved true that the disease was a result of failure in a project. Four *qian* of Radix Panacis Ginseng (*Ren Shen*) and 2 *qian* of Caulis Akebiae Mutong (*Mu Tong*) were boiled and taken with *Long Hui Wan* (Gentiana & Aloe Pills). A number of doses later, recovery ensued.

A person had pain in the spleen (and) arm.[2] (They were given) *Er Chen Tang* (Two Aged Decoction) plus wine-soaked Radix Scutellariae Baicalensis (*Huang Qin*), Rhizoma Atractylodis (*Cang Zhu*), and Radix Et Rhizoma Notopterygii (*Qiang Huo*. Besides) Folium Impatientis Balsaminae (*Feng Xian Ye*) was pounded and applied to the painful places.

Chapter Forty-eight

Arm Pain

This is due to dampness in the upper burner running wildly in the channels and connecting vessels. The treatment is to use *Er Chen Tang* (Two Aged Decoction) plus Rhizoma Atractylodis (*Cang Zhu*), Rhizoma Cyperi Rotundi (*Xiang Fu*), Radix Clematidis Chinensis (*Wei Ling Xian*), wine-processed Radix Scutellariae Baicalensis (*Huang Qin*), Rhizoma

---

[1] The heart is connected with the small intestine in an interior/exterior relationship. Both correspond to fire. While the liver is connected with the gallbladder, both corresponding to wood. The scapulas are traversed by the path of the small intestine channel, while the chest and lateral costal regions are traversed by the gallbladder channel. One should also note that the gallbladder holds the office of decision. When thought and worry are excessive, it is up to the gallbladder to resolve them.

[2] The translator suspects that "upper" should be read for "spleen (and)".

Arisaematis (*Nan Xing*), and Rhizoma Atractylodis Macrocephalae (*Bai Zhu*). Boil the above with fresh Rhizoma Zingiberis (*Sheng Jiang*) and take. A (variant) formula includes in addition Radix Angelicae Sinensis (*Dang Gui*) and Radix Et Rhizoma Notopterygii (*Qiang Huo*) and is called *Huo Luo Tang* (Quicken the Connecting Vessel Decoction).

(Pain) in the left side is ascribed to wind dampness. (For this, use) Radix Bupleuri (*Chai Hu*), Rhizoma Ligustici Wallichii (*Chuan Xiong*), Radix Angelicae Sinensis (*Dang Gui*), Radix Et Rhizoma Notopterygii (*Qiang Huo*), Radix Angelicae Duhuo (*Du Huo*), Rhizoma Pinelliae Ternatae (*Ban Xia*), Rhizoma Atractylodis (*Cang Zhu*), Rhizoma Cyperi Rotundi (*Xiang Fu*), and Radix Glycyrrhizae (*Gan Cao*), (while pain) in the right is ascribed to phlegm dampness. (For it, use) Rhizoma Arisaematis (*Nan Xing*), Rhizoma Atractylodis (*Cang Zhu*), and the like.

Chapter Forty-nine

Painful Wind[1] with Itching Appended

(This is classified into) wind heat, wind dampness, blood vacuity, or existence of phlegm (types). The great method is to use Rhizoma Atractylodis (*Cang Zhu*), Rhizoma Arisaematis (*Nan Xing*), Rhizoma Ligustici Wallichii (*Chuan Xiong*), Radix Angelicae Sinensis (*Dang Gui*), Radix Angelicae (*Bai Zhi*), and wine-processed Radix Scutellariae Baicalensis (*Huang Qin*. If the evil is located) above, add Radix Et Rhizoma Notopterygii (*Qiang Huo*), Radix Clematidis Chinensis (*Wei Ling Xian*), and Ramulus Cinnamomi (*Gui Zhi*. If it is located) below, add Radix Achyranthis Bidentatae (*Niu Xi*), Radix Stephaniae Tetrandrae (*Fang Ji*), Caulis Akebiae Mutong (*Mu Tong*), and Cortex Phellodendri (*Huang Bai*).

---

[1] This is also known as painful *bi* or white tiger articular wind and is manifest by acute pain in the joints which is fixed and worsens with cold weather.

For blood vacuity, mostly use Rhizoma Ligustici Wallichii (*Chuan Xiong*) and Radix Angelicae Sinensis (*Dang Gui*) in large quantities. As assistants, (use) Semen Pruni Persicae (*Tao Ren*) and Flos Carthami Tinctorii (*Hong Hua*). In case of wind dampness, (use) Rhizoma Atractylodis (*Cang Zhu*), Rhizoma Atractylodis Macrocephalae (*Bai Zhu*), and the like plus qi-moving medicinals as assistants, such as Succus Bambusae (*Zhu Li*) and Succus Zingiberis (*Jiang Zhi*). In case of wind heat, (use) medicinals such as Radix Et Rhizoma Notopterygii (*Qiang Huo*) and Radix Ledebouriellae Sesloidis (*Fang Feng*) plus qi-moving medicinals as assistants. (And) in case of phlegm, (use) *Er Chen* (Two Aged [Decoction]) plus Rhizoma Arisaematis (*Nan Xing*), etc.

Herba Menthae (*Bo He*) and Ramulus Cinnamomi (*Gui Zhi*) treat painful wind. They are flavorless or thin (of flavor) and, (as such,) they are only able to penetrate throughout the hands and arms, leading Rhizoma Arisaematis (*Nan Xing*), Rhizoma Atractylodis (*Cang Zhu*), etc. to the painful places. In order to lead Rhizoma Arisaematis, Rhizoma Atractylodis, etc. downwards, use stir-fried Cortex Phellodendri (*Huang Bai*) in the treatment.

A formula for the treatment of painful wind in the upper, middle and lower (part of the body consists of) ginger-processed Rhizoma Arisaematis (*Nan Xing*), 2 *liang*, Rhizoma Ligustici Wallichii (*Tai Xiong*), 1 *liang*, Radix Angelicae (*Bai Zhi*), 5 *qian*, Semen Pruni Persicae (*Tao Ren*), 5 *qian*, Massa Medica Fermentata (*Shen Qu*), 3 *qian*, Ramulus Cinnamomi (*Gui Zhi*), 3 *qian*, which penetrates throughout the hand and arm, Radix Stephaniae Tetrandrae (*Han Fang Ji*), 5 *qian*, which goes downward, Radix Gentianae Scabrae (*Long Dan Cao*), 5 *qian*, which goes downward, Rhizoma Atractylodis (*Cang Zhu*), soaked with rice water overnight and stir-fried, 2 *liang*, wine-fried Cortex Phellodendri (*Huang Bai*), 1 *liang*, wine-washed Flos Carthami Tinctorii (*Hong Hua*), 1 *qian*, Radix Et Rhizoma Notopterygii (*Qiang Huo*), 3 *qian*, which travels throughout and penetrates all the joints in the body, [A {variant} version gives {this ingredient} at 3 *liang*. {later editor}], and wine-washed (and) stemmed Radix Clematidis Chinensis (*Wei Ling Xian*), 3 *qian*, which goes upward. Powder the above, make into pills with Massa Medica Fermentata (*Shen Qu*) paste, and take 100 pills with boiled water before a meal.

Zhang Zi-yuan's[2] formula treats painful wind with dual vacuity of the qi and blood, existence of phlegm, turbid urine, and yin fire. (It consists of) Radix Panacis Ginseng (*Ren Shen*), 1 *liang*, Rhizoma Atractylodis Macrocephalae (*Bai Zhu*), 2 *liang*, prepared Radix Rehmanniae (*Shu Di Huang*), 2 *liang*, Radix Dioscoreae Oppositae (*Shan Yao*), 1 *liang*, good quality Pumice (*Hai Shi*), 1 *liang*, Cortex Phellodendri (*Huang Bai*), stir-fried to black, 2 *liang*, Herba Cynomorii Songarici (*Suo Yang*), 5 *qian*, Rhizoma Arisaematis (*Nan Xing*), 1 *liang*, wine-fried vanquished (*i.e.*, processed) Plastrum Testudinis (*Bai Gui Ban*), 2 *liang* and, dry Rhizoma Zingiberis (*Gan Jiang*), 5 *qian*, ash-burnt to rid it of its penetrating nature. Powder the above, make into pills with gruel, and take.

A formula for painful wind (consists of) 1 cup of glutinous rice, a handful of Radix Rhododendri Mollei (*Huang Zhi Zhu Gen*), and one half cupful of black soybeans (*Hei Dou*). Boil the above in 1 bowl each of wine and water and take little by little. If violent vomiting and violent diarrhea (are induced), do not take a second dose, and one's ability to move about will be restored. *Kong Xian Dan* (Control Drool Elixir) treats migratory pain all over the body, including the lateral costal regions. In case of phlegm embracing dead blood, add smashed Semen Pruni Persicae (*Tao Ren*) and make into pills. In case of phlegm with damp heat, first administer *Zhou Che Wan* (Boat & Coach Pills)[3]

---

[2] A.k.a. Zhang Zi-he; see Note 21, Ch. 1, Bk. 1.

[3] This consists of Radix Et Rhizoma Rhei (*Da Huang*), 2 *liang*, Radix Euphorbiae Kansui (*Gan Sui*), Herba Cirsii Japonici (*Da Ji*), Flos Daphnis Genkwae (*Yuan Hua*), Pericarpium Viridis Citri Reticulatae (*Qing Pi*), and Pericarpium Citri Reticulatae (*Chen Pi*), 1 *liang* for each of the above, Semen Pharbitidis (*Qian Niu Zi*), 4 *liang*, and Radix Saussureae Seu Vladimiriae (*Mu Xiang*), one half *liang*.

or the water-conducting *Shen Xiong Wan* (Divine Ligusticum Pills).[4] Afterwards, administer *Chen Tong San* (Soothe Pain Powder). The ingredients in that formula are Gummum Olibani (*Ru Xiang*), Myrrha (*Mo Yao*), Semen Pruni Persicae (*Tao Ren*), Flos Carthami Tinctorii (*Hong Hua*), Radix Angelicae Sinensis (*Dang Gui*), Radix Rehmanniae (*Di Huang*), wine-fried Feces Trogopterori Seu Pteromi (*Wu Ling Zhi*), winesoaked Radix Achyranthis Bidentatae (*Niu Xi*), Radix Et Rhizoma Notopterygii (*Qiang Huo*), Rhizoma Cyperi Rotundi (*Xiang Fu*), and urinesoaked Radix Glycyrrhizae (*Sheng Gan Cao*). In case of phlegm heat, (add) wine-processed Radix Scutellariae Baicalensis (*Huang Qin*) and wine-processed Cortex Phellodendri (*Huang Bai*). Powder the above and take 2 *qian* brewed with wine.

Er Miao San (Two Miracles Powder) treats aching and pain in the sinews and bones due to the existence of heat and dampness. In case of qi (depression), add qi(-moving) medicinals. In case of blood vacuity, add blood-supplementing medicinals. In case of severe pain, it is necessary to take this with heated, pungent, native juice[5] from Rhizoma Zingiberis (*Jiang*. This formula consists of) stir-fried Cortex Phellodendri (*Huang Bai*) and stir-fried Rhizoma Atractylodis (*Cang Zhu*). Strip off the skin and powder. Grind Rhizoma Zingiberis (*Jiang*), put in boiling water, boil with the above two ingredients, and take. These two ingredients are both possessed of vigorous and dynamic qi. In case of exterior repletion, add a small amount of wine as an assistant.

Long Hu Dan (Dragon Tiger Elixir) treats migratory aches and pain, numbness and paraplegia, or hemilateral pain: Rhizoma Atractylodis (*Cang Zhu*), 1 *liang*, Radix Angelicae (*Bai Zhi*), 1 *liang*, Radix Aconiti (*Cao Wu*), 1 *liang*, the above three powdered coarsely, dampened with water, fermented (*fa re*, literally, giving off heat) in a container before

---

[4] This consists of Radix Et Rhizoma Rhei (*Da Huang*), Radix Scutellariae Baicalensis (*Huang Qin*), Talcum (*Hua Shi*), and Semen Pharbitidis (*Qian Niu Zi*). Note that this formula does not actually include Rhizoma Ligustici Wallichii (*Chuan Xiong*).

[5] So-called native juice is juice not mixed with water.

use, Gummum Olibani (*Ru Xiang*), 2 *qian*, Myrrha (*Mo Yao*), 2 *qian*, Radix Angelicae Sinensis (*Dang Gui*), 5 *qian*, and Radix Achyranthis Bidentatae (*Niu Xi*), 5 *qian*. Powder all the above, make into pills the size of pellets with wine paste, dissolve in warm wine, and take.

Ba Zhen Wan (Eight Pearls Pills) treat all kinds of painful wind, foot qi, and head wind. (They consist of) Gummum Olibani (*Ru Xiang*), 3 *qian*, Myrrha (*Mo Yao*), 3 *qian*, Hematitum (*Dai Zhe Shi*), 3 *qian*, Squama Manitis (*Chuan Shan Jia*), 3 *qian* used raw, Radix Aconiti (*Chuan Wu*) from Sichuan, 1 *liang*, with the skin and tips preserved and used raw, wild Radix Aconiti (*Cao Wu Tou*), 5 *qian*, with skins and tips preserved and used raw, Radix Et Rhizoma Notopterygii (*Qiang Huo*), 5 *qian*, and dried Buthus Martensi (*Quan Xie*), 21 pieces, intact with head and tail preserved. Powder the above and make into pills the size of Chinese parasol tree seeds with vinegar paste; 11 pills per dose.

To treat painful wind migratory pain, (use) wine-fried Cortex Phellodendri (*Huang Bai*), 2 *qian*, and wine-fried Rhizoma Atractylodis (*Cang Zhu*), 2 *qian*. (Take) all the above as one dose, powder and boil ready for use. Obtain powdered Radix Clematidis Chinensis (*Wei Ling Xian*) as the sovereign, carbonized Cornu Caprae Hircis (*Yang Jiao Hui*) as the minister, Herba Xanthii Sibirici (*Cang Er*) as the assistant, and Semen Sinapis Albae (*Jie Zi*) as the envoy. Put 1 slice of ginger into 1 *qian* of the powder, pound finely, and take with the above decoction warm.

For painful wind damp aching due to drinking of wine, (use) wine-fried Cortex Phellodendri (*Huang Bai*), 5 *fen*, powdered wine-fried Radix Clematidis Chinensis (*Wei Ling Xian*), 5 *fen*, stir-fried Rhizoma Atractylodis (*Cang Zhu*), 2 *qian*, Pericarpium Citri Reticulatae (*Chen Pi*), 1 *qian*, Radix Paeoniae Lactiflorae (*Shao Yao*), 1 *qian*, Radix Glycyrrhizae (*Gan Cao*), 3 *qian*, and Radix Et Rhizoma Notopterygii (*Qiang Huo*), 2 *qian*. Powder the above and take.

Post-dysentery flaccid feet with pain in the bones and swollen knees is (due to) collapse of yin. Rhizoma Ligustici Wallichii (*Chuan Xiong*), Radix Angelicae Sinensis (*Dang Gui*), Radix Rehmanniae (*Di Huang*), and other such supplementing medicinals are appropriate for treating this. In case of qi vacuity, add Radix Panacis Ginseng (*Ren Shen*) and

Radix Astragali Membranacei (*Huang Qi*). In case of embraced wind dampness, add Radix Et Rhizoma Notopterygii (*Qiang Huo*), Radix Ledebouriellae Sesloidis (*Fang Feng*), Rhizoma Atractylodis Macrocephalae (*Bai Zhu*), etc. If this is treated as wind, yin will be dried contrarily.

A formula for pain in the joints of the bones with qi repletion and exterior repletion (consists of) Talcum (*Hua Shi*), 6 *qian*, Radix Glycyrrhizae (*Gan Cao*), 1 *qian*, Rhizoma Cyperi Rotundi (*Xiang Fu*), 3 *qian*, and Radix Scutellariae Baicalensis (*Pian Qin*), 3 *qian*. Powder the above and make into pills with Succus Zingiberis (*Jiang Zhi*) paste. To treat pain in the shoulder and leg with food accumulation, (use) wine-processed Plastrum Testudinis (*Gui Ban*), 1 *liang*, wine-processed Folium Campsis Grandiflorae (*Ling Xiao Ye*), 5 *qian*, Rhizoma Cyperi Rotundi (*Xiang Fu*), 5 *qian*, hot (*i.e.*, acrid, pungent) Semen Sinapis Albae (*Jie Zi*), and *Ling Bai Hua* (identification unknown; possibly a typographical error since there is no amount given [trans.]). Make into pills with wine-paste. Take with a decoction of *Si Wu Tang* (Four Materials Decoction) plus Pericarpium Citri Reticulatae (*Chen Pi*) and Radix Glycyrrhizae (*Gan Cao*).

In terms of the treatment of swelling and pain in the joints of the limbs, because pain is ascribed to fire and swelling to dampness, (this) is a disease caused by damp heat. Moreover, because of external contraction of wind cold which launches (an offensive) and stirs inside the channels and connecting vessels, damp heat streams endlessly into the joints of the limbs. (For this, use) Rhizoma Atractylodis (*Cang Zhu*), 5 *fen*, Herba Ephedrae (*Ma Huang*), 1 *qian*, stripped of its roots and joints, Radix Ledebouriellae Sesloidis (*Fang Feng*), 5 *fen*, Herba Seu Flos Schizonepetae Tenuifoliae (*Jing Jie Sui*), 5 *fen*, Radix Et Rhizoma Notopterygii (*Qiang Huo*), 5 *fen*, Radix Angelicae Duhuo (*Du Huo*), 5 *fen*, Radix Angelicae (*Bai Zhi*), 5 *fen*, hair of Radix Angelicae Sinensis (*Gui Xu*), 3 *fen*, Radix Rubrus Paeoniae Lactiflorae (*Chi Shao*), 1 *qian*, Radix Clematidis Chinensis (*Wei Ling Xian*), 5 *fen*, Radix Scutellariae Baicalensis (*Pian Qin*), 5 *fen*, Fructus Immaturus Citri Seu Ponciri (*Zhi Shi*), 5 *fen*, Radix Platycodi Grandiflori (*Jie Geng*), 5 *fen*, Radix Puerariae Lobatae (*Ge Gen*), 5 *fen*, Rhizoma Ligustici Wallichii (*Chuan Xiong*), 5 *fen*, Radix Glycyrrhizae (*Gan Cao*), 3 *fen*, and Rhizoma Cimicifugae

(*Sheng Ma*), 3 *fen*. Boil the above and take. If the disease is located below, add wine-fried Cortex Phellodendri (*Huang Bai*). For females, add wine-processed Flos Carthami Tinctorii (*Hong Hua*). In case of much swelling, add Semen Arecae Catechu (*Bing Lang*), Pericarpium Arecae (*Da Fu Pi*), and Rhizoma Alismatis (*Ze Xie*). Take before a meal. This (formula) is particularly remarkable if 1 *qian* of Myrrha (*Mo Yao*), which can settle the pain, is added.

For aching pain and wind dampness all over the body, (use) Radix Clematidis Chinensis (*Wei Ling Xian*), 1 *qian*, Radix Rubrus Paeoniae Lactiflorae (*Chi Shao Yao*), 1 *qian*, Herba Ephedrae (*Ma Huang*), stripped of its joints, 1 *qian*, Radix Et Rhizoma Notopterygii (*Qiang Huo*), Radix Angelicae Duhuo (*Du Huo*), hair of Radix Angelicae Sinensis (*Gui Xu*), Rhizoma Ligustici Wallichii (*Chuan Xiong*), Radix Ledebouriellae Sesloidis (*Fang Feng*), Radix Angelicae (*Bai Zhi*), and Radix Saussureae Seu Vladimiriae (*Mu Xiang*), 1.5 *qian* for each of the above, Rhizoma Atractylodis (*Cang Zhu*), 1 *qian*, Semen Pruni Persicae (*Tao Ren*), 7 pieces, and Radix Glycyrrhizae (*Gan Cao*), 3 *fen*. Boil the above and take.

For vexing pain in the joints of the limbs, heavy shoulder and upper back, inhibited chest and diaphragm, aching pain all over the body, and (dampness) streaming down into the feet and lower legs causing swelling and pain, (use) *Dang Gui Nian Tong Tang* (*Dang Gui* Stifle Pain Decoction).[6]

In deep autumn, a male, aged 36 and a farmer by occupation living in poverty, suddenly had body heat with pain in the upper and lower arms, wrists, feet, and hips as if being burnt in a furnace. (This) would

---

[6] This consists of Rhizoma Atractylodis Macrocephalae (*Bai Zhu*), 1.5 *qian*, Radix Panacis Ginseng (*Ren Shen*), wine-fried Radix Sophorae Flavescentis (*Ku Shen*), Rhizoma Cimicifugae (*Sheng Ma*), Radix Puerariae Lobatae (*Ge Gen*), and Rhizoma Alismatis (*Ze Xie*), 2 *qian* for each of the above, Radix Ledebouriellae Sesloidis (*Fang Feng*), wine-washed Rhizoma Anemarrhenae (*Zhi Mu*), Rhizoma Alismatis (*Ze Xie*), stir-fried Radix Scutellariae Baicalensis (*Huang Qin*), Sclerotium Polypori Umbellati (*Zhu Ling*), Radix Angelicae Sinensis (*Dang Gui*), 3 *qian* for each of the above, mix-fried Radix Glycyrrhizae (*Zhi Gan Cao*), wine-fried Herba Artemisiae Capillaris (*Yin Chen*), and Radix Et Rhizoma Notopterygii (*Qiang Huo*), 3 *qian* for each of the above.

abate during the day but got worse at night. The (attending) physician administered wind medicinals only which made his pain worse. Blood medicinals (also) proved ineffective. (The patient) was just waiting for death. The pulses on both hands were choppy and rapid, worse on the right hand than on the left. (His) food intake was normal and his form was wirily emaciated due to the pain. (I) prescribed Rhizoma Atractylodis (*Cang Zhu*), 1.5 *qian*, Radix Aconiti (*Sheng Fu*), 1 slice, Radix Glycyrrhizae (*Sheng Gan Cao*), 2 *qian*, Herba Ephedrae (*Ma Huang*), 5 *fen*, ground Semen Pruni Persicae (*Tao Ren*), 9 pieces, and wine-processed Cortex Phellodendri (*Huang Bai*), 1.5 *qian*. All the above (should be taken) as one dose, boiled with a little Succus Zingiberis (*Jiang Zhi*) put in to make (the decoction) pungent. After 4 doses were administered, Radix Aconiti was deleted and 1 *qian* of Radix Achyranthis Bidentatae (*Niu Xi*) was added. Eight doses later, there arose qi ascension rapid dyspneic breathing with inability to sleep, but the pain was improved. (I) thought that the blood vacuity must be the result of taking excessive Herba Ephedrae and (that consequently) yang had become vacuous and dwindled, stirring and running upwards.

(Therefore,) it was necessary to supplement the blood to settle (yang). Then (I) prescribed *Si Wu Tang*, subtracting Rhizoma Ligustici Wallichii (*Chuan Xiong*) but adding 5 *qian* of Radix Panacis Ginseng (*Ren Shen*) and 12 pieces of Fructus Schizandrae Chinensis (*Wu Wei Zi*) to astringe and collect the upward counterflow of qi with its sour flavor. This was taken as one dose and, following another dose, the dyspnea was settled and (the qi) became quiet. Three days later, the pulse reduced by more than a half in terms of its rapidness but still remained as choppy as before. When asked, the patient said that the pain was not improved. However, his groan was heard no more. On examination, his qi seemed weak, but he himself said otherwise. Then (I) added Radix Achyranthis Bidentatae (*Niu Xi*), Rhizoma Atractylodis Macrocephalae (*Bai Zhu*), Radix Panacis Ginseng (*Ren Shen*), Semen Pruni Persicae (*Tao Ren*), Pericarpium Citri Reticulatae (*Chen Pi*), Radix Glycyrrhizae (*Gan Cao*), and Semen Arecae Catechu (*Bing Lang*) to *Si Wu Tang*. These were boiled with 3 slices of fresh Rhizoma Zingiberis (*Sheng Jiang*). After taking 50 doses, recovery was affected. (Later) the pain recurred with reduced food intake as a result of lifting weights. The same formula was prescribed with 3 *qian* of Radix Astragali

Membranacei (*Huang Qi*) added and, not till another 10 doses were taken, was complete recovery realized.

In most cases, painful wind is due to blood subjected to heat. An old person with quick temper taxed himself and (therefore) suffered from severe pain in the legs. A woman who (also) had quick temper and (lived on) thick flavors suffered from painful wind for several months. A young person had dysentery and then took astringing medicinals resulting in painful wind. [All these are discussed in the *Yi Yao* {*Essentials of Medicine*. later editor}]. A person who suffered from pain in the heels and had phlegm and blood heat was treated with *Si Wu Tang* plus Cortex Phellodendri (*Huang Bai*), Rhizoma Anemarrhenae (*Zhi Mu*), Radix Achyranthis Bidentatae (*Niu Xi*), etc. For body vacuity itching and pain, (use) *Si Wu Tang* plus Radix Scutellariae Baicalensis (*Huang Qin*). Boil and take with powdered Folium Spirodelae Polyrrhizae (*Fu Ping*).

In treating painful wind, treatment should vary depending on whether it is in the upper or lower (part of the body). For that due to wind, *Xiao Xu Ming Tang* (Minor Reinforce Destiny Decoction) is extremely effective. That due to dampness (requires) Rhizoma Atractylodis (*Cang Zhu*), Rhizoma Atractylodis Macrocephalae (*Bai Zhu*), and the like with qi-moving medicinals as assistants. For that due to phlegm, *Er Chen Tang* should be used with additions and subtractions.

The various kinds of itching are ascribed to vacuity. Itching arises because the blood fails to nurture the muscle interstices. (Therefore,) it is necessary to introduce enriching and supplementing medicinals to nourish yin blood. When blood becomes harmonious in the muscle interstices, itching automatically stops.

Chapter Fifty

Food Damage

Aversion to food is (due to some) substance retained in the chest. (To treat this,) conduct phlegm and supplement the spleen with *Er Chen Tang* (Two Aged Decoction) plus Rhizoma Atractylodis Macrocephalae (*Bai Zhu*), Fructus Crataegi (*Shan Zha*), Rhizoma Ligustici Wallichii (*Chuan Xiong*), and Rhizoma Atractylodis (*Cang Zhu*. However,) damage by drink and food (requires) strengthening the stomach and dispersing food. For qi vacuity, (use) *Zhi Zhu Wan* (Immature Aurantium & Atractylodes Pills).[1] In case of wine causing a disease of vomiting and retching or abdominal distention, use *Ge Hua Jie Cheng Tang* (Kudzu Blossom Resolve Hangover Decoction).[2] In case of repeated damage by drink and food giving rise to glomus and fullness with inability to take in food, (use) *Kuan Zhong Jin Shi Wan* (Loose the Center & Promote Food Intake Pills).[3]

---

[1] This consists of Fructus Immaturus Citri Seu Ponciri (*Zhi Shi*) stir-fried with bran, 1 *liang*, and Rhizoma Atractylodis Macrocephalae (*Bai Zhu*), 2 *liang*. Make into pills with rice cooked with lotus leaves as a wrapping.

[2] This consists of Radix Saussureae Seu Vladimiriae (*Mu Xiang*), 5 *fen*, Pericarpium Citri Reticulatae (*Ju Pi*), Radix Panacis Ginseng (*Ren Shen*), Sclerotium Polypori Umbellati (*Zhu Ling*), and Sclerotium Poriae Cocoris (*Fu Ling*), 1.5 *qian*, stir-fried Massa Medica Fermentata (*Shen Qu*), Rhizoma Alismatis (*Ze Xie*), dry Rhizoma Zingiberis (*Gan Jiang*), and Rhizoma Atractylodis Macrocephalae (*Bai Zhu*), 2 *qian* for each of the above, Pericarpium Viridis Citri Reticulatae (*Qing Pi*), 3 *qian*, Fructus Cardamomi (*Bai Dou Kou Ren*), Fructus Amomi (*Sha Ren*), and Flos Puerariae Lobatae (*Ge Hua*), 5 *qian* for each of the above.

[3] This consists of vinegar-calcined Hematitum (*Dai Zhe Shi*), slightly stir-fried Radix Angelicae Sinensis (*Dang Gui*), water-ground Cinnabar (*Zhu Sha*), bran-fried Fructus Citri Seu Ponciri (*Zhi Qiao*), and Radix Saussureae Seu Vladimiriae (*Mu Xiang*), one half *liang* for each of the above, Secretio Moschi Moschiferi (*She Xiang*), 1 *fen*, and Pulvis Semenis Crotonis (*Ba Dou Shuang*), one half *fen*.

A person was frequently feverish due to wine and meat. (They were prescribed) Pulvis Indigonis (*Qing Dai*), Semen Trichosanthis Kirlowii (*Gua Lou Ren*), and Succus Zingiberis (*Jiang Zhi*). These three flavors (*i.e.*, ingredients) were powdered (and) a number of spoonfuls were taken each day. Recovery occurred (after) three days.

An(other) person who suffered from internal damage with vomiting of blood, fever, and headache as a result of (over)eating wheat flour (products) was prescribed Rhizoma Atractylodis Macrocephalae (*Bai Zhu*), 1.5 *qian*, Radix Albus Paeoniae Lactiflorae (*Bai Shao Yao*), 1 *qian*, Pericarpium Citri Reticulatae (*Chen Pi*), 1 *qian*, Rhizoma Atractylodis (*Cang Zhu*), 1 *qian*, Sclerotium Poriae Cocoris (*Fu Ling*), 5 *fen*, Rhizoma Coptidis Chinensis (*Huang Lian*), 5 *fen*, Radix Scutellariae Baicalensis (*Huang Qin*), 5 *fen*, Radix Panacis Ginseng (*Ren Shen*), 5 *fen*, and Radix Glycyrrhizae (*Gan Cao*), 5 *fen*. The above, all as one dose, were boiled with 3 slices of Rhizoma Zingiberis (*Jiang*). In case of thirst, add 2 *qian* of Radix Puerariae Lobatae (*Ge Gen*). To regulate and rectify (the stomach) further, (prescribe) Rhizoma Atractylodis Macrocephalae (*Bai Zhu*), 1.5 *qian*, Radix Achyranthis Bidentatae (*Niu Xi*), 2.5 *qian*, Pericarpium Citri Reticulatae, 1.5 *qian*, Radix Panacis Ginseng, 1 *qian*, Radix Albus Paeoniae Lactiflorae (*Bai Shao Yao*), 1 *qian*, Radix Glycyrrhizae (*Gan Cao*), 2 *fen*, and Sclerotium Poriae Cocoris (*Fu Ling*), 5 *fen*. To regulate (and rectify) the stomach still further, (use) Rhizoma Atractylodis Macrocephalae (*Bai Zhu*), 2 *qian*, Radix Albus Paeoniae Lactiflorae (*Bai Shao Yao*), 1.5 *qian*, Radix Panacis Ginseng (*Ren Shen*), 1 *qian*, Radix Angelicae Sinensis (*Dang Gui*), 1 *qian*, stir-fried Pericarpium Citri Reticulatae (*Chen Pi*), 1 *qian*, Radix Scutellariae Baicalensis (*Huang Qin*), 5 *fen*, Radix Bupleuri (*Chai Hu*), 3 *fen*, Rhizoma Cimicifugae (*Sheng Ma*), 2 *fen*, and Radix Glycyrrhizae (*Gan Cao*), a small amount.

(Yet) an(other) person, as a result of eating wheat flour (products), suffered from generalized aching and fever with coughing and phlegm. (They) were prescribed Rhizoma Atractylodis (*Cang Zhu*), 1.5 *qian*, Pericarpium Citri Reticulatae (*Chen Pi*), 1 *qian*, Rhizoma Pinelliae Ternatae (*Ban Xia*), 1 *qian*, Radix Et Rhizoma Notopterygii (*Qiang Huo*), 5 *fen*, Sclerotium Poriae Cocoris (*Fu Ling*), 5 *fen*, Radix Ledebouriellae Sesloidis (*Fang Feng*), 5 *fen*, Radix Scutellariae Baicalensis (*Huang Qin*), 5 *fen*, Rhizoma Ligustici Wallichii (*Chuan Xiong*), 5 *fen*, and Radix

Glycyrrhizae (*Gan Cao*), 2 *fen*. The above, all as one dose, were boiled with 3 slices of ginger and taken (while) half full, half hungry, (*i.e.*, between meals).

(And still) an(other) person of advanced age suffered from retching and vomiting of phlegm and rheum, great fullness of the chest, and (alternating) cold and heat arising as a result of food damage. (They were prescribed) Rhizoma Pinelliae Ternatae (*Ban Xia*), Pericarpium Citri Reticulatae (*Chen Pi*), and Sclerotium Poriae Cocoris (*Fu Ling*) to conduct rheum, Rhizoma Atractylodis Macrocephalae (*Bai Zhu*) to supplement the spleen, Radix Bupleuri (*Chai Hu*), Radix Glycyrrhizae (*Sheng Gan Cao*), and Radix Scutellariae Baicalensis (*Huang Qin*) to abate cold and heat, Rhizoma Atractylodis (*Cang Zhu*) added to dissipate exterior cold, and Fructus Amomi (*Suo Sha Ren*) to settle retching and precipitate qi.

A formula for food damage (consists of) Fructus Crataegi (*Tang Qiu*), 3 *liang*, Rhizoma Pinelliae Ternatae (*Ban Xia*), 1 *liang*, Sclerotium Poriae Cocoris (*Fu Ling*), 1 *liang*, Fructus Forsythiae Suspensae (*Lian Qiao*), 5 *qian*, Pericarpium Citri Reticulatae (*Chen Pi*), 5 *qian*, and Semen Raphani Sativi (*Lai Fu Zi*), 5 *qian*. Make the above into pills with gruel and take.

Chapter Fifty-one

Glomus

Fullness below the heart without pain is called glomus. For glomus below the heart due to food accumulation complicated by dampness, use Fructus Immaturus Citri Seu Ponciri (*Zhi Shi*) and Rhizoma Coptidis Chinensis (*Huang Lian*). If glomus embracing phlegm develops into a gathering mass, use Semen Pruni Persicae (*Tao Ren*), Flos Carthami Tinctorii (*Hong Hua*), Rhizoma Cyperi Rotundi (*Xiang Fu*), Radix Et Rhizoma Rhei (*Da Huang*), and the like. For glomus arising below the heart following eating, (use) *Ju Pi Zhi Zhu Wan* (Orange Peel, Immature Aurantium & Atractylodes Pills).[1]

A formula to treat glomus fullness (consists of) wine-soaked Radix Scutellariae Baicalensis (*Huang Qin*), 1 *liang*, wine-soaked Cortex Phellodendri (*Huang Bai*), 1 *liang*, Talcum (*Hua Shi*), 5 *qian*, and Radix Glycyrrhizae (*Gan Cao*), 2 *qian*. Powder the above and make into pills with water. (However, for) not eating or sleeping from the noon till night, (use) *Zhi Pi Zhi Zhu Wan* (Treat Glomus Immature Aurantium & Atractylodes Pills): Rhizoma Atractylodis Macrocephalae (*Bai Zhu*), 2 *liang*, Fructus Immaturus Citri Seu Ponciri (*Zhi Shi*), 1 *liang*, Rhizoma Pinelliae Ternatae (*Ban Xia*), 1 *liang*, Massa Medica Fermentata (*Shen Qu*), 1 *liang*, Fructus Germinatus Hordei Vulgaris (*Mai Ya*), 1 *liang*, Fructus Crataegi (*Shan Zha*), 1 *liang*, Rhizoma Curcumae (*Jiang Huang*), 5 *qian*, Pericarpium Citri Reticulatae (*Chen Pi*), 5 *qian*, and Radix Saussureae Seu Vladimiriae (*Mu Xiang*), 2.5 *qian*. Powder the above and make into pills with rice cooked with lotus leaves as a wrapping. In addition, *Zhi Zhu Wan* assist the stomach in dispersing food and loosen the center to rid glomus fullness. (These consist of) Rhizoma Atractylodis Macrocephalae (*Bai Zhu*), 4 *liang*, and Fructus Immaturus Citri Seu Ponciri (*Zhi Shi*), 2 *liang*. Powder and make into pills with rice cooked with lotus leaves as a wrapping.

Da Xiao Pi Wan (Major Disperse Glomus Pills, consist of) stir-fried Rhizoma Coptidis Chinensis (*Huang Lian*), 6 *qian*, Radix Scutellariae Baicalensis (*Huang Qin*), 6 *qian*, Rhizoma Curcumae (*Jiang Huang*), 1 *liang*, Rhizoma Atractylodis Macrocephalae (*Bai Zhu*), 1 *liang*, Radix Panacis Ginseng (*Ren Shen*) and Pericarpium Citri Reticulatae (*Chen Pi*), 2 *qian* each, Rhizoma Alismatis (*Ze Xie*), 2 *qian*, mix-fried Radix Glycyrrhizae (*Zhi Gan Cao*) and Fructus Amomi (*Sha Ren*), 1 *qian* each, fresh Rhizoma Zingiberis (*Sheng Jiang*), 1 *qian*, stir-fried Massa Medica Fermentata (*Shen Qu*), 1 *qian*, stir-fried Fructus Immaturus Citri Seu Ponciri (*Zhi Shi*), 1 *qian*, Rhizoma Pinelliae Ternatae (*Ban Xia*), 4 *qian*,

---

[1] This consists of Rhizoma Atractylodis Macrocephalae (*Bai Zhu*), 2 *liang*, and Pericarpium Citri Reticulatae (*Ju Pi*) and Fructus Immaturus Citri Seu Ponciri (*Zhi Shi*), 1 *liang* each.

Cortex Magnoliae Officinalis (*Hou Po*), 3 *qian*, and Sclerotium Polypori Umbellati (*Zhu Ling*), 1.5 *qian*. Powder the above and make into pills with steamed cake.

For repeated damage by drink and food giving rise to enduring fullness and inability to take in food, use *Kuan Zhong Jin Shi Wan* (Loosen the Center & Promote Food Intake Pills. But for) glomus below the heart, use (the above) *Xiao Pi Wan* (Disperse Glomus Pills). Lack of hunger (long) after eating is ascribed to cold in any case. This is due to decrepit *wu* earth[2] which is unable to putrefy (*i.e.*, ferment) and cook water and grains. (For this) use *Ding Xiang Lan Fan Wan* (Clove Well-Done Pills).[3] For spleen damaged by summer depression[4] with no desire for food, (use) stir-fried Rhizoma Coptidis Chinensis (*Huang Lian*), wine-processed Radix Paeoniae Lactiflorae (*Shao Yao*), powdered Herba Typhae Angustatae (*Sheng Suo*), and *Qing Liu* (Cyan Six [Pills]) in powdered form. Make into pills with Succus Zingiberis (*Jiang Zhi*) cake.

For damp phlegm and qi stagnation with no liking for grains, (use) *San Bu Wan* (Three Supplement Pills) with Rhizoma Atractylodis (*Cang Zhu*) added and Rhizoma Cyperi Rotundi (*Xiang Fu*) in double amount, (while) *Hui Ling Wan* (Reverse the Season Pills) drain liver fire, move dampness which generates heat, and are even able to open glomus bind. As an indirect assistant, (they are also able) to treat liver evils and supplement the spleen. (They are composed of) Rhizoma

---

[2] According to the five phase theory, *wu*, S5 or the fifth heavenly stem, is associated with earth. Thus, TCM doctors often use *wu* earth as a compound to refer to the earth phase.

[3] This consists of Flos Caryophylli (*Ding Xiang*), Rhizoma Curcumae Zedoariae (*Peng E Zhu*), Rhizoma Sparganii (*San Leng*), Radix Saussureae Seu Vladimiriae (*Mu Xiang*), Radix Glycyrrhizae (*Gan Cao*), Radix Seu Rhizoma Nardostachys Chinensis (*Gan Song*), Fructus Alpiniae Oxyphyllae (*Yi Zhi*), Pericarpium Citri Reticulatae (*Guang Pi*), Fructus Amomi (*Sha Ren*), and Rhizoma Cyperi Rotundi (*Xiang Fu*). Grind finely, soak in water, steam, and make into pills.

[4] This refers to overwhelming damp heat in summer.

Coptidis Chinensis (*Huang Lian*), 6 *liang*, and Fructus Evodiae Rutecarpae (*Wu Zhu Yu*), 1 *liang*. Powder the above and make into pills with gruel.

A person suffered from excessive food accumulation internally with constant inflating distention in the cardiac and abdominal regions. (They were prescribed) ginger-processed Rhizoma Arisaematis (*Nan Xing*), Trichosanthes-processed Rhizoma Pinelliae Ternatae (*Ban Xia*), 1.5 *liang*, the processing method (consisting of) moistening (the Pinellia) with ground Fructus Trichosanthis Kirlowii (*Gua Lou Ren*), Rhizoma Cyperi Rotundi (*Xiang Fu*), soaked with child's urine, 1 *liang*, Chlorite Schist (*Qing Meng Shi*), calcined with Nitre (*Xiao*), 1 *liang*, steamed Semen Raphani Sativi (*Luo Fu Zi*), 5 *qian*, Pericarpium Citri Rubri (*Ju Hong*), 5 *qian*, and a tiny amount of Secretio Moschi Moschiferi (*She Xiang*). Powder the above and make into pills with Massa Medica Fermentata (*Shen Qu*) paste.

An alcoholic suffered from great fullness of the stomach, fever, and delirious speech (during sleep) at night. (This was) a quasi-cold damage (pattern). Their pulse was less large on the right hand than on the left. (They were prescribed) *Bu Zhong Yi Qi Tang* (Supplement the Center & Boost the Qi Decoction) with Radix Astragali Membranacei (*Huang Qi*), Radix Bupleuri (*Chai Hu*), and Rhizoma Cimicifugae (*Sheng Ma*) removed and Rhizoma Pinelliae Ternatae (*Ban Xia*) added. The reason for these subtractions is that Radix Astragali Membranacei supplements, resulting in (even more) fullness, while Radix Bupleuri and Rhizoma Cimicifugae are capable of upbearing. After recovery thanks to the administration of this formula, heart pain arose as a result of eating cold food. (Based on this,) several grains of Semen Alpiniae Katsumadai (*Cao Dou Kou*) were added to the above formula.

A female suffered from glomus bind, inflating distention (of the abdomen) with block, and restlessness whether sitting or lying down. (She) was administered powdered Fructus Germinatus Hordei Vulgaris (*Mai Ya*) brewed with wine. (Eventually, the qi) freed itself after a long time.

Chapter Fifty-two

Eructation

(This is due to) the existence of fire and phlegm in the stomach. Rhizoma Arisaematis (*Nan Xing*), Rhizoma Pinelliae Ternatae (*Ban Xia*), Rhizoma Cyperi Rotundi (*Xiang Fu*), and soft Gypsum (*Ruan Shi Gao*, should be) introduced into formulas for the treatment (of this condition). Take (in the form of) either decoction or pill. Another formula (consists of) stir-fried Fructus Gardeniae Jasminoidis (*Shan Zhi*). Belching and acid regurgitation are ascribed to food depression and the existence of heat with fire qi upsurging and stirring. (For this) use Radix Scutellariae Baicalensis (*Huang Qin*) as the sovereign, Rhizoma Arisaematis (*Nan Xing*) and Rhizoma Pinelliae Ternatae (*Ban Xia*) as the ministers, and Pericarpium Citri Rubri (*Ju Hong*) as the assistant. In case of abundant heat, add Pulvis Indigonis (*Qing Dai*).

Chapter Fifty-three

Acid Regurgitation

When damp heat has been depressed and has accumulated for a long (time) in the liver, it is unable to gush out on its own and is confined somewhere between the lungs and stomach. (In that case, one) must take coarse foods and vegetables to nurture oneself and use Fructus Evodiae Rutecarpae (*Zhu Yu*) to comply with the nature (of the disease)[1] in order to thwart it. This is a counterassisting method.

---

[1] Fructus Evodiae Rutecarpae (*Wu Zhu Yu*) is hot in qi and the cause of the disease is also heat. Therefore, according to the logic of TCM, this is a contrary treatment.

A formula (to treat) acid swallowing (consists of) Fructus Evodiae Rutecarpae (*Zhu Yu*), 5 *qian*, stemmed, boiled for a short time, soaked for half a day, and dried in the sun for use, Pericarpium Citri Reticulatae (*Chen Pi*), 5 *qian*, Rhizoma Atractylodis (*Cang Zhu*), 7.5 *qian*, soaked with rice water, Rhizoma Coptidis Chinensis (*Huang Lian*), 1 *liang*, stir-fried with old wall clay which is removed afterwards, and Radix Scutellariae Baicalensis (*Huang Qin*), 5 *qian*, also stir-fried with old wall clay which is removed afterwards. Powder the above and make into pills with Massa Medica Fermentata (*Shen Qu*) paste.

To treat acid regurgitation, use Rhizoma Coptidis Chinensis (*Huang Lian*) and Fructus Evodiae Rutecarpae (*Zhu Yu*), both stir-fried separately, as the assistant or envoy depending on the season[2], and Rhizoma Atractylodis (*Cang Zhu*) and Sclerotium Poriae Cocoris (*Fu Ling*) as the adjuncts. Soak with boiled water, prepare into cakes by steaming, make into small pills, and take. Still, one should take vegetables to nurture oneself. Then the disease will be easy to overcome.

Zhu Yu Wan (Evodia Pills) treat damp heat with qi (depression), and, in case of severe damp heat, they are used as a guide, treating acid regurgitation above and loosening the bowels below. (They are comprised of) 1 dose of *Liu Yi San* (Six To One Powder) with 1 *liang* of boiled Fructus Evodiae Rutecarpae (*Wu Zhu Yu*). There is (also) another formula in which Fructus Evodiae Rutecarpae is replaced by dry Rhizoma Zingiberis (*Gan Jiang*. This) is called *Wen Qing San* (Warm & Clear Pills). A (variant) formula (consists of) 7 *qian* of *Liu Yi San* and 3 *qian* of Fructus Evodiae Rutecarpae. It disperses phlegm.

For several years, a person suffered from intermittent retching and vomiting of acid water with inhibited defecation and rumbling intestines. (They were prescribed) Rhizoma Atractylodis Macrocephalae

---

[2] Rhizoma Coptidis Chinensis (*Huang Lian*) is cold in nature. Therefore, in summer which is a hot season, it should be used in large amounts as the assistant. Since Fructus Evodiae Rutecarpae (*Wu Zhu Yu*) is hot in nature, in the summer, it should be used in small amounts as the envoy. In winter, the relative proportions of these two ingredients should be reversed.

(*Bai Zhu*), Fructus Immaturus Citri Seu Ponciri (*Zhi Shi*), Fructus Evodiae Rutecarpae (*Zhu Yu*), Rhizoma Atractylodis (*Cang Zhu*), Fructus Amomi (*Suo Sha*), Pericarpium Citri Reticulatae (*Chen Pi*), Sclerotium Poriae Cocoris (*Fu Ling*), Rhizoma Cyperi Rotundi (*Xiang Fu*), Bulbus Fritillariae (*Bei Mu*), Radix Glycyrrhizae (*Sheng Gan Cao*), Fructus Cardamomi (*Bai Dou Kou*), and Talcum (*Hua Shi*). Boil the above and take.

Chapter Fifty-four

Clamoring Stomach

(This is due to) phlegm stirring because of fire with the (possible) existence of food and the existence of heat. Stir-fried Fructus Gardeniae Jasminoidis (*Zhi Zi*) and Ginger-fried Rhizoma Coptidis Chinensis (*Huang Lian*) are indispensable (medicinals). For the existence of heat in the venter, (use) stir-fried Fructus Gardeniae Jasminoidis (*Shan Zhi*) and Radix Scutellariae Baicalensis (*Huang Qin*) as the sovereigns and Rhizoma Arisaematis (*Nan Xing*), Rhizoma Pinelliae Ternatae (*Ban Xia*), Pericarpium Citri Reticulatae (*Chen Pi*), and Radix Glycyrrhizae (*Gan Cao*) as the assistants. In case of abundant heat, add Pulvis Indigonis (*Qing Dai*).

For clamoring stomach in fat people, the appropriate (medicinals) are *Er Chen* (Two Aged [Decoction]) plus Rhizoma Atractylodis (*Cang Zhu*), Rhizoma Atractylodis Macrocephalae (*Bai Zhu*), Fructus Gardeniae Jasminoidis (*Zhi Zi*), and Rhizoma Ligustici Wallichii (*Chuan Xiong*. But for) water cold qi in the cardiac region, abdomen, and middle venter with a clamoring stomach below the heart, rumbling intestines, frequent vomiting of clear water which runs out continually, acute distention and pain in the region of the free ribs, inability to take in food, and a wiry, slow, thin pulse, (use) *Ban Xia Wen Fei Tang* (Pinellia Warm the Lungs Decoction): Herba Cum Radice Asari Sieboldi (*Xi Xin*), Pericarpium Citri Reticulatae (*Chen Pi*), Rhizoma Pinelliae

Ternatae (*Ban Xia*), Cortex Cinnamomi (*Gui Xin*), Flos Inulae (*Xuan Fu Hua*), Radix Glycyrrhizae (*Gan Cao*), and Radix Platycodi Grandiflori (*Jie Geng*), 5 *qian* for each of the above, Pericarpium Rubrum Poriae Cocoris (*Chi Fu Ling*), 3 *qian*, Radix Paeoniae Lactiflorae (*Shao Yao*), 5 *qian*, and fresh Rhizoma Zingiberis (*Sheng Jiang*), 7 slices. The above is the ruling (formula) for treating stomach qi vacuity and cold.

Chapter Fifty-five

Consumption

This is an extreme yin vacuity (condition, as well as) a disease of phlegm and blood. Usually there are also worms (*i.e.*, parasites). Vacuity taxation with a thin body is ascribed to fire. This is a result of fire burning and wasting away (the flesh. If) there is severe desertion of flesh, it is difficult to treat. Those rejecting supplementation are (also) difficult to treat. The ruling method of treatment is to administer great supplementation with *Si Wu Tang* (Four Materials Decoction) plus Succus Bambusae (*Zhu Li*), child's urine, and Succus Zingiberis (*Jiang Zhi*). A (variant edition) adds stir-fried Cortex Phellodendri (*Huang Bai*. But for) yang vacuity, (use) *Si Jun Zi Tang* (Four Gentlemen Decoction) plus Tuber Ophiopogonis Japonicae (*Mai Dong*), Fructus Schizandrae Chinensis (*Wu Wei Zi*), Pericarpium Citri Reticulatae (*Chen Pi*), stir-fried Cortex Phellodendri (*Huang Bai*), Succus Bambusae (*Zhu Li*), child's urine, and Succus Zingiberis (*Jiang Zhi*).

Vacuity taxation is the product of accumulated heat. At the beginning when (the patient is still) strong, (Zhang) Zi-he's methods[1] can be employed. At the later stage when there is emaciation and fatigue,

---

[1] Zhang Zi-he was the founder of the School of Attack and Purgation. His three methods (*san fa*) consisted of diaphoresis, ejection, and precipitation.

(administer) *Si Wu Tang* with *Xiao Ji Wan* (Disperse Accumulation Pills)[2] with additions and subtractions. Heat assists the qi and is not the cause of yang vacuity. Steaming fever is most likely a disease of accumulation.

Among formulas to regulate the tripod[3], *Zi He Che Wan* (Placenta Pills)[4] treat cadaverous transmission consumption[5] and *Qing Hao Jian* (Artemisia Qinghao Decoction)[6] treats consumption. [The above two formulas are both given in the *Yi Yao* {*Essentials of Medicine* later editor}]. For cadaverous transmission consumption (manifested by) alternating attacks of cold and heat, enduring cough, hacking up of blood, and increasing emaciation, first administer *San Niu Tang* (Three Negatives Decoction) and then *Lian Xin San* (Lotus Seed Powder).[7]

---

[2] This consists of Flos Caryophylli (*Ding Xiang*), 9 pieces, Fructus Amomi (*Sha Ren*), 20 pieces, Fructus Pruni Mume (*Wu Mei Rou*), 3 pieces, and de-oiled Semen Crotonis (*Ba Dou*), 2 pieces.

[3] In ancient times, a tripod was a ceremonial appliance used on grave occasions, often as a container of burning incense. Hence, tripods also came to symbolize something burning or great heat itself. However, *tiao ding*, regulate the tripod, might also be the name of a formula, in which case its ingredients are unknown to the translator.

[4] The ingredients in this formula can be found in the text of Ch. 17, Bk. 1.

[5] The modern translation of this term is (pulmonary) tuberculosis. The translation, cadaverous transmission, however, implies the communicable nature of this disease.

[6] This formula consists of Herba Artemisiae Apiaceae (*Qing Hao*) and Carapax Amydae (*Bie Jia*), 2 *liang* each, Radix Gentianae Scabrae (*Long Dan Cao*), 3.5 *fen*, Fructus Gardeniae Jasminoidis (*Zhi Zi Ren*), and Rhizoma Anemarrhenae (*Zhi Mu*), 3 *fen* each, Rhizoma Coptidis Chinensis (*Huang Lian*), Radix Astragali Membranacei (*Huang Qi*), Cortex Radicis Mori Albi (*Sang Bai Pi*), and Rhizoma Atractylodis Macrocephalae (*Bai Zhu*), 1 *liang* for each of the above, Cortex Radicis Lycii (*Di Gu Pi*), mix-fried Radix Glycyrrhizae (*Zhi Gan Cao*), one half *liang* each, and Radix Bupleuri (*Chai Hu*), 1.5 *liang*.

[7] This is the powdered core of Semen Nelumbinis Nuciferae (*Lian Zi*).

A man suffered from consumption with weakness, tidal fever, and coughing with blood in the sputum which was better during the day and worse at night, a desiccated and languid appearance, and no taste for drink or food. (This was) severe kidney vacuity. (For this, he was prescribed) Radix Panacis Ginseng (*Ren Shen*), Radix Astragali Membranacei (*Huang Qi*), Rhizoma Atractylodis Macrocephalae (*Bai Zhu*), and Carapax Amydae (*Bie Jia*), 1 *qian* for each of the above, Radix Angelicae Sinensis (*Dang Gui*), Fructus Schizandrae Chinensis (*Wu Wei*), stir-fried Radix Scutellariae Baicalensis (*Huang Qin*), stir-fried Cortex Phellodendri (*Huang Bai*), Radix Bupleuri Scorzonerifolii (*Ruan Chai*), Cortex Radicis Lycii (*Di Gu Pi*), Radix Gentianae Macrophyllae (*Qin Jiao*), stir-fried Rhizoma Coptidis Chinensis (*Huang Lian*), Sclerotium Poriae Cocoris (*Fu Ling*), and Rhizoma Pinelliae Ternatae (Ban Xia), 5 *fen* for each of the above, and Tuber Ophiopogonis Japonicae (*Mai Dong*), 7.5 *fen*. These were boiled with Rhizoma Zingiberis (*Jiang*) and taken with *San Bu Wan* (Three Supplements Pills).

A woman suffering from consumption (was prescribed) *Si Wu [Tang]* plus Radix Panacis Ginseng (*Ren Shen*), Radix Astragali Membranacei (*Huang Qi*), Radix Bupleuri (*Chai Hu*), Radix Scutellariae Baicalensis (*Huang Qin*), Carapax Amydae (*Bie Jia*), Cortex Radicis Lycii (*Di Gu*), dry Radix Puerariae Lobatae (*Gan Ge*), Fructus Schizandrae Chinensis (*Wu Wei*), and Radix Glycyrrhizae (*Gan Cao*). These were boiled in water and taken.

People with vacuity taxation and great heat who are unable to bear cold medicinals, such as Radix Scutellariae Baicalensis (*Huang Qin*) and Rhizoma Coptidis Chinensis (*Huang Lian*), may be prescribed Radix Panacis Ginseng (*Ren Shen*), Radix Astragali Membranacei (*Huang Qi*), Radix Angelicae Sinensis (*Dang Gui*), Rhizoma Atractylodis Macrocephalae (*Bai Zhu*), Radix Bupleuri (*Chai Hu*), Cortex Radicis Lycii (*Di Gu*), Tuber Ophiopogonis Japonicae (*Mai Dong*), Fructus Schizandrae Chinensis (*Wu Wei*), Radix Gentianae Macrophyllae (*Qin Jiao*), Radix Paeoniae Lactiflorae (*Shao Yao*), Herba Artemisiae Apiaceae (*Qing Hao*), Rhizoma Pinelliae Ternatae (*Ban Xia*), Radix Glycyrrhizae (*Gan Cao*), and Rhizoma Picrorrhizae (*Hu Lian*). Boil the above with fresh

Rhizoma Zingiberis (*Sheng Jiang*) and Fructus Pruni Mume (*Wu Mei*) and take.

A person, aged 35, suffered from vacuity detriment with cold in the mornings and heat in the evenings. (They were prescribed) *Si Jun Zi Tang* plus Radix Bupleuri Scorzonerifolii (*Ruan Chai Hu*), Radix Scutellariae Baicalensis (*Huang Qin*), Radix Angelicae Sinensis (*Dang Gui*), Radix Paeoniae Lactiflorae (*Shao Yao*), Rhizoma Ligustici Wallichii (*Chuan Xiong*), Cortex Radicis Lycii (*Di Gu Pi*), and Radix Gentianae Macrophyllae (*Qin Jiao*).

An(other) person suffered from dual vacuity of the qi and blood with steaming bones, alternating cold and heat, normal defecation, a thin, rapid pulse, and low food intake. (They were prescribed) *Ba Wu Tang* (Eight Materials Decoction) plus Radix Bupleuri (*Chai Hu*), Rhizoma Anemarrhenae (*Zhi Mu*), and Cortex Phellodendri (*Huang Bai*).

Chapter Fifty-six

Various Kinds of Vacuity

Da Bu Wan (Great Supplement Pills) rid the kidney channel of fire, dry dampness in the lower burner, and treat flaccid sinews and bones. (They should be) taken with qi-supplementing medicinals in case of qi vacuity or with blood-supplementing medicinals in case of blood vacuity. (They are composed of) Cortex Phellodendri (*Huang Bai*). Stir-fry with wine till brown, powder, make into pills with water, and take.

Wu Bu Tang (Five Supplements Decoction) supplements the heart, liver, spleen, lungs, and kidneys. (It consists of) pitted Semen Nelumbinis Nuciferae (*Lian Rou*), steamed dry Radix Dioscoreae Oppositae (*Gan Shan Yao*), Fructus Lycii Chinensis (*Gou Qi Zi*), and wine-washed Herba Cynomorii Songarici (*Suo Yang*), all in equal amounts. Powder the above, put in a small amount of butter (*Su You*), and take little by little with boiled water.

Chen Xiang Bai Bu Wan (Eaglewood Hundred Supplements Pills) consist of wine-washed prepared Radix Rehmanniae (*Shu Di*), 6 *liang*, Cortex Phellodendri (*Huang Bai*), stir-fried with wine, Rhizoma Anemarrhenae (*Zhi Mu*), stir-fried with wine, and Radix Panacis Ginseng (*Ren Shen*), 2 *liang* for each of the above, stir-fried Cortex Eucommiae Ulmoidis (*Du Zhong*) and Radix Angelicae Sinensis (*Dang Gui*), 3 *liang* each, wine soaked Semen Cuscutae (*Tu Si*), 4 *liang*, and Lignum Aquilariae Agallochae (*Chen Xiang*), 1 *liang*. Powder the above, make into pills with honey, and take with boiled saltwater.

The lower burner supplementing formula, *Long Hu Wan* (Dragon & Tiger Pills) is very efficacious: vinegar-fried Carapax Amydae (*Shang Jia*), 6 *liang*, Semen Germinatus Dioscoreae Oppositae (*Yao Miao*), steamed with wine and baked dry, 2 *liang*, Cacumen Biotae Orientalis (*Ce Bai*), 2 *liang*, Cortex Phellodendri (*Huang Bai*), stir-fried with wine, one half *jin*, Rhizoma Anemarrhenae (*Zhi Mu*), stir-fried with salt and wine, 2 *liang*, prepared Radix Rehmanniae (*Shu Di Huang*), 2 *liang*, Radix Paeoniae Lactiflorae (*Shao Yao*), 2 *liang*, Herba Cynomorii Songarici (*Suo Yang*), pounded with wine, 5 *qian*, wine-soaked Radix Angelicae Sinensis (*Dang Gui*), 5 *qian*, Pericarpium Citri Reticulatae (*Chen Pi*), stripped of the white (inner) skin, 2 *liang*, Os Tigridis (*Hu Gu*), soaked with wine and crisp-fried, 1 *liang*, and Plastrum Testudinis (*Gui Ban*), soaked with wine and crisp-fried, 4 *liang*. Powder the above and make into pills with wine-cooked mutton. In winter months, add dry Rhizoma Zingiberis (*Gan Jiang*).

Bu Shen Wan (Supplement the Kidneys Pills) treat severe atony inversion due to dissipation in wine and sex. They are taken with the same envoy soup as *Da Bu Wan*. In winter months, the formula is as follows (below), but in spring and summer, dry Rhizoma Zingiberis (*Gan Jiang*) should be removed: dry Rhizoma Zingiberis (*Gan Jiang*) 1 *qian*, stir-fried Cortex Phellodendri (*Huang Bai*), 1.5 *liang*, wine-fried Plastrum Testudinis (*Gui Ban*), 1.5 *liang*, wine-baked Radix Achyranthis Bidentatae (*Niu Xi*), 1 *liang*, and Pericarpium Citri Reticulatae (*Chen Pi*), one half *liang*, stripped of its pulp. Powder the above and make into pills with ginger paste or wine; 80-90 pill per dose.

Bu Tian Wan (Supplement Heaven Pills) can supplement dual vacuity of qi and blood when used in combination with *Bu Shen Wan* and should be assisted by bone-steaming medicinals in case of vacuity taxation fever. The formula (consists of) washing Placenta Hominis (*Zi He Che*) clean, drying with a cloth, and pounding (this) finely together with *Bu Shen Wan*. (Then) bake dry, grind, and make into pills with wine and rice paste. In summer, add one half *liang* of Fructus Schizandrae Chinensis (*Wu Wei Zi*).

Hu Qian Wan (Tiger In Hiding Pills) treat atony the same way *Bu Shen Wan* do. (They are composed of) Cortex Phellodendri (*Huang Bai*), stir-fried with wine, one half *jin*, crisp-fried Plastrum Testudinis (*Gui Ban*), 4 *liang*, Rhizoma Anemarrhenae (*Zhi Mu*), stir-fried with wine, 3 *liang*, prepared Radix Rehmanniae (*Shu Di Huang*), 2 *liang*, Pericarpium Citri Reticulatae (*Chen Pi*), 2 *liang*, Radix Albus Paeoniae Lactiflorae (*Bai Shao Yao*), 2 *liang*, Herba Cynomorii Songarici (*Suo Yang*), 1.5 *liang*, processed Os Tigridis (*Hu Gu*), 1 *liang*, and dry Rhizoma Zingiberis (*Gan Jiang*), one half *liang*. Powder the above and make into pills with wine paste or gruel. In a (variant) formula, 10 foils of native gold (*Jin Bo*) are added, while in another (variant) formula, Radix Rehmanniae (*Sheng Di Huang*) is added. In case of disinclination to speak, add Radix Dioscoreae Oppositae (*Shan Yao*).

Bu Xue Wan (Supplement Blood Pills, consist of) stir-fried Cortex Phellodendri (*Huang Bai*), wine-fried Rhizoma Anemarrhenae (*Zhi Mu*), and crisp-fried Plastrum Testudinis (*Gui Ban*), all in equal amounts, dry Rhizoma Zingiberis (*Gan Jiang*), 1/3 (in quantity). Powder the above and make into pills with wine paste.

Bu Xu Wan (Supplement Vacuity Pills, consist of) Radix Panacis Ginseng (*Ren Shen*), Rhizoma Atractylodis Macrocephalae (*Bai Zhu*), Radix Dioscoreae Oppositae (*Shan Yao*), Fructus Lycii Chinensis (*Qi Zi*), and Herba Cynomorii Songarici (*Suo Yang*). Powder and make into pills.

Bu Yin Wan (Supplement Yin Pills, consist of) Cacumen Biotae Orientalis (*Ce Bai*), 2 *liang*, Cortex Phellodendri (*Huang Bai*), 2 *liang*, Radix Dioscoreae Oppositae (*Shan Yao*), 2 *liang*, wine-fried Plastrum Testudinis (*Gui Ban*), 3 *liang*, Rhizoma Coptidis Chinensis (*Huang Lian*), one half *liang*, and Radix Sophorae Flavescentis (*Ku Shen*), 3 *liang*. Powder the above and make into pills with *Di Huang Gao* (Rehmannia Paste).[1] Add dry Rhizoma Zingiberis (*Gan Jiang*) in winter and Fructus Amomi (*Suo Sha*) in summer.

Another formula consists of Plastrum Amydae (*Xia Jia*), 2 *liang*, Cortex Phellodendri (*Huang Bai*), 5 *qian*, Radix Achyranthis Bidentatae (*Niu Xi*), 5 *qian*, Radix Panacis Ginseng (*Ren Shen*), 5 *qian*, Rhizoma Cyperi Rotundi (*Xiang Fu*), 1 *liang*, Radix Albus Paeoniae Lactiflorae (*Bai Shao Yao*), 1 *liang*, Radix Glycyrrhizae (*Gan Cao*), 3 *qian*, and Fructus Amomi (*Suo Sha*), 3 *qian*, not used in spring. Powder the above and make into pills with wine paste. (Still) another formula: Plastrum Amydae (*Xia Jia*), 3 *liang*, and Cortex Phellodendri (*Huang Bai*), 1 *liang*. Cut Radix Rehmanniae (*Di Huang*) finely, steam with wine, pestle, and make into pills (with the above two ingredients. Yet) another formula: wine-processed Plastrum Testudinis (*Gui Ban*), 2 *liang*, Cortex Phellodendri (*Huang Bai*), 7.5 *qian*, Rhizoma Anemarrhenae (*Zhi Mu*), one half *liang*, Radix Panacis Ginseng (*Ren Shen*), 3.5 *qian*, and Radix Cyathulae (*Chuan Niu Xi*), 1 *liang*. Powder the above and make into pills with wine paste. (And still) another formula: wine-processed Plastrum Testudinis (*Gui Ban*), 1 *liang*, Cortex Phellodendri (*Huang Bai*), one half *liang*, Rhizoma Anemarrhenae (*Zhi Mu*), 3 *qian*, and Fructus Schizandrae Chinensis (*Wu Wei Zi*), 2 *qian*. Powder the above and make into pills with wine paste.

For depression bind refusing to disperse, (use) Plastrum Amydae (*Xia Jia*), 5 *liang*, Cacumen Biotae Orientalis (*Ce Bai*), 1.5 *liang*, and Rhizoma Cyperi Rotundi (*Xiang Fu*), 2 *liang*. Powder the above, make into pills

---

[1] This refers to the resulting thick paste that occurs when one boils a medicinals down over a long period of time, similar to reducing apple cider to apple jelly or maple sap to maple syrup.

with *Di Huang Gao* (Rehmannia Paste) soaked with Succus Zingiberis (*Jiang Zhi*), and take on an empty stomach.

San Bu Wan (Three Supplements Pills) treat accumulated heat in the upper burner and drain fire from the five viscera. (They are composed of) Radix Scutellariae Baicalensis (*Huang Qin*), Rhizoma Coptidis Chinensis (*Huang Lian*), and Cortex Phellodendri (*Huang Bai*). Powder the above and make into pills with cake.

Another formula for excessive dissipation in wine and sex damaging the *shao yin* (consists of) stir-fried Cortex Phellodendri (*Huang Bai*), 1.5 *liang*, stir-fried Rhizoma Coptidis Chinensis (*Huang Lian*), 1 *liang*, stir-fried Radix Scutellariae Baicalensis (*Tiao Qin*), one half *liang*, and wine-fried Plastrum Testudinis (*Gui Ban*), 3 *liang*. Powder the above. In winter, add 3 *qian* of black-fried Rhizoma Zingiberis (*Jiang*). In summer, add 3 *qian* of Fructus Amomi (*Suo Sha*) and one half *liang* of Fructus Schizandrae Chinensis (*Wu Wei Zi*). Make into pills the size of Chinese parasol tree seeds with steamed cake; 30 pills per dose taken before a meal with boiled water.

To treat yin vacuity, (one can use) Radix Panacis Ginseng (*Ren Shen*), 7 *qian*, Rhizoma Atractylodis Macrocephalae (*Bai Zhu*), 3 *qian*, Tuber Ophiopogonis Japonicae (*Mai Men Dong*), one half *liang*, and Pericarpium Citri Reticulatae (*Chen Pi*), 1 *qian*, all as one dose. Boil and take with *San Bu Wan*.

To treat a weak yet fat body with blood vacuity but a large pulse, (use) Plastrum Testudinis (*Gui Ban*), 3 *liang*, Cacumen Biotae Orientalis (*Ce Bai*), steamed with wine, 7.5 *qian*, Radix Rehmanniae (*Sheng Di Huang*), 1.5 *liang*, stir-fried Radix Albus Paeoniae Lactiflorae (*Bai Shao Yao*), 1 *liang*, and Folium Linderae Strychnifoliae (*Wu Yao Ye*), steamed with wine, 7.5 *qian*. Powder the above. (Then) boil Radix Rehmanniae (*Sheng Di Huang*) down to a paste, pound with the (above) powdered medicinals, and make into pills. Boil 4 *qian* of Rhizoma Atractylodis Macrocephalae (*Bai Zhu*) and 1.5 *qian* of Rhizoma Cyperi Rotundi (*Xiang Fu*) and swallow the pills with this decoction.

To boost the blood of the *shao yin* channel and resolve bound qi in the five viscera, the following formula offers a very rapid result. Stir-fry Fructus Gardeniae Jasminoidis (*Shan Zhi Zi*) till 2/10 black, powder, boil in water together with Succus Zingiberis (*Jiang Zhi*), and take.

Wu Bu Wan (Five Supplements Pills, consist of) Fructus Lycii Chinensis (*Gou Qi*), 5 *qian*, Herba Cynomorii Songarici (*Suo Yang*), 5 *qian*, Radix Dipsaci (*Xu Duan*), 1 *liang*, slightly stir-fried Fructus Cnidii Monnieri (*She Chuang Zi*), 1 *liang*, and Radix Aconiti (*Liang Tou Jian*), 2.5 *qian*. Powder the above finely and make into pills with wine paste. Take 36 pills with bland saltwater.

Suo Yang Wan (Lock Yang Pills, consist of) wine-fried Plastrum Testudinis (*Gui Ban*), 1 *liang*, Rhizoma Anemarrhenae (*Zhi Mu*), stir-fried with wine, 1 *liang*, Cortex Phellodendri (*Huang Bai*), stir-fried with wine, 1 *liang*, wine-fried Os Tigridis (*Hu Gu*), 2.5 *qian*, Cortex Eucommiae Ulmoidis (*Du Zhong*), stir-fried with Succus Zingiberis (*Jiang Zhi*), one half *liang*, wine-soaked Herba Cynomorii Songarici (*Suo Yang*), one half *liang*, Radix Angelicae Sinensis (*Dang Gui*), one half *liang*, Radix Rehmanniae (*Di Huang*), one half *liang*, wine-soaked Radix Achyranthis Bidentatae (*Niu Xi*), 2.5 *qian*, Fructus Psoraleae Corylifoliae (*Po Gu Zhi*), 2.5 *qian*, and wine-soaked Radix Dipsaci (*Xu Duan*), 2.5 *qian*. In order to supplement essence, one must introduce blood(-nourishing) medicinals into the various formulas that supplement the life gate because it is the *dao* that yang arises when yin grows. Yang(-supplementing) medicinals are quite capable of dispersing fire.

Bu Xin Wan (Supplement the Heart Pills, consist of) Cinnabar (*Zhu Sha*), 2.5 *qian*, Fructus Trichosanthis Kirlowii (*Gua Lou*), one half *liang*, Rhizoma Coptidis Chinensis (*Huang Lian*), 3 *qian*, and Radix Angelicae Sinensis (*Dang Gui Shen Wei*), 3.5 *qian*. Powder the above and make into pills with the blood from a pig's heart.

Ning Xin Yi Zhi Wan (Tranquilize the Heart & Boost the Orientation [*i.e.*, Will or Intelligence] Pills, consist of) Radix Panacis Ginseng (*Ren Shen*), Sclerotium Pararadicis Poriae (*Fu Shen*), Concha Ostreae (*Mu Li*), Radix Polygalae Tenuifoliae (*Yuan Zhi*), Semen Zizyphi Spinosae (*Suan Zao Ren*), and Fructus Alpiniae Oxyphyllae (*Yi Zhi Ren*), 5 *qian* for each of the above, and Cinnabar (*Chen Sha*), 2.5 *qian*. Powder the above and make into pills with Fructus Zizyphi Jujubae (*Zao Rou*).

An Shen Wan (Calm the Spirit Pills) consist of Cinnabar (*Zhu Sha*), 1 *qian*, wine-processed Rhizoma Coptidis Chinensis (*Huang Lian*), 1.5 *qian*, mix-fried Radix Glycyrrhizae (*Gan Cao Zhi*), one half *qian*, Radix Rehmanniae (*Sheng Di Huang*), 5 *fen*, and Radix Angelicae Sinensis (*Dang Gui*), 1 *qian*. Powder the above and make into pills with cake.

To supplement and boost vacuity weakness of the spleen, stomach, and kidneys in males, (use) blast-fried Radix Praeparatus Aconiti Carmichaeli (*Chuan Fu*), 1 *liang*, Radix Panacis Ginseng (*Ren Shen*), Rhizoma Atractylodis Macrocephalae (*Bai Zhu*), Fructus Schizandrae Chinensis (*Wu Wei Zi*), Radix Angelicae Sinensis (*Dang Gui*), Radix Dipsaci (*Xu Duan*), stemmed Fructus Corni Officinalis (*Shan Zhu Yu*), Fructus Psoraleae Corylifoliae (*Po Gu Zhi*), wine-soaked Herba Cistanchis (*Rou Cong Rong*), stir-fried Radix Albus Paeoniae Lactiflorae (*Bai Shao Yao*), and Semen Nelumbinis Nuciferae (*Lian Rou*), 1 *liang* for each of the above, Semen Cuscutae (*Tu Si Zi*), 2 *liang*, crisp-fried Cornu Cervi Parvum (*Lu Rong*), Lignum Aquilariae Agallochae (*Chen Xiang*), and Cortex Cinnamomi (*Rou Gui*), 2 *qian* for each of the above. Powder the above, make into pills with wine paste, and take on an empty stomach with boiled saltwater.

Bu Yin Wan (Supplement Yin Pills, consist of) wine-washed prepared Radix Rehmanniae (*Shu Di*), 8 *liang*, wine-washed Cortex Phellodendri (*Huang Bai*), 4 *liang*, wine-washed Radix Angelicae Sinensis (*Dang Gui*), Semen Cuscutae (*Tu Si Zi*), wine-washed Herba Cistanchis (*Rou Cong Rong*), wine-washed Rhizoma Anemarrhenae (*Zhi Mu*), and Fructus Lycii Chinensis (*Gou Qi*), 3 *liang* for each of the above, Tuber Asparagi Cochinensis (*Tian Men Dong*), crisp-fried Plastrum Testudinis (*Gui Ban*), and Radix Dioscoreae Oppositae (*Shan Yao*), 2 *liang* for each of the above, and Fructus Schizandrae Chinensis (*Wu Wei*), 1.5 *liang*. Powder the above. Boil 4 *liang* of Radix Panacis Ginseng (*Ren Shen*) and 8 liang of Radix Astragali Membranacei (*Huang Qi*) down to a paste. Cook pig's kidneys in wine and then pound thoroughly. Mix (all the above) and make into pills.

Gu Ben Wan (Secure the Root Pills, consist of) Radix Panacis Ginseng (*Ren Shen*), Radix Rehmanniae (*Sheng Di*), prepared Radix Rehmanniae (*Shu Di*), Tuber Asparagi Cochinensis (*Tian Dong*), and Tuber Ophiopogonis Japonicae (*Mai Dong*), 2 *liang* for each of the above, Cortex Phellodendri (*Huang Bai*), Rhizoma Anemarrhenae (*Zhi Mu*), Radix Achyranthis Bidentatae (*Niu Xi*), Cortex Eucommiae Ulmoidis (*Du Zhong*), Plastrum Testudinis (*Gui Ban*), Fructus Schizandrae Chinensis (*Wu Wei*), Sclerotium Pararadicis Poriae Cocoris (*Fu Shen*), and Radix Polygalae Tenuifoliae (*Yuan Zhi*), 1 *liang* for each of the above. Powder all the above and make into pills with wine paste. [In case of timorous {*i.e.*, weakened} spleen and stomach, add Rhizoma Atractylodis Macrocephalae {*Bai Zhu*}; to brighten the eyes, add Fructus Lycii Chinensis {*Gou Qi Zi*. later editor}]

Chapter Fifty-seven

Cold and Heat

The disease of (alternating) cold and heat is difficult to treat if it is due to yin vacuity. In enduring (*i.e*, chronic) disease, (if there is) aversion to cold, normally use resolving depression. For aversion to cold due to yang vacuity, use Radix Panacis Ginseng (*Ren Shen*) and Radix Astragali Membranacei (*Huang Qi*), and the like, and in severe cases, add a small amount of Radix Praeparatus Aconiti Carmichaeli (*Fu Zi*) to move the qi of Radix Panacis Ginseng and Radix Astragali Membranacei. Severe aversion of the back to cold with a floating and large yet weak pulse is (due to) yang vacuity. Vacuity taxation with worse aversion to cold in winter months may be treated with precipitation if the qi is replete. Simultaneously, it is (also) appropriate to resolve the exterior with Radix Bupleuri (*Chai Hu*) and Radix Puerariae Lobatae (*Ge Gen*). Rhizoma Atractylodis (*Cang Zhu*) should not be used for fear of its dryness. For yin vacuity fever, (use) *Si Wu Tang* (Four Materials Decoction) plus stir-fried Cortex Phellodendri (*Huang Bai*). If complicated by qi vacuity, add Radix

Panacis Ginseng (*Ren Shen*), Rhizoma Atractylodis Macrocephalae (*Bai Zhu*), and Radix Astragali Membranacei (*Huang Qi*). For yang vacuity fever, (use) *Bu Zhong Yi Qi Tang* (Supplement the Center & Boost the Qi Decoction).[1] For damp phlegm fever arising at night, (use) *San Bu Wan* (Three Supplements Pills) plus Radix Albus Paeoniae Lactiflorae (*Bai Shao Yao*). (And) for qi vacuity fever, (use) *Shen Su Yin* (Ginseng & Perilla Drink).

For fever at night in enduring disease with yin vacuity and qi depression, (use) wine-processed Radix Paeoniae Lactiflorae (*Shao Yao*), 1.2 *liang*, Rhizoma Cyperi Rotundi (*Xiang Fu*), 1 *liang*, Rhizoma Atractylodis (*Cang Zhu*), 5 *qian*, Radix Scutellariae Baicalensis (*Pian Qin*), 3 *qian*, and Radix Glycyrrhizae (*Gan Cao*), 1.5 *qian*. Steam as cake, make into pills, and take. (But) for intermittent fever arising at night and ceasing during the day, arising during the day and ceasing at night, or arising during *si* and *wu* or *shen* and *wei*[2], (use) *Xiao Chai Hu Tang* (Minor Bupleurum Decoction) plus Radix Panacis Ginseng (*Ren Shen*) and Rhizoma Atractylodis Macrocephalae (*Bai Zhu*). In case of thirst, add Radix Trichosanthis Kirlowii (*Gua Lou Gen*). If the pulse remains weak after administration of this formula, (prescribe) *Bu Zhong Yi Qi Tang* with Radix Panacis Ginseng (*Ren Shen*), Radix Astragali Membranacei (*Huang Qi*), Radix Angelicae Sinensis (*Dang Gui*), and Rhizoma Atractylodis Macrocephalae (*Bai Zhu*) doubled in amount. (After) numerous (doses) have been administered, recuperation will occur by itself.

For fever with aversion to cold it is appropriate to resolve the exterior. For the fever, use Radix Bupleuri (*Chai Hu*); for the aversion to cold, use Rhizoma Atractylodis (*Cang Zhu*). In case of mild vacuity of qi with

---

[1] This consists of Radix Panacis Ginseng (*Ren Shen*), Folium Perillae Frutescentis (*Zi Su Ye*), Radix Puerariae Lobatae (*Ge Gen*), washed, stir-fried with Succus Zingiberis (*Jiang Zhi*), Rhizoma Pinelliae Ternatae (*Ban Xia*), Radix Peucedani (*Qian Hu*). and Sclerotium Poriae Cocoris (*Fu Ling*), 3 *fen* for each of the above, Radix Saussureae Seu Vladimiriae (*Mu Xiang*), bran-fried Fructus Citri Seu Ponciri (*Zhi Qiao*), Radix Platycodi Grandiflori (*Jie Geng*), mix-fried Radix Glycyrrhizae (*Zhi Gan Cao*), and Pericarpium Citri Reticulatae (*Chen Pi*), one half *liang* for each of the above. Powder all the above; 4 *qian* per dose. Boil with 7 slices of ginger.

[2] *Si* (B6), 9-11 AM; *wu* (B7), 11 AM-1 PM; *shen* (B9), 3-5 PM; *wei* (B8), 1-3 PM

steaming bones, fever or cold, inhibited defecation, a replete pulse, and ability to eat, heat will be removed once defecation is disinhibited. (Therefore, prescribe) *Chai Hu Yin Zi* (Bupleurum Drink)[3]. (However,) for qi repletion with exterior heat, ability to eat, a wiry pulse, absence of sweating, and ability to sleep, or phlegm accumulation cold and heat, (use) *Xiao Chai Hu Tang.*

In the sixth month, a person contracted aversion to cold with dry, bound stools and fear of exposure to wind. This person was fat and sturdy and (their) daily life activities were normal. (They were prescribed) *Da Cheng Qi Tang* (Major Support the Qi Decoction).

A female with aversion to cold was prescribed 1 *qian* each of powdered Radix Sophorae Flavescentis (*Ku Shen*) and Semen Phaseoli Calcarati (*Chi Xiao Dou*) with pickle water as emetics. After that, (she) was administered Rhizoma Ligustici Wallichii (*Chuan Xiong*), Rhizoma Atractylodis (*Cang Zhu*), Rhizoma Arisaematis (*Nan Xing*), and wine-processed Radix Scutellariae Baicalensis (*Huang Qin,* all the above) made into pills with wine paste and Massa Medica Fermentata (*Shen Qu*).

A male, aged 23, ran a fever as a result of drinking wine. (He) was prescribed Pulvis Indigonis (*Qing Dai*) and Fructus Trichosanthis Kirlowii (*Gua Lou Ren.* These) were ground, mixed with Succus Zingiberis (*Jiang Zhi*), and drunk, several spoonfuls a day. Three days later, recovery ensued.

An(other) person (caught) a slight cold at daybreak and, from then onward, (had) fever lasting till night. Once the two armpits sweat and the hands and feet became very hot, there arose chest fullness and hypertonicity. The stools were solid with ability to eat. Apparently, it was a taxation vacuity disease, but the pulse was not rapid. (Rather) it was wiry, thin, and deep. Questioning revealed that this resulted from angry qi. Then *Da Chai*

---

[3] This consists of Radix Bupleuri (*Chai Hu*), Radix Scutellariae Baicalensis (*Huang Qin*), Radix Panacis Ginseng (*Ren Shen*), Radix Angelicae Sinensis (*Dang Gui*), Radix Paeoniae Lactiflorae (*Shao Yao*), Radix Et Rhizoma Rhei (*Da Huang*), and Radix Glycyrrhizae (*Gan Cao*), one half *liang* for each of the above; 3 *qian* per dose. Boil in water with 3 slices of ginger and take 3 times per day.

Hu Tang (Major Bupleurum Decoction) alone was administered, and only the hypertonicity of the chest and back remained to be eliminated. Then *Er Chen Tang* (Two Aged Decoction) was prescribed plus Radix Et Rhizoma Notopterygii (*Qiang Huo*), Radix Ledebouriellae Sesloidis (*Fang Feng*), Radix Scutellariae Baicalensis (*Huang Qin*), and Flos Carthami Tinctorii (*Hong Hua*).

Advanced Scholar[4] Zhou Ben-dao, who was more than 30 years of age, contracted a disease (characterized by) fear of cold. He asked (me) for treatment when his condition deteriorated after the administration of several hundred (*liang*) of Radix Praeparatus Aconiti Carmichaeli (*Fu Zi*). His pulse was wiry and seemed retarded. I administered river water tea with Succus Zingiberis (*Jiang Zhi*) and a small amount of sesame oil put in. (This) induced vomiting of about 1 *sheng* of phlegm. (His symptoms) abated by more than half, and then I prescribed *Fang Feng Tong Sheng San* (Ledebouriella Communicate with the Divinity Powder) with Radix Et Rhizoma Rhei (*Da Huang*) and Mirabilitum (*Mang Xiao*) deleted and Radix Rehmanniae (*Di Huang*) added. A little more than 100 doses and (his symptoms) were calmed. Zhou was very delighted, but the master said: (Your condition) is not yet overcome and dry heat has done much damage to (your) blood. Therefore, (you) must necessarily take food of bland (flavor) to nurture (your) stomach and introspect to nurture (your) spirit. Only then can water be engendered and fire downborne. (However,) vigorously seeking promotion at that time, (the patient) was too fully engaged in social activities to abide by these prohibitions. I observed that security might be insured to a small degree provided blood-supplementing, cool medicinals were administered in large amounts. With disquietude both internally and externally, kidney water would not engender and hidden toxins were sure to awake a disease. After the relief (of his symptoms), he secured an appointment in Wu Town[5] and had to be on night patrol. His cold stomach could be cured by nothing but Radix

---

[4]   In feudal China, a successful candidate in the national examination was called *jin shi*, advanced scholar. He was then qualified for a position as a government official.

[5]   This is a county in Jiangxi Province.

Praeparatus Aconiti Carmichaeli (*Fu Zi*). Because (Radix Praeparatus Aconiti Carmichaeli) fears fresh Rhizoma Zingiberis (*Sheng Jiang*), it had to be boiled with sliced pig's kidneys. After 3 doses, recovery ensued. Knowing that the hidden toxins might easily break out (again), I advised him to return home without delay. He, (however,) thought (my advice) was (overly) fastidious. Half a year later, it turned out that *ju*[6] broke out on his back, (eventually) ending in death.

In the ninth month, a person, who was more than 20 years of age, had fever with headache and wildly declared seeing ghosts. The (attending) physician administered him more than 10 doses of *Xiao Chai Hu Tang*, and his fever became all the more severe. He had a fat form with a wiry, large, rapid pulse, larger by far on the left (hand). Then he was treated as a vacuity (pattern) with Radix Panacis Ginseng (*Ren Shen*) and Rhizoma Atractylodis Macrocephalae (*Bai Zhu*) as the sovereigns, Sclerotium Poriae Cocoris (*Fu Ling*) and Radix Paeoniae Lactiflorae (*Shao Yao*) as the ministers, Radix Astragali Membranacei (*Huang Qi*) as the assistant, and 1 slice of Radix Praeparatus Aconiti Carmichaeli (*Fu Zi*) as the envoy. Two doses were administered, but his condition did not improve. Because there was mania, fever, and great thirst with a large, rapid pulse, some may assume that Radix Praeparatus Aconiti Carmichaeli may have been abused. The master said: Extreme vacuity, inappropriate administration of cool and cold medicinals, fatness, and a pulse which is larger on the left than on the right (all point to) a critical situation. What else but 1 slice of Radix Praeparatus Aconiti Carmichaeli to move Radix Panacis Ginseng and Rhizoma Atractylodis Macrocephalae can rescue (such a) crisis? Only after another dose was administered, did I delete Radix Praeparatus Aconiti Carmichaeli and prescribe a large dose. After more than 50 doses were administered, massive sweating was induced which was followed by recovery. (The patient) carried out self-supplementation and self-nurturing for 2 more months, and his qi and body were still not (quite) sound.

---

[6] This refers to a suppurative inflammation with overlying skin of normal color, absence of heat, and little pain.

One day, a male, aged 19, who had no fear of taxation (*i.e.*, was accustomed to the hardest labor) in farming, suddenly had great fever with thirst. He drank several bowls of water at a time to his heart's content and, the next morning, the fever abated. However, he was no longer able to recognize people. He spoke nonsense, telling (people) that he was unable to turn his belly, was unable to take in drink or food, and was unable to turn over his body. After another 2 days, (I) was asked for emergency help. The pulse at both hands was choppy and large and more so on the right hand. (I) moxaed 30 cones at *Qi Hai* (CV 6)[7] and prescribed 2 *qian* of Rhizoma Atractylodis Macrocephalae (*Bai Zhu*), 2 *qian* of Radix Astragali Membranacei (*Huang Qi*), 1 slice of Radix Praeparatus Aconiti Carmichaeli (*Fu Zi*), and one half *qian* of Pericarpium Citri Reticulatae (*Chen Pi*. However, after) 10 doses had been taken, no effect was seen. What's more, moderate thirst appeared with the other conditions persisting. Nonetheless, (he) was able to eat a little gruel. This showed that (his) qi had become loosened and harmonious but that (his) blood had not yet responded. The preceding formula (was used) with Radix Praeparatus Aconiti Carmichaeli replaced by wine-processed Radix Angelicae Sinensis (*Dang Gui*) to harmonize the blood, and, on account of the presence of heat, 1.5 *qian* of Radix Panacis Ginseng (*Ren Shen*) was (also) added. (After) 30 doses were administered, recovery ensued.

In early autumn, elder brother (*i.e.*, friend) Zheng, who was more than 20 years of age, had fever with thirst and delirious speech. (This seemed like) a disease due to ghost evils. Eight days later, his pulse on both sides was surging, rapid, and forceful. He had a fat form with a white complexion and slightly prominent sinews and bones. The pulse striking the (feeling) hand (forcefully) must be a result of cool medicinals. This was a disease of taxation fatigue and warming and supplementing would calm it automatically. After 7-8 doses of *Chai Hu*

---

[7]   Sea of Qi

(Bupleurum [Decoction])[8] were taken, no effect was seen. Therefore, (he) was prescribed *Huang Qi Fu Zi Tang* (Astragalus & Aconite Decoction)[9] and was made to drink this when cooled. After 3 doses were taken, moderate sweating was induced which was followed by sleep. Moreover, the pulse became softer. Then, (administration of) *Huang Qi Bai Zhu Tang* (Astragalus & Atractylodes Decoction)[10] succeeded in regulating and supplementing (further). Ten days later, relief ensued. After that, Pericarpium Citri Reticulatae (*Chen Pi*) was added. The administration was carried on for half a month more and there was full recovery.

A relative (of mine) named Lu frequently drank wine without control. In addition, he was lustful and a half hundred (years old). One day, he had great aversion to cold and shivering with thirst. Yet he drank a little water. The pulse was large and weak. The right *guan* was a bit replete and a little rapid. It (also) felt choppy when pressure was applied. Because wine heat was depressed internally, exterior repletion had developed into lower vacuity. (He) was prescribed two times as much Radix Astragali Membranacei (*Huang Qi*) as dry Radix Puerariae Lobatae (*Gan Ge*. These) were boiled and taken. After 5 or 6 doses were taken, massive sweating was induced, followed by calming (of his symptoms).

---

[8] There are two versions of *Chai Hu Tang*, the major (*da*) and minor (*xiao*). The author may be referring to a modified form of either of these or a combination of both. See Note 5, Ch. 13, Bk. 1 and Note 7, Ch. 17, Bk. 1.

[9] This consists of honey-fried Radix Astragali Membranacei (*Huang Qi*), prepared Radix Rehmanniae (*Shu Di*), Radix Albus Paeoniae Lactiflorae (*Bai Shao Yao*), Fructus Schizandrae Chinensis (*Wu Wei*), and Tuber Ophiopogonis Japonicae (*Mai Men Dong*), 3 *fen* for each of the above, Sclerotium Poriae Cocoris (*Fu Ling*), 1 *fen*, mix-fried Radix Glycyrrhizae (*Zhi Gan Cao*), one half *liang*, and Radix Praeparatus Aconiti Carmichaeli (*Fu Zi*).

[10] This formula is the same as in Note 17 above except that Rhizoma Atractylodis Macrocephalae (*Bai Zhu*) is used instead of Radix Praeparatus Aconiti Carmichaeli (*Fu Zi*).

A female who was vacuous and emaciated suffered from thief sweating and aversion to cold. (She) was prescribed Fructus Evodiae Rutecarpae (*Wu Zhu Yu*), the size of a hen's egg, which was soaked for half a day in 3 *sheng* of wine, boiled, and taken.

(As far as) cold or heat in the face (is concerned), cold in the face is (a sign of) stomach heat. (This) is heat due to depressed cold. (While) heat in the face is (a sign of) fire rising. (This) is heat from depressed (fire). People who are diseased mostly die if red spots suddenly appear on their face.

Book Five

Chapter Fifty-eight

Coughing of Blood

If there is exuberant phlegm with body heat, (coughing of blood) is usually due to blood vacuity. The medicinals to be introduced are Pulvis Indigonis (*Qing Dai*), Fructus Trichosanthis Kirlowii (*Gua Lou Ren*), Fructus Terminaliae Chebulae (*He Zi*), Pumice (*Hai Shi*), and Fructus Gardeniae Jasminoidis (*Shan Zhi*). Powder the above, make into pills with Succus Zingiberis (*Jiang Zhi*) and honey (*Mi*), and melt in the mouth. In case of severe cough, add Semen Pruni Armeniacae (*Xing Ren*) and then apply regulation and rectification with *Ba Wu Tang* (Eight Materials Decoction). If there are threads of blood in the phlegm, use child's urine and Succus Bambusae (*Zhu Li*). Spitting of red (blood) followed by phlegm is usually ascribed to yin vacuity and fire counterflow (causing) ascension of phlegm. Prescribe the ingredients of *Si Wu Tang* (Four Materials Decoction) as the basis and add phlegm fire (removing) medicinals. (Whereas,) coughing of phlegm followed by red (blood) is usually ascribed to phlegm accumulation heat, and it is urgent to downbear phlegm fire. (And) fat persons with coughing, (alternating) cold and heat, and spitting of blood should be prescribed *Qiong Yu Gao* (Fine Jade Paste).

As a result of worry, a person suffered from the disease of coughing and spitting of blood with a dusky, dark facial complexion. After 10 days of medication, he showed no improvement. (I) said to his elder brother, First on the Bulletin Chen[1], that this disease resulted from frustration and despondency injuring the kidneys and that only by delighting could it be resolved. Thereupon he found his brother a place with abundant supplies of clothing and food. (The patient) was very pleased, and, on the spot, the (ill) complexion disappeared. Recovery ensued without any medication. It is justified to say that to

---

[1] *Zhang yuan* refers to the first successful candidate in the imperial examination.

treat disease, the root must be sought out. Even though the medicinals chosen are indicated by the qi of the disease, a formula may fail to bring any effect if the emotional (factors) that lead to that disease are not remedied.

Chapter Fifty-nine

Vomiting Blood

Fire carrying blood upward (leads to) menstrual bleeding or blood running frenetically (in which case) a large pulse indicates fever, and sore throat is due to qi vacuity. (In this case,) use Radix Panacis Ginseng (*Ren Shen*), Radix Astragali Membranacei (*Huang Qi*), honey-fried Cortex Phellodendri (*Huang Bai*), Herba Seu Flos Schizonepetae Tenuifoliae (*Jing Jie*), Radix Rehmanniae (*Sheng Di Huang*), and Radix Angelicae Sinensis (*Dang Gui*). For retching of blood, drink Succus Allii Tuberosi (*Jiu Zhi*), child's urine, Succus Zingiberis (*Jiang Zhi*), and rubbed Tuber Curcumae (*Yu Jin.*) For fire carrying blood upward, running in the wrong course and in a frenetic way, use *Si Wu Tang* (Four Materials Decoction) plus stir-fried Fructus Gardeniae Jasminoidis (*Shan Zhi*), child's urine, and Succus Zingiberis (*Jiang Zhi*). Flos Camelliae Japonicae (*Shan Cha Hua*) and powdered Tuber Curcumae (*Yu Jin*) mixed with child's urine, Succus Zingiberis (*Jiang Zhi*), and wine can treat vomiting of blood. (While) counterflow of menstrual blood giving rise to vomiting, spitting, or nasal discharge of blood or a fishy, bloody smell can be cured instantly by administering Succus Allii Tuberosi (*Jiu Zhi*).

In case of threads of blood in phlegm, use child's urine and Succus Bambusae (*Zhu Li*) and, afterwards, *Xi Jiao Di Huang Wan* (Rhinoceros

Horn & Rehmannia Decoction).[1] Another formula (consists of) obtaining two ingredients: Succus Allii Tuberosi (*Jiu Zhi*) and child's urine. Finely grind Tuber Curcumae (*Yu Jin*), put in the above two ingredients, and take. The blood will naturally be cleared. Another formula that treats vomiting of blood and nosebleed due to ascension of blood (is made by) powdering Tuber Curcumae (*Yu Jin*) and mixing this with Succus Zingiberis (*Jiang Zhi*), child's urine, and good wine. (Then) take. If Tuber Curcumae is not available, Flos Camelliae Japonicae (*Shan Cha Hua*) may be used instead.

In case of vomiting of blood embracing (*i.e.*, containing) as much as 1 or even 2 bowlsful of phlegm, just supplement yin and downbear fire with such formulas as *Si Wu Tang* plus fire-(downbearing) medicinals. If phlegm is embraced, the use of blood(-stanching) medicinals may cause stagnation and non-circulation. But if fire is treated, (blood) will naturally be stanched, since vomiting of blood is a disease of fire. (Even though) 1 or 2 bowlsful of purple blood is suddenly vomited, there is no need to worry. This vomiting is a good thing, for this is blood damaged by heat and (consequently is already) dead in the center. (For this) use *Si Wu Tang* plus toxin-resolving medicinals.

For incessant vomiting of blood, stir-fry powdered dry Rhizoma Zingiberis (*Gan Jiang*) till black and take brewed with child's urine. For phlegm and blood (coming out from) the throat, use *Jing Jie San* (Schizonepeta Powder).[2] For blood exiting for no reason like threads on the tongue, stir-fry Flos Immaturus Sophorae Japonicae (*Huai Hua*) and grind into powder. Apply dry (to the tongue. Whereas,) clear

---

[1] This consists of Cornu Rhinoceroris (*Xi Jiao*), 1 *liang*, Radix Rehmanniae (*Sheng Di Huang*), 8 *liang*, Radix Paeoniae Lactiflorae (*Shao Yao*), 3 *liang*, and Cortex Radicis Moutan (*Dan Pi*), 2 *liang*.

[2] There are several different versions of this formula with the same name, but none of them are designed for internal bleeding. It is, therefore, possible that the name is wrong. A formula with a similar name that does treat this disease is given below but only for reference. *Jing Jie Yin* (Schizonepeta Drink): Herba Seu Flos Schizonepetae Tenuifoliae (*Jing Jie Sui*), Fructus Gardeniae Jasminoidis (*Zhi Zi Ren*), Radix Scutellariae Baicalensis (*Huang Qin*), and Pollen Typhae (*Pu Huang*), 1 *liang* each.

blood in the stomach cannot be removed but by Fructus Polygoni Tinctorii (*Lan Shi*). Fructus Gardeniae Jasminoidis (*Shan Zhi*) is most able to clear blood from the venter.

Vomiting of purple blood that is preceded by a sensation of qi obstructing and ascending in the chest should be treated by precipitating (the blood) with *Tao Ren Cheng Qi Tang* (Persica Support the Qi Decoction. Another way) to treat vomiting of blood is to powder 5 *qian* of Ramulus Cinnamomi (*Gui*), put in cold water, and take. Blood in the phlegm and drool is clear blood from the stomach opening, driven out by steaming heat. In severe cases, use Fructus Gardeniae Jasminoidis (*Shan Zhi*), and in mild cases, use Fructus Polygoni Tinctorii (*Lan Shi*. One can also) treat vomiting of blood by obtaining 1 *fen* of child's urine and one half *fen* of wine. Pound Folium Cupressi Funebris (*Bai Ye*, with the above) and drink (the juice) after warming it. Wine is an indispensable agent. In case of coughing and vomiting of blood, take *Ji Su (i.e., Shui Su) Wan* (Stachys Baicalensis Pills)[3] in the shape of either pills or decoction.

For blood moving frenetically, (use) *Jie Du Si Wu Tang* (Resolve Toxins Four Materials Decoction).[4] In severe cases, introduce a number of slices of stir-fried dry Rhizoma Zingiberis (*Gan Jiang*). For vomiting of blood, administer powdered Rhizoma Cyperi Rotundi (*Xiang Fu*) or powdered Rhizoma Bletillae Striatae (*Bai Ji*) brewed with child's urine. For vomiting of blood with coughing, (use) Flos Carthami Tinctorii

---

[3] This consists of Folium Stachysis Baicalensis (*Ji Su Ye*), Radix Astragali Membranacei (*Huang Qi*), Radix Rehmanniae (*Sheng Di Huang*), Gelatinum Corii Asini (*E Jiao*), Rhizoma Imperatae Cylindricae (*Bai Mao Gen*), Radix Platycodi Grandiflori (*Jie Geng*), Tuber Ophiopogonis Japonicae (*Mai Men Dong*), stir-fried Pollen Typhae (*Pu Huang*), Bulbus Fritillariae (*Bei Mu*), and mix-fried Radix Glycyrrhizae (*Zhi Gan Cao*).

[4] This consists of prepared Radix Rehmanniae (*Shu Di Huang*), Radix Albus Paeoniae Lactiflorae (*Bai Shao Yao*), Radix Angelicae Sinensis (*Dang Gui*), Rhizoma Ligustici Wallichii (*Chuan Xiong*), Radix Scutellariae Baicalensis (*Huang Qin*), Rhizoma Coptidis Chinensis (*Huang Lian*), Cortex Phellodendri (*Huang Bai*), Fructus Gardeniae Jasminoidis (*Zhi Zi*), and Radix Rehmanniae (*Sheng Di Huang*), 1 *qian* for each of the above.

(*Hong Hua*), Semen Pruni Armeniacae (*Xing Ren*), tip-nipped and skinned, Folium Eriobotryae Japonicae (*Pi Ba Ye*), stir-fried with ginger and stripped of hair, Radix Asteris Tatarici (*Zi Wan Rong*), Cornu Cervi Parvum (*Lu Rong*), mix-fried Cortex Radicis Mori Albi (*Sang Bai Pi*), and Caulis Akebiae Mutong (*Mu Tong*), 1 *liang* for each of the above, and Radix Et Rhizoma Rhei (*Da Huang*), one half *liang*. Make into pills with honey and melt in the mouth.

Blood exiting through the upper (portals) is always due to exuberant yang and vacuous yin. Because of ascending without descending[5] and of exuberant yang and vacuous yin, blood is unable to flow down and is forced by upflaming (yang to also move) upward and exit. (In such cases,) the pulse must be large and hollow. Largeness shows heat, while hollowness shows stasis and loss of blood. The great method is to supplement water to suppress fire in order to restore the (blood to its proper) position. (For this purpose, use) *Si Wu Tang* plus stir-fried Fructus Gardeniae Jasminoidis (*Shan Zhi Ren*), child's urine, Succus Zingiberis (*Jiang Zhi*), Tuber Curcumae (*Yu Jin*), and Succus Bambusae (*Zhu Li*). *Si Sheng Wan* (Four Raw [Ingredient] Pills)[6] in the *Da Quan Liang Fang (The Great Collection of Fine Formulas)* is very remarkable (in order to accomplish this). As for blood oozing from between the teeth or from under the tongue in the mouth without coughing or spitting of blood, (I) have always treated this by boosting kidney water and draining ministerial fire. Cure is achieved in never more than 10 days.

A person in the prime of his life suffered from cough... [This has already been discussed in the *Yi Yao {Essentials of Medicine}*.]

---

[5] This implies that yang, which is exuberant, keeps ascending, while yin, which is depleted, is unable to descend as it does in the normal state.

[6] This consists of raw Folium Nelumbinis Nuciferae (*He Ye*), raw Folium Artemisiae Argyii (*Ai Ye*), raw Cacumen Biotae Orientalis (*Bai Ye*), and raw Radix Rehmanniae (*Di Huang*), all in equal amounts.

Chapter Sixty

Hacking of Blood

(For this condition) use Succus Zingiberis (*Jiang Zhi*), child's urine, and Pulvis Indigonis (*Qing Dai*) introduced into blood medicinals (*i.e.,* formulas) such as *Si Wu Tang* (Four Materials Decoction), *Di Huang Gao* (Rehmannia Paste)[1], and *Niu Xi Gao* (Achyranthes Paste).[2] (To treat) cadaverous transmission consumption with alternating attacks of cold and heat, enduring cough and hacking of blood, and increasing emaciation, first administer *San Niu Tang* (Three Negatives Decoction) boiled together with *Lian Xin San* (Lotus Heart Powder). This never fails to offer a cure out of ten thousand cases. Another treatment for hacking of blood (consists of) boiling and taking black soybean (*Hei Dou*), Pericarpium Citri Reticulatae (*Chen Pi*), and Radix Glycyrrhizae (*Gan Cao*).

---

[1] There are several different formulas with this same name. Among these, the most likely one consists of pounded Radix Rehmanniae (*Sheng Di Huang*), 10 *jin* of the juice thus extracted being used, Radix Angelicae Sinensis (*Dang Gui*), 1 *jin*, Radix Paeoniae Lactiflorae (*Shao Yao*) and Fructus Lycii Chinensis (*Gou Qi Zi*), one half *jin* each, Tuber Asparagi Cochinensis (*Tian Men Dong*) and Tuber Ophiopogonis Japonicae (*Mai Men Dong*), 6 *liang* each, Rhizoma Ligustici Wallichii (*Chuan Xiong*) and Cortex Radicis Moutan (*Dan Pi*), 2 *liang* each, Semen Nelumbinis Nuciferae (*Lian Rou*), 4 *liang*, Rhizoma Anemarrhenae (*Zhi Mu*) and Cortex Radicis Lycii (*Di Gu Pi*), 3 *liang* each, and Radix Panacis Ginseng (*Ren Shen*) and Radix Glycyrrhizae (*Gan Cao*), 1 *liang* each. However, because this is a blood- supplementing formula, another equally if not more probable formula consists of just a paste of Radix Rehmanniae (*Sheng Di Huang*).

[2] This consists of tipped, skinned, stir-fried Semen Pruni Persicae (*Tao Ren*) and wine-washed Radix Angelicae Sinensis (*Dang Gui*), 1 *liang* each, wine-soaked Radix Achyranthis Bidentatae (*Niu Xi*), 4 *liang*, Radix Rubrus Paeoniae Lactiflorae (*Chi Shao Yao*) and wine-washed Radix Rehmanniae (*Sheng Di Huang*), 1.5 *liang*, and Rhizoma Ligustici Wallichii (*Chuan Xiong*), 5 *qian*. Powder the above, boil, and then put in a small amount of Secretio Moschi Moschiferi (*She Xiang*).

Chapter Sixty-one

Nosebleed

What is true of vomiting of blood is largely true (of nosebleeding as well). Roughly speaking, it is due to blood compelled by heat qi to ascend along with it. It should be treated by qi-dissipating and heat-abating as the ruling (methods) and by blood-cooling and moving (also) as the ruling (methods). Introduced into the formula are (the ingredients of) *Xi Jiao Di Huang Tang* (Rhinoceros Horn & Rehmannia Decoction), Cornu Rhinoceroris (*Xi Jiao*), Radix Rubrus Paeoniae Lactiflorae (*Chi Shao Yao*), Cortex Radicis Moutan (*Mu Dan Pi*), and Radix Rehmanniae (*Sheng Di Huang*) plus Tuber Curcumae (*Yu Jin*). If Cornu Rhinoceroris is not available, Rhizoma Cimicifugae (*Sheng Ma*) can be substituted. For erratic movement of the menstrual blood giving rise to a fishy, bloody smell, vomiting of blood, or spitting of blood, take Succus Allii Tuberosi (*Jiu Zhi*) and instant effect follows. In most cases, toxins can be resolved by Cornu Rhinoceroris (*Xi Jiao*). For incessant nosebleed, boil and take *Yang Wei Tang* (Nurture the Stomach Decoction).[1] One dose will result in a cure. For nosebleeding and retching of blood as well as forced diaphoresis when treating the *shao yin* pattern of cold damage[2], (use) *Xi Jiao Di Huang Tang* plus Radix Scutellariae Baicalensis (*Huang Qin*. However, for a) cold damage pattern similar to internal damage disease with incessant, massive nosebleeding following diaphoresis and precipitation, (use) *Zhen Wu*

---

[1] There are several versions of *Yang Wei Tang* existent, but none of them is indicated for nosebleed. The following is a typical one, given only for reference: Cortex Magnoliae Officinalis (*Hou Po*), Rhizoma Atractylodis (*Cang Zhu*), Rhizoma Pinelliae Ternatae (*Ban Xia*), Herba Agastachis Seu Pogostemi (*Huo Xiang*), Fructus Amomi Tsao-ko (*Cao Guo Ren*), Sclerotium Poriae Cocoris (*Fu Ling*), Radix Panacis Ginseng (*Ren Shen*), Radix Glycyrrhizae (*Gan Cao*), and Pericarpium Citri Rubri (*Ju Hong*).

[2] The *shao yin* pattern of cold damage does not permit diaphoresis even in case of sweat refusing to exude. If diaphoresis is administered, various kinds of bleeding may arise.

Tang (Turtle & Snake Decoction). If vexation and agitation, thirst, a deep, thin, faint pulse, cold feet, and a red and white, desertion facial complexion arise, this is yang desertion and yin vacuity.

Chapter Sixty-two

Hematuria

(This disease) is ascribed to (either) heat or blood vacuity. (To treat) hematuria ascribed to heat, boil and take stir-fried Fructus Gardeniae Jasminoidis (*Shan Zhi*) or Herba Cephalanoploris Segeti (*Xiao Ji*) and Succinum (*Hu Po*). If there is blood vacuity, (use) *Si Wu Tang* (Four Materials Decoction) plus *Niu Xi Gao* (Achyranthes Paste). Blood in the urine (due to) repletion calls for precipitation. *Dang Gui Cheng Qi Tang* (Dang Gui Support the Qi Decoction) is capable of this. Afterwards, administer *Si Wu Tang* plus stir-fried Fructus Gardeniae Jasminoidis (*Shan Zhi*). For hematuria in females for no (known) reason, (use) Os Draconis (*Long Gu*), 1 *liang*. Mix a 1 *cun* square coin[1] with wine. In general, hematuria, bloody *lin* or strangury, and blood in the stool are (all) of a kind in terms of the nature of the disease even though (the blood) exits from different (portals, *i.e.,*) the front or the back private (organs). Therefore their treatment is the same in terms of differentiation of root and branch. (The medicinals) used to scatter the blood and stop bleeding are no more than several tens in range. Somewhat different are those that serve best as their ushers, conductors, assistants, and envoys.

---

[1] This refers to a coinlike container, 1 *cun* or inch square. This is used simultaneously as a tool and unit for weighing medicinals. In terms of liquid, it amounted to 2.74 ml.

Chapter Sixty-three

Hemafecia

(This disease is due to either) heat or vacuity. To treat bleeding, it is inappropriate to use only cool and cold medicinals. One must make use of cold by virtue of heat, (in other words,) to combine cool and cold medicinals with acrid-flavored upbearing and warming ones. An example is to soak and stir-fry cool medicinals with wine or to boil *Huang Lian Wan* (Coptis Pills)[1] with wine. If there is heat, (use) *Si Wu Tang* (Four Materials Decoction) plus stir-fried Fructus Gardeniae Jasminoidis (*Shan Zhi*), Rhizoma Cimicifugae (*Sheng Ma*), Radix Gentianae Macrophyllae (*Qin Jiao*), and Gelatinum Corii Bovis Seu Equi (*Jiao Zhu*). For large intestine damp heat hemafecia which, over time, is categorized as (type of) vacuity, usually one should warm and dissipate with *Si Wu Tang* plus blast-fried Rhizoma Zingiberis (*Pao Jiang*) and Rhizoma Cimicifugae (*Sheng Ma*). An(other) formula (consists of) powdered Radix Angelicae (*Bai Zhi*) and Galla Rhi Chinensis (*Wu Bei Zi*). Make into pills with rice. (Yet) an(other) formula (is made by) burning dried Fructus Diosphyroris Kaki (*Gan Shi*) to ash (while) preserving its nature. Take 2-3 *qian* with thin gruel.

For blood in the stools due to accumulated heat, (use) Rhizoma Atractylodis (*Cang Zhu*), 1.5 *liang*, Pericarpium Citri Reticulatae (*Chen Pi*), 1.5 *liang*, Rhizoma Coptidis Chinensis (*Huang Lian*), Cortex Phellodendri (*Huang Bai*), and Radix Scutellariae Baicalensis (*Tiao Qin*), 7.5 *qian* for each of the above, and Fructus Forsythiae Suspensae (*Lian Qiao*), 5 *qian*. Powder the above and make into pills with paste (made from) 6 *liang* of Radix Rehmanniae (*Sheng Di Huang*). An(other) formula (consists of) Rhizoma Atractylodis (*Cang Zhu*) and Radix Rehmanniae (*Di Huang*). Pound the above into fine powder and make

---

[1]   This consists of Rhizoma Coptidis Chinensis (*Huang Lian*) and Gelatinum Corii Asini (*E Jiao*).

into pills with cooked rice. (During their preparation, these medicinals) should be kept off iron utensils.

To treat excessive blood in stools, (use) *Si Wu Tang* plus Corium Erinacei Europae (*Wei Pi*). An(other) formula (is made by) burning Pediculus Solani Melongenae (*Qie Di*) to ash while preserving its nature. (Then) stir-fry and grind Fructus Gardeniae Jasminoidis (*Shan Zhi*). Make into pills with cooked rice; 100 pills per dose taken with thin gruel early in the morning.

If hemafecia has lasted in a person so long as to damage blood and (hence) give rise to (blood) vacuity with a numb, wind(like) face growing tinea sores, (use) Plastrum Testudinis (*Gui Ban*), Rhizoma Cimicifugae (*Sheng Ma*), and Rhizoma Cyperi Rotundi (*Xiang Fu*), 5 *qian* for each of the above, Radix Albus Paeoniae Lactiflorae (*Bai Shao Yao*), 1.5 *qian*, Cacumen Biotae Orientalis (*Ce Bai*), 1 *liang*, and Cortex Cedrelae (*Chun Gen Pi*), 7.5 *qian*. Powder the above, make into pills with gruel, and take with a decoction of *Si Wu Tang* plus Rhizoma Atractylodis Macrocephalae (*Bai Zhu*), Rhizoma Coptidis Chinensis (*Huang Lian*), Radix Glycyrrhizae (*Gan Cao*), and Pericarpium Citri Reticulatae (*Chen Pi*).

A large, moderate (*i.e.*, relaxed/retarded) pulse with thirst, blood in the stools, and purple menstrual discharge is due to taxation damage embracing dampness. (In that case, use) Rhizoma Atractylodis Macrocephalae (*Bai Zhu*), 5 *qian*, Radix Rehmanniae (*Di Huang*), 3 *qian*, stir-fried Cortex Phellodendri (*Huang Bai*), 3 *qian*, Radix Albus Paeoniae Lactiflorae (*Bai Shao Yao*), Rhizoma Cyperi Rotundi (*Xiang Fu*), and Radix Sanguisorbae (*Di Yu*), 2 *qian* for each of the above, and Radix Scutellariae Baicalensis (*Huang Qin*), 1 *qian*. Powder the above and make into pills with cake. *Di Yu San* (Sanguisorba Powder)[2] from the

---

[2] This consists of Radix Sanguisorbae (*Di Yu*), stir-fried Radix Angelicae Sinensis (*Dang Gui*), Os Draconis (*Long Gu*), Rhizoma Ligustici Wallichii (*Chuan Xiong*), Gelatinum Corii Asini (*E Jiao*), and Os Sepiae Seu Sepiellae (*Wu Zei Gu*), 3 *fen* for each of the above, blast-fried Rhizoma Zingiberis (*Pao Jiang*), 1 *fen*, stir-fried Folium Artemisiae Argyii (*Ai Ye*), Rhizoma Atractylodis Macrocephalae (*Bai Zhu*), and Pollen Typhae (*Pu Huang*), one half *liang* each, and prepared Radix Rehmanniae (*Shu Di*) and

Xuan Ming Fang (Enlightening Formulas)[3] is a remarkably effective formula for the treatment of blood in the stools. (However,) people with yang vacuity and yin destitution who suffer from years long hemafecia with a face occasionally tinged the color of Cortex Phellodendri (*Huang Bai*, should be prescribed) *Li Zhong Tang* (Rectify the Center Pills) plus Radix Praeparatus Aconiti Carmichaeli (*Fu Zi*) and Pulvis Fumi Carbonisati (*Bai Cao Shuang*). Make into pills and take.

Dai comments: Coughing of blood is coughing of phlegm mixed with blood. Retching of blood means retching entirely of blood. Hacking of blood is discharge entirely of bloody lumps whenever hacked. Nosebleed is discharge of blood from the nose. Hematuria is discharge of blood with urination. Hemafecia is discharge of blood with defecation. Despite differences in names and colors, they are all heat patterns. They only differ (in terms of) vacuity and repletion, new and old (*i.e.*, recent or chronic onset). In any case, recklessly saying that they are cold is wrong.

---

carbonized Cornu Bovis Tauri (*Niu Jiao Hui*), 1 *liang* each.

[3] *I.e., Xuan Ming Fang Lun (Treatise on Enlightening Formulas)* in full. This book was written by Liu Wan-su, a.k.a. Liu He-jian, of the Jin Dynasty (1115-1234 CE). As mentioned above, Liu was the founder of the School of Cold & Cool (Medicine), one of the four great schools of the Jin/Yuan.

Chapter Sixty-four

Intestinal Wind[1]

(In this case, blood) exits solely from the stomach and large intestine. One should mostly use Radix Scutellariae Baicalensis (*Huang Qin*), Radix Gentianae Macrophyllae (*Qin Jiao*), Fructus Sophorae Japonicae (*Huai Jiao*), Rhizoma Cimicifugae (*Sheng Ma*), and Pulvis Indigonis (*Qing Dai*. However, if) complicated by wind, (use) Rhizoma Atractylodis (*Cang Zhu*), Radix Gentianae Macrophyllae (*Qin Jiao*), Radix Paeoniae Lactiflorae (*Shao Yao*), and Rhizoma Cyperi Rotundi (*Xiang Fu*).

One formula for intestinal wind (consists of) Rhizoma Atractylodis (*Cang Zhu*), Talcum (*Hua Shi*), Radix Angelicae Sinensis (*Dang Gui*), Radix Rehmanniae (*Sheng Di*), Radix Scutellariae Baicalensis (*Huang Qin*), and Radix Glycyrrhizae (*Gan Cao*). This is often used to settle intestinal pain. An(other) formula (consists of) roasted Radix Et Rhizoma Rhei (*Da Huang*), 3 *qian*, Radix Angelicae Sinensis (*Dang Gui*), one half *liang*, Semen Pruni Persicae (*Tao Ren*), 3 *qian*, tip-nipped and skinned, roasted Corium Erinacei Europae (*Wei Pi*), 1 *liang*, stir-fried Rhizoma Coptidis Chinensis (*Huang Lian*), 1 *liang*, Radix Gentianae Macrophyllae (*Qin Jiao*), 1 *liang*, Semen Sophorae Japonicae (*Huai Jiao Zi*), 1 *liang*, Semen Arecae Catechu (*Bing Lang*), one half *liang*, Semen Gleditschiae Sinensis (*Zao Jiao Ren*), one half *qian*, Cortex Phellodendri (*Huang Bai*), and Herba Seu Flos Schizonepetae Tenuifoliae (*Jing Jie Sui*), 5 *qian* each and stir-fried, and Fructus Citri Seu Ponciri (*Zhi Qiao*), 5 *qian*. Powder the above and make into pills the size of Chinese parasol tree seeds with paste; 50 pills per dose taken before a meal

---

[1] This disease is due to invasion of the stomach and intestines by wind evils which then transform into heat. It is characterized by bright bleeding from the anus during a bowel movement but preceding the actual passage of stool. Typically there is no swelling around the anus but there may be various gastrointestinal complaints.

with boiled water. In case of discharge of fresh blood, add carbonized Petriolus Trachycarpi (*Zong Mao Hui*) and carbonized Receptaculum Nelumbinis Nuciferae (*Peng Fang Hui*). The above (formulas) are specific against blood in the stools due to visceral toxins.

Intestinal *pi* with blood in the stools (due to) dual affection of dampness and heat and lack of regularity in daily life activities may develop into the swill diarrhea intestinal *pi*. (For this use) *Liang Xue Di Huang Tang* (Cool the Blood Rehmannia Decoction).[2] (But,) for blood in the stools due to damp toxins, (use) *Dang Gui He Xue San* (Dang Gui Harmonize the Blood Powder).[3] (While to treat) prolapse of the anus with intestinal wind, bake dry and powder 5-7 turtledoves and mix with vinegar. Sweep this onto (the prolapsed anus).

---

[2] This consists of Radix Scutellariae Baicalensis (*Huang Qin*), Herba Seu Flos Schizonepetae Tenuifoliae (*Jing Jie Sui*), and Fructus Viticis (*Man Jing Zi*), 1 *fen* for each of the above, Cortex Phellodendri (*Huang Bai*), Rhizoma Anemarrhenae (*Zhi Mu*), Radix Et Rhizoma Ligustici Sinensis (*Gao Ben*), Herba Cum Radice Asari Sieboldi (*Xi Xin*), and Rhizoma Ligustici Wallichii (*Chuan Xiong*), 2 *fen* for each of the above, Rhizoma Coptidis Chinensis (*Huang Lian*), Radix Et Rhizoma Notopterygii (*Qiang Huo*), Radix Bupleuri (*Chai Hu*), Rhizoma Cimicifugae (*Sheng Ma*), and Radix Ledebouriellae Sesloidis (*Fang Feng*), 3 *fen* for each of the above, Radix Rehmanniae (*Sheng Di Huang*) and Radix Angelicae Sinensis (*Dang Gui*), 5 *fen* each, Radix Glycyrrhizae (*Gan Cao*), 1 *qian*, and a small amount of Flos Carthami Tinctorii (*Hong Hua*).

[3] This consists of Radix Angelicae Sinensis (*Dang Gui*) and Rhizoma Cimicifugae (*Sheng Ma*), 2 *qian* each, Flos Immaturus Sophorae Japonicae (*Huai Hua*), Pericarpium Viridis Citri Reticulatae (*Qing Pi*), Herba Seu Flos Schizonepetae Tenuifoliae (*Jing Jie*), Rhizoma Atractylodis Macrocephalae (*Bai Zhu*), and prepared Radix Rehmanniae (*Shu Di*), 6 *fen* for each of the above, and Rhizoma Ligustici Wallichii (*Chuan Xiong*), 4 *fen*.

Chapter Sixty-five

Piles & Fistulas

(In the treatment of these conditions,) the rule is to exclusively cool the blood. In case of fistulas, first administer a large dose of a supplementing formula to generate qi and blood. Panacis Ginseng (*Ren Shen*), Radix Astragali Membranacei (*Huang Qi*), Radix Angelicae Sinensis (*Dang Gui*), Rhizoma Atractylodis Macrocephalae (*Bai Zhu*), and Rhizoma Ligustici Wallichii (*Chuan Xiong*) are the rulers (in such a formula). As an external treatment, mix powdered Radix Praeparatus Aconiti Carmichaeli (*Fu Zi*) with saliva, make into a cake a coin thick, place on the affected area, and moxa (over it), making (the place moxaed) moderately hot (but) without causing pain. When (the cake) is dry, change it. (One can) grind the dried cake and reshape it for further moxaing as explained above. When (the patient) becomes tired and sleepy, stop moxaing till the next day. Continue this practice till the flesh grows level. After that, boil the preceding qi and blood supplementing medicinals down into a paste and apply as a plaster. Slices of Radix Praeparatus Aconiti Carmichaeli (*Fu Zi*) can also be used for moxaing (on top of). This is also an appropriate method for (treating) *yong* and *ju*, sores and boils on the limbs (or) trunk whose openings have refused to close for a long time.

The great method for (treating) piles is to use Radix Scutellariae Baicalensis (*Tiao Qin*) to cool the large intestine, Radix Panacis Ginseng (*Ren Shen*), Rhizoma Coptidis Chinensis (*Huang Lian*), Radix Rehmanniae (*Sheng Di*), and Fructus Sophorae Japonicae (*Huai Jiao*) to cool and generate blood, Rhizoma Ligustici Wallichii (*Chuan Xiong*) and Radix Angelicae Sinensis (*Dang Gui*) to harmonize the blood, Fructus Citri Seu Ponciri (*Zhi Qiao*) to loosen the intestines, and Rhizoma Cimicifugae (*Sheng Ma*) to upraise. Externally, wash and steam with a decoction of Galla Rhi Chinensis (*Wu Bei*), slaked lime (*Po Xiao*), Ramus Loranthi Seu Visci (*Sang Ji Sheng*), and ptaculum Nelumbinis Nuciferae (*Lian Peng*). In case of swelling, apply powdered Semen Momordicae

Cochinensis (*Mu Bie Zi*) and Galla Rhi Chinensis (*Wu Bei Zi*) as a dressing. An(other) formula (is made by) boiling 2 *liang* of Rhizoma Coptidis Chinensis (*Huang Lian*) down into a paste. Then put in the same amount of Mirabilitum (*Mang Xiao*) and 1 *qian* of Borneolum (*Bing Pian*). Apply on the piles and they will soon disappear.

Around the anus, a new lump may grow over an existing hemorrhoid or fistula with thickened skin and swelling, issuing pus through the hemorrhoid opening. This should be treated as a downpouring of food accumulation. (To treat this, use) Rhizoma Coptidis Chinensis (*Huang Lian*), Resina Ferulae Asafoetidae (*A Wei*), Massa Medica Fermentata (*Shen Qu*), Fructus Crataegi (*Shan Zha*), Fructus Pruni Persicae (*Tao Ren*), Fructus Forsythiae Suspensae (*Lian Qiao*), Fructus Sophorae Japonicae (*Huai Jiao*), and Cornu Rhinoceroris (*Xi Jiao*). Make into pills and take. If the hemorrhoid head (grows) upwards, this is extreme heat of the large intestine which makes it contract and turn upwards. (In this case,) *Si Wu Tang* (Four Materials Decoction, can be used to) resolve toxins to which should be added Fructus Citri Seu Ponciri (*Zhi Qiao*), Rhizoma Atractylodis Macrocephalae (*Bai Zhu*), Fructus Sophorae Japonicae (*Huai Jiao*), and Radix Gentianae Macrophyllae (*Qin Jiao*. Also) use Herba Seu Flos Schizonepetae Tenuifoliae (*Jing Jie*), slaked lime (*Po Xiao*), and Ramus Loranthi Seu Visci (*Sang Ji Sheng*) as a wash. This settles pain, dispels wind, resolves toxins, and cools heat of the large intestine. In case of swelling, add Galla Rhi Chinensis (*Wu Bei Zi*) and Semen Momordicae Cochinensis (*Mu Bie Zi*).

(When treating) hemorrhoidal fistulas, cool the blood and loosen the large intestine (by) stripping Fructus Citri Seu Ponciri (*Zhi Qiao*) of pulp. (Then) fill (this with) Semen Crotonis (*Ba Dou*) and tie with iron wire. After cooking thoroughly, remove the Semen Crotonis. If this is introduced via pill, pound well (before) using. If it is introduced via decoction, dry in the sun (before) using.

A formula for fistulas (consists of) Rhizoma Ligustici Wallichii (*Chuan Xiong*), 5 *qian*, Herba Cum Radice Asari Sieboldi (*Xi Xin*), and Radix Angelicae (*Bai Zhi*), 2.5 *qian* each. Powder the above, make into a decoction, and take daily. If the disease is located in the lower, take before a meal. If it is located in the upper, take after a meal. Based on the size of the fistula, obtain Radix Corchori Capsularis (*Mai Huang Gen*) from the previous year, scrape off the bark, twist into a thread, (the thickness) depending on the size (of the fistula), and insert into the opening (of the fistula) all the way till (the thread) can go no further. If the lesion is not old, apply an ointment over this.

A person grew hemorrhoids around (their) anus whose openings refused to close. There were three needle-sized holes (discharging of) pus on taxation and labor. (For this I prescribed) Radix Scutellariae Baicalensis (*Huang Qin*), Fructus Forsythiae Suspensae (*Lian Qiao*), and Radix Gentianae Macrophyllae (*Qin Jiao*, all) the above powdered and made into pills with Massa Medica Fermentata (*Shen Qu*).

An(other) formula to treat piles (is made by) thoroughly mixing and applying (as a dressing) Arsenolitum (*Xiong Dan*) and Borneolum (*Pian Nao*). To treat blooming hemorrhoids, make a decoction of Herba Seu Flos Schizonepetae Tenuifoliae (*Jing Jie*), Radix Ledebouriellae Sesloidis (*Fang Feng*), and slaked lime (*Po Xiao*) and wash (with it). Then grind Semen Momordicae Cochinensis (*Mu Bie Zi*) and Tuber Curcumae (*Yu Jin*), put in a small amount of Borneolum (*Long Nao*), mix with water, and apply (as a dressing). Another method (consists of) obtaining a slice of Bulbus Allii Sativi (*Da Suan*), make dandruff (*Tou Gou*) into a cake, place the cake over the head of the hemorrhoid, lay the slice of Bulbus Allii Sativi over (this), and moxa.

To cure a rotten bone with enduring *ju* as well as hemorrhoidal fistulas with holes, obtain the leg bones of a black-boned chicken (*Wu Gu Ji*). Fill in (the cavities with) good quality Arsenicum (*Pi Shuang*), seal with salty mud, and calcine with fire till red hot. (Then) take out from the fire, set on the ground to rid of fire toxins, remove the mud, and grind finely. Make into pills the size of millet with cooked rice. Insert (one pill) into the (hemorrhoid) hole with a rolled piece of paper. Finally, apply an ointment.

Chapter Sixty-six

Dream Emission

(This disease) is exclusively governed by heat. Seminal loss, vaginal discharge, and dream emission[1] (can all be treated) in the same way (with) Pulvis Indigonis (*Qing Dai*), Pumice (*Hai Shi*), and Cortex Phellodendri (*Huang Bai*). (If there is) internal damage of the qi and blood (with) inability to secure (*i.e.*, consolidate one's semen), swallow *Chun Gen Wan* (Cedrela Bark Pills)[2] with *Ba Wu Tang* (Eight Materials Decoction) with additions and subtractions. If due to thought and yearning, the disease is located in the heart. (In this case,) it is appropriate to calm the spirit combined with supplementation. Cold contributes to hardening and congelation, while heat to free flowing. This is why seminal emission is exclusively governed by heat. Use stir-fried Cortex Phellodendri (*Huang Bai*), Concha Mactrae Quadrangularis (*He Fen*), and Pulvis Indigonis (*Qing Dai*). In case of dream emission, add Rhizoma Anemarrhenae (*Zhi Mu*). If recurrent, dream emission with turbid urine is ascribed to heart vacuity. (Use) *Zhen Zhu Fen Wan* (Pearl Powder Pills) with *Ding Zhi Wan* (Settle the Orientation [*i.e.*, Mind] Pills)[3] from the *Ju Fang* (*Collected Formulas*).

One formula, *Bu Shen Wan* (Supplement the Kidney Pills, consists of) Pericarpium Citri Reticulatae (*Chen Pi*), one half *liang*, stir-fried Cortex Phellodendri (*Huang Bai*), 1.5 *liang*, Radix Achyranthis Bidentatae (*Niu*

---

[1] Dream emission is defined as ejaculation during dreams of sexual intercourse during sleep, while seminal loss is defined as discharge of semen without dreaming of sex.

[2] This is composed of Cortex Cedrelae (*Chun Gen Bai Pi*), Fructus Citri Seu Ponciri (*Zhi Qiao*), and Rhizoma Atractylodis (*Cang Zhu*).

[3] This consists of Rhizoma Acori Graminei (*Shi Chang Pu*) and Radix Polygalae Tenuifoliae (*Yuan Zhi*), 2 *liang* each, and Sclerotium Poriae Cocoris (*Fu Ling*) and Radix Panacis Ginseng (*Ren Shen*), 3 *liang* each.

Xi), 1 *liang*, wine-fried, vanquished (*i.e.*, prepared) Plastrum Testudinis (*Bai Gui Ban*), 1.5 *liang*, and dry Rhizoma Zingiberis (*Gan Jiang*), 2 *qian*, not used in spring and summer. Powder the above and make into pills with a paste of Succus Zingiberis (*Jiang Zhi*).

Zheng Shu-lu, more than 20 years of age, (suffered from) excessive taxation of the heart. While in pursuit of (his) studies for provincial official examination, he sat up every day reading till the fourth drum striking.[4] (Then) suddenly, he contracted a disease. Whenever his yin (*i.e.*, genitals) touched anything during sleep, he would dream of sexual intercourse and have seminal discharge. When (his yin) were suspended (with nothing touching them), he would dream no dream. His food intake reduced day by day accompanied by fatigue, lassitude, and diminished qi. Because (he) exploited his heart to an extreme degree, two fires[5] broke out (simultaneously, thus) causing sleeplessness in the night. Blood failed to return to the kidneys, and kidney water became insufficient. (Thus) fire, taking advantage of yin vacuity, intruded into the lower burner, stirring the chamber of semen so that the semen could not gather or be stored but (rather) desired to escape. As a result, during sleep, whenever the yin touched something, dreams of sexual intercourse were provoked because of the intrusion of inverted qi. Accordingly, medicinals were prescribed to supplement the heart and calm the spirit in the upper, to regulate the spleen and stomach in the middle to upbear yang, and to boost essence, engender yin, and secure yang in the lower. In less than 3 months, the disease was overcome.

There (once) was a case of yin evil fixity. The son of Premier Jiang had dreams every night. I was sent to examine (him). For two days running, (I) examined his pulse and observed his behavior, but never once did he raise his head. He just kept looking down without turning his eyes towards other people. This was an obsession by an yin evil.

---

[4] In olden times, from midnight till dawn was divided into five periods and, at the beginning of each period, a watch struck a gong or drum to tell the time.

[5] *I.e.*, heart fire and kidney fire

When asked (about this), he would not let out a word concerning the ghost with which he had communicated. Therefore, (I) had to question his attending servants, and they told (me) that one day (he) went to a temple and caught sight of a statue of a maiden. He had caressed its body with his hands. Three to five days later, they learned that he had contracted this disease. Thereupon (I) bid some people to go to the temple and demolish the statue. (When they did this, they) found that the lower abdomen of the statue was all wet. After that, the disease was soon overcome.

Chapter Sixty-seven

Seminal Efflux[1]

(This condition) is exclusively governed by damp heat. Stir-fried Cortex Phellodendri (*Huang Bai*) strengthens the kidneys. Rhizoma Anemarrhenae (*Zhi Mu*) downbears fire. (And) Concha Ostreae (*Mu Li*) and Concha Mactrae Quadrangularis (*He Fen*) dry dampness. One formula to treat seminal efflux (consists of) Rhizoma Alpiniae Officinari (*Liang Jian*), 3 *qian*, Radix Paeoniae Lactiflorae (*Shao Yao*) and Cortex Phellodendri (*Huang Bai*), 2 *qian* each, burnt with (their) nature preserved, and Cortex Cedrelae (*Chun Gen Bai Pi*), 1.5 *liang*. Powder the above and make into pills with paste; 30 pills per dose.

---

[1] This condition is defined as the uncontrollable, spontaneous discharge of semen when awake and without sex.

Chapter Sixty-eight

Turbidity

(This condition) is (also) governed by damp heat. Although it is differentiated into red and white (types), it is never classified as cold and heat (varieties. Liu) He-jian says: In hot weather, water turns turbid, while in cold days, it becomes clear and cool. Looking from this (point of view), it is obvious that turbidity is a disease of damp heat. Red turbidity is ascribed to blood and heat, and white turbidity is ascribed to qi and phlegm. The red comes from the small intestine because it is ascribed to fire. The white comes from the large intestine because it is ascribed to metal. Turbid urine is (due to) heat. The red is (due to) heart vacuity, usually as a result of thought and worry. The white is ascribed to kidney vacuity as a result of excessive desire for sex. The treatment method is to dry dampness and downbear fire. *Zhen Zhu Fen Wan* (Pearl Powder Pills) are very good (at this). In addition, there is an uplifting method which is also very remarkable.

Cold leads to hardening and congelation, while heat leads to free flow. In general, (turbidity) is streaming damp phlegm. (Therefore,) it is appropriate to dry the dampness in the central palace. (For this purpose,) use *Er Chen Tang* (Two Aged Decoction) plus Rhizoma Atractylodis (*Cang Zhu*) and Rhizoma Atractylodis Macrocephalae (*Bai Zhu*) to dry the dampness. The red is dampness damaging blood. (For this) add Radix Albus Paeoniae Lactiflorae (*Bai Shao Yao*). Again, use *Zhen Zhu Fen Wan* plus Cortex Cedrelae (*Chun Gen Pi*), Talcum (*Hua Shi*), Pulvis Indigonis (*Qing Dai*), etc. Make into pills with Massa Medica Fermentata (*Shen Qu*) paste. A (variant) formula adds dry Rhizoma Zingiberis (*Gan Jiang*) which should be stir-fried to black so that it settles rather than penetrates. *Zhen Zhu Fen Wan* consists of Margarita (*Zhen Zhu*), 2 *liang*, true Concha Mactrae Quadrangularis (*He Fen*), 1 *jin*, and Cortex Phellodendri (*Huang Bai*), 1 *jin*, stir-fried to a red color on a new tile. Powder the above and make into pills the size of Chinese parasol tree seeds; 100 pills per dose taken on an empty stomach with warm wine. A wiry pulse indicates liver disease. (For this,) use Pulvis Indigonis (*Qing Dai*) to drain the liver.

Ban Ling Wan (Pinellia & Poria Pills) treat white turbidity. (They consist of) stir-fried Rhizoma Pinelliae Ternatae (*Ban Xia*) to dry dampness and Sclerotium Poriae Cocoris (*Fu Ling*) to separate water. A (variant) edition gives Sclerotium Polypori Umbellati (*Zhu Ling*, instead of Sclerotium Poriae Cocoris).

If white turbidity has not been cured for a long (time), this is due to fire not keeping to (its position. Therefore use) stir-fried Rhizoma Anemarrhenae (*Zhi Mu*), stir-fried Cortex Phellodendri (*Huang Bai*), and Radix Praeparatus Aconiti Carmichaeli (*Fu Zi*), all in equal amounts. Powder the above and make into pills with water. (However,) for vacuity taxation, use *Bu Yin Wan* (Supplement Yin Pills).[1] Generally speaking, neither cool nor hot medicinals should be used. If the patient is white and fat, there must be abundant damp phlegm. Use *Er Chen Tang* to remove dampness. If there is weak stomach, simultaneously use Radix Panacis Ginseng (*Ren Shen*). Radix Bupleuri (*Chai Hu*) and Rhizoma Cimicifugae (*Sheng Ma*) can be used to upbear the qi in the stomach. Use Pulvis Indigonis (*Qing Dai*), Cortex Phellodendri (*Huang Bai*), stir-fried to a slightly brown color, stir-fried Talcum (*Hua Shi*), dry Rhizoma Zingiberis (*Gan Jiang*), stir-fried to slightly black, Concha Mactrae Quadrangularis (*He Fen*) as medicinals for pills. Powder the above and make into pills.

For damp, turbid qi in the stomach flowing down resulting in red and white turbidity, add Radix Bupleuri (*Chai Hu*), Rhizoma Cimicifugae (*Sheng Ma*), Rhizoma Atractylodis (*Cang Zhu*), and Rhizoma Atractylodis Macrocephalae (*Bai Zhu*) to *Er Chen Tang*. Boil and take. As pill medicinals it is appropriate to use powdered Cortex Ailanthi Altissimae (*Chu Gen Mo*), Concha Mactrae Quadrangularis (*He Fen*), dry Rhizoma Zingiberis (*Gan Jiang*), and stir-fried Cortex Phellodendri (*Huang Bai*. While) the ruling (medicinals) specific for turbid qi in the stomach flowing down into the urinary bladder are Pulvis Indigonis (*Qing Dai*)

---

[1]   The ingredients in this formula can be found in the text of Ch. 56, Bk. 4.

and Concha Mactrae Quadrangularis (*He Fen*).

One formula to treat red and white turbidity (consists of) Cortex Phellodendri (*Huang Bai*), stir-fried to black, 1 *liang*, fresh Cortex Phellodendri (*Sheng Huang Bai*), 2.5 *qian*, Pumice (*Hai Shi*), 3 *liang*, and Massa Medica Fermentata (*Shen Qu*), one half *liang*. Powder the above and make into pills with water. In the presence of heat, (use) Cortex Phellodendri (*Huang Bai*), Talcum (*Hua Shi*), Pulvis Indigonis (*Qing Dai*), and the like. Powder the above and make into pills with water. A formula to dry damp phlegm (consists of) equal amounts of Rhizoma Arisaematis (*Nan Xing*), Pumice (*Hai Shi*), Massa Medica Fermentata (*Shen Qu*), and Rhizoma Pinelliae Ternatae (*Ban Xia*). Make into pills with Pulvis Indigonis (*Qing Dai*) as coating. Zhang Zi-yuan (has offered a formula to treat) dual vacuity of the qi and blood, the existence of phlegm, occasional fits of painful wind, recurrent breaking out of yin fire, and whitish turbid urine or red and white vaginal discharge. The formula is given in the preceding (chapter on) painful wind (*i.e.*, Ch. 49). To treat red turbidity, combine *Wu Ling San* with *Miao Xiang Wan* (Miraculous Fragrant Powder)[2] and take *Er Dong Tang* (Two Winters Decoction)[3] with *Ding Zhi Wan* (Settle Orientation [*i.e.*, the Mind] Pills). Their formula is composed of Radix Polygalae Tenuifoliae (*Yuan Zhi*), pitted, stripped of sprouts, 2 *liang*, Rhizoma Acori Graminei (*Shi Chang Pu*), 3 *liang*, Radix Panacis Ginseng (*Ren*

---

[2]   This is composed of Secretio Moschi Moschiferi (*She Xiang*), ground separately, 1 *qian*, roasted Radix Saussureae Seu Vladimiriae (*Mu Xiang*), 2.5 *liang*, Radix Dioscoreae Oppositae (*Shan Yao*), Sclerotium Poriae Cocoris (*Fu Ling*), Sclerotium Pararadicis Poriae Cocoris (*Fu Shen*), Radix Astragali Membranacei (*Huang Qi*), and Radix Polygalae Tenuifoliae (*Yuan Zhi*), 1 *liang* for each of the above, Radix Panacis Ginseng (*Ren Shen*), Radix Platycodi Grandiflori (*Jie Geng*), and mix-fried Radix Glycyrrhizae (*Zhi Gan Cao*), one half *liang* for each of the above, and Cinnabar (*Zhu Sha*), 3 *qian*, ground separately.

[3]   This is composed of pitted Tuber Asparagi Cochinensis (*Tian Men Dong*), 2 *qian*, pitted Tuber Ophiopogonis Japonicae (*Mai Men Dong*), 3 *qian*, Radix Trichosanthis Kirlowii (*Tian Hua Fen*), Radix Scutellariae Baicalensis (*Huang Qin*), Rhizoma Anemarrhenae (*Zhi Mu*), and Folium Nelumbinis Nuciferae (*He Ye*), 1 *qian* for each of the above, and Radix Panacis Ginseng (*Ren Shen*) and Radix Glycyrrhizae (*Gan Cao*), 5 *fen* each.

Shen), 3 *liang*, and skinned Sclerotium Poriae Cocoris (*Bai Fu Ling*), 3 *liang*. Powder the above, make into pills the size of Chinese parasol tree seeds with honey, and coat with Cinnabar (*Zhu Sha*); 20 pills per dose taken before a meal with thin gruel. Increase (gradually) to 30 pills.

Turbid qi is, without exception, damp phlegm. The medicinals to be introduced into a pill formula are Pulvis Indigonis (*Qing Dai*), powdered Cortex Ailanthi Altissimae (*Chu Pi Mo*), Concha Mactrae Quadrangularis (*He Fen*), Talcum (*Hua Shi*), stir-fried dry Rhizoma Zingiberis (*Gan Jiang*) and brown-fried Cortex Phellodendri (*Huang Bai*). Make the above into pills with paste of stir-fried Massa Medica Fermentata (*Shen Qu*). These pills for drying damp phlegm can also be used to treat the disease of vaginal discharge. Master Dai explains: Talcum (*Hua Shi*) disinhibits the portals. Cortex Phellodendri (*Huang Bai*) treats damp heat. Pulvis Indigonis (*Qing Dai*) resolves heat. Concha Mactrae Quadrangularis (*He Fen*, being) salty and cold, enters the kidneys. And stir-fried dry Rhizoma Zingiberis (*Gan Jiang*, being) bitter in flavor, leads lung qi downward. To generate yin blood, dry Rhizoma Zingiberis should be processed with salt.

A person who had suffered from turbid urine for half a year with frequent dream emission and a thin form was treated mainly as heart vacuity. (He was prescribed) *Ding Zhi Wan* taken together with *Zhen Zhu Fen Wan*. Another person had impaired memory and white turbidity. The treatment method was the same.

(I) often heard the master[4] explain that white turbidity usually develops from damp qi flowing down into the urinary bladder. The *Ling Shu Jing (The Spiritual Pivot Classic)* states in (slightly) different words: Red and white turbidity is (an abnormal) change of urine due to insufficient central qi. It is necessary first to supplement and upraise the central qi and then to give treatment based on the (involved)

---

[4] Zhu Dan-xi was the master, the lecturer, while the audience were his pupils. This style of presentation supports the hypothesis that the present work was written by the pupils of Zhu rather than by him personally.

viscus or bowel, qi or blood, red or white, vacuity or repletion. Like damage done by other kinds of evil heat, it truly requires draining heat and supplementing vacuity. If there is severe kidney qi vacuity or extreme hyperactive fire heat, it is not appropriate to use only cool and cold (medicinals). This needs to be treated with a counterassistant method.[5] What is essential is to weigh the severe against the light.

Chapter Sixty-nine

Strangury

Strangury is divided into five types, all ascribed to heat. (Therefore,) resolving heat and disinhibiting urination are the ruling (methods). Boil and take such medicinals as Fructus Gardeniae Jasminoidis (*Shan Zhi Zi*) with Radix Polygoni Cuspidati (*Hu Zhang*) and Radix Glycyrrhizae (*Gan Cao*). *Xiao Ji Tang* (Cephalanoplos Decoction)[1] treats blood strangury due to heat bound in the lower burner. One may also have strangury due to extreme kidney vacuity. (In that case,) it is necessary to supplement kidney essence and disinhibit urination, and it is not allowed to only drain. (In the treatment of) strangury pattern, diaphoresis is not acceptable since diaphoresis (in this case) is bound to result in hematuria. Old people may also have qi vacuity (strangury. In that case, use) Radix Panacis Ginseng (*Ren Shen*) and Rhizoma Atractylodis Macrocephalae (*Bai Zhu*) together with Caulis Akebiae Mutong (*Mu Tong*) and Fructus Gardeniae Jasminoidis (*Shan Zhi Zi*).

---

[5] This implies the use of warming and supplementing formulas.

[1] This consists of Radix Rehmanniae (*Sheng Di Huang*), 4 *liang*, Herba Seu Radix Cephalanoploris Segeti (*Xiao Ji*), Talcum (*Hua Shi*), Medulla Tetrapanacis Papyriferi (*Tong Cao*), stir-fried Pollen Typhae (*Pu Huang*), Herba Lophatheri Gracilis (*Dan Zhu Ye*), Rhizoma Nelumbinis Nuciferae (*Ou Jie*), Radix Angelicae Sinensis (*Dang Gui*), Fructus Gardeniae Jasminoidis (*Zhi Zi Ren*), and mix-fried Radix Glycyrrhizae (*Zhi Gan Cao*), one half *liang* for each of the above.

In addition, one may have strangury due to dead blood. *Niu Xi Gao* (Achyranthis Paste, is effective for this but is) capable of damaging the stomach, thus giving rise to an inability to take in food. (Therefore) it should not be administered in great quantities.

To treat strangury, (use) skinned, stir-fried Fructus Gardeniae Jasminoidis (*Shan Zhi*), 1 *liang*. Take with boiled water. To treat qi vacuity strangury, (use) *Ba Wu Tang* (Eight Materials Decoction) plus Radix Astragali Membranacei (*Huang Qi*) as well as Radix Polygoni Cuspidati (*Hu Zhang*) and Radix Glycyrrhizae (*Gan Cao*). Boil and take with Radix Achyranthis Bidentatae (*Niu Xi*) added. One formula consists of *Yi Yuan San* (Boost the Origin Powder) plus Fructus Gardeniae Jasminoidis (*Shan Zhi*) and Caulis Akebiae Mutong (*Mu Tong*). In summer months, boil Fructus Foeniculi Vulgaris (*Hui Xiang*), brew with *Yi Yuan San*, and take. For phlegm heat obstructed and stagnated in the middle burner (giving rise to) dribbling and inhibited urination, (use) Sodium Sulfate (*Xuan Ming Fen*). For heat existing in the qi and blood, (use) *Ba Wu Tang* plus Cortex Phellodendri (*Huang Bai*) and Rhizoma Anemarrhenae (*Zhi Mu*). And for dribbling urinary block in males and females alike when blood medicinals prove ineffective, (use) Cortex Phellodendri (*Huang Bai*), baked on a new tile, and fire-calcined Concha Ostreae (*Mu Li*). Powder the above finely and take before a meal or brewed with Fructus Foeniculi Vulgaris (*Xiao Hui Xiang*) soup.

Chapter Seventy

Urinary Incontinence

Urinary incontinence or enuresis is ascribed to (either) heat or vacuity. (Li) Dong-yuan states: (If) lung qi is vacuous, it is appropriate to calm the spirit and nurture the qi, and taxation and toil are prohibited. To calm the spirit and nurture qi, use Radix Panacis Ginseng (*Ren Shen*) and Radix Astragali Membranacei (*Huang Qi*). If supplementation fails to achieve a cure, there is heat. (In that case,) add Cortex Phellodendri (*Huang Bai*) and Radix Rehmanniae (*Sheng Di*).

Chapter Seventy-one

Urinary Stoppage

(This may be due to) qi vacuity, blood vacuity, repletion heat, or the existence of phlegm. Perform ejection to uplift the qi, and, when qi is upborne, water will naturally be downborne. (This is) because qi conveys and contains water. For qi vacuity, (use) Radix Panacis Ginseng (*Ren Shen*), Radix Astragali Membranacei (*Huang Qi*), Rhizoma Cimicifugae (*Sheng Ma*), etc. Administration (of these) can (then) be followed by ejection. Or perform mechanical emesis in the course of (taking) Radix Panacis Ginseng and Radix Astragali Membranacei. (However, for) blood vacuity, (use) *Si Wu Tang* (Four Materials Decoction). Administration (of this) can (also) be followed by ejection. In addition, *Xiong Gui Tang* (Ligusticum & Dang Gui Decoction)[1] can also be used with mechanical emesis. For copious phlegm, (use) mechanical emesis with *Er Chen Tang* (Two Aged Decoction) plus Caulis Akebiae Mutong (*Mu Tong*) and Rhizoma Cyperi Rotundi (*Xiang Fu*. But) repletion heat requires disinhibition (of urination).

A female suffered from fecal and urinary stoppage following pain in her spleen. This was phlegm obstructing the middle burner and qi gathering in the lower burner. *Er Chen Tang* plus Caulis Akebiae Mutong (*Mu Tong*) was prescribed. (The decoction) was taken after a first boil. Then mechanical emesis was performed after a decoction made of the dregs was (also) taken.

---

[1] A.k.a. *Fo Shou San* (Buddha's Hand Powder). This consists of equal amounts of Radix Angelicae Sinensis (*Dang Gui*) and Rhizoma Ligustici Wallichii (*Chuan Xiong*).

For people with strong qi and replete heat, (use) *Ba Zheng San* (Eight Righteous Powder).[2] When the bowels are loosened, the urine will flow freely by itself. For urinary stoppage due to depressive heat, (use) Sclerotium Rubrum Poriae Cocoris (*Chi Fu Ling*), Radix Scutellariae Baicalensis (*Huang Qin*), Rhizoma Alismatis (*Ze Xie*), Semen Plantaginis (*Che Qian Zi*), Tuber Ophiopogonis Japonicae (*Mai Men Dong*), Cortex Cinnamomi (*Gui*), Talcum (*Hua Shi*), Caulis Akebiae Mutong (*Mu Tong*), and Apex Radicis Glycyrrhizae (*Gan Cao Xiao*). In case of qi vacuity pain, add Radix Saussureae Seu Vladimiriae (*Mu Xiang*) and Radix Astragali Membranacei (*Huang Qi*). In case of strangury pain, add Cortex Phellodendri (*Huang Bai*) and Radix Rehmanniae (*Sheng Di Huang.* And) in summer months, brew with *Yi Yuan San* (Boost the Origin Powder).

For phlegm obstructed in the middle burner, boil a large bowl of decocted *Er Chen Tang* and take all at once to provoke vomiting for the purpose of regulating the true qi. Or brew 2 *qian* of powdered, sifted Semen Pharbitidis (*Qian Niu*) with granulated sugar solution and take (to also provoke) vomiting. After cold damage, in case of urinary stoppage as a result of yang desertion, brew Fructus Foeniculi Vulgaris (*Hui Xiang*) with undiluted Succus Zingiberis (*Sheng Jiang Zhi*), apply onto the lower abdomen, and take *Yi Zhi Hui Xiang Wan* (Boost Orientation [*i.e.*, the Mind] Fennel Pills)[3] in combination with *Yi Yuan San.*

A person's lower burner was damaged by dry heat and, consequently, they had inhibited urination. It was necessary to nurture yin with

---

[2] This consists of equal amounts of Semen Plantaginis (*Che Qian Zi*), Herba Dianthi (*Qu Mai*), Herba Polygoni Avicularis (*Bian Xu*), Talcum (*Hua Shi*), Fructus Gardeniae Jasminoidis (*Zhi Zi Ren*), mix-fried Radix Glycyrrhizae (*Zhi Gan Cao*), Caulis Akebiae Mutong (*Mu Tong*), and Radix Et Rhizoma Rhei (*Da Huang*); 2 *qian* per dose.

[3] This consists of Rhizoma Atractylodis Macrocephalae (*Bai Zhu*), Sclerotium Poriae Cocoris (*Fu Ling*), stir-fried Fructus Foeniculi Vulgaris (*Hui Xiang*), Fructus Evodiae Rutecarpae (*Wu Zhu Yu*), Semen Litchi Chinensis (*Li Zhi He*), and Semen Crataegi (*Shan Zha He*), 1 *liang* for each of the above, Semen Citri (*Ju He*), 3 *liang*, and Fructus Immaturus Citri Seu Ponciri (*Zhi Shi*), 8 *qian*.

Radix Angelicae Sinensis (*Dang Gui*), Radix Rehmanniae (*Di Huang*), Rhizoma Anemarrhenae (*Zhi Mu*), Cortex Phellodendri (*Huang Bai*), Radix Achyranthis Bidentatae (*Niu Xi*), Sclerotium Poriae Cocoris (*Fu Ling*), Radix Glycyrrhizae (*Sheng Gan Cao*), Rhizoma Atractylodis Macrocephalae (*Bai Zhu*), Pericarpium Citri Reticulatae (*Chen Pi*), and others.

A female, aged 50, suffered from inhibited urination. After administering *Ba Zheng San*, her lower abdomen became tense with distention, (urinary) stoppage, and a nettle-pricking sensation over (her whole) body. Thinking that the evil dampness of continual rain with which she had been affected was in the upper and the exterior, I prescribed Rhizoma Atractylodis (*Cang Zhu*) as the sovereign and Radix Praeparatus Aconiti Carmichaeli (*Fu Zi*) as the assistant to effuse the exterior. One dose resulted in perspiration and her urination was instantly unblocked.

A male, aged 80, suffered from short, inhibited voiding of urine and later developed urinary block without voiding a drop of urine. This was the result of taking excessive (water-)separating and disinhibiting medicinals. Thinking that excessive drink and food had damaged his stomach causing the qi to sink in the lower burner, I prescribed *Bu Zhong Yi Qi Tang* (Supplement the Center & Boost the Qi Decoction). After taking 1 dose, his urination was unblocked. Because too many disinhibitors had been taken, the kidney qi had been damaged. Therefore, urinary incontinence followed unblocking of urination with incessant voidings for a whole night. (Complete) recovery was achieved after the kidneys were supplemented. The existence of heat requires clearing. The existence of dampness requires drying. The existence of qi bound below requires upbearing.

There are (also) passing over to the second and passing over to the third (methods of) treatment.[4] For example, in case of failure to

---

[4] The underlying logic is that kidney/bladder water is the child of lung metal. While the latter is the child of spleen earth. Treating urinary disorders by treating the kidney/bladder is a primary or direct method. Treating lung metal is a secondary

engender water as a result of dry lungs, lung metal should be cleared. This is (a species) of passing over to the second. If the cause is not lung dryness but (rather) the existence of heat in the urinary bladder, urinary bladder fire should be drained straight away. This is a direct treatment. If the lungs are unable to engender water because spleen dampness is not moved and the essential qi does not ascend, then it is necessary to dry the spleen. This is (a species of) passing over to the third. To clear the lungs, use Semen Plantaginis (*Che Qian Zi*), Sclerotium Poriae Cocoris (*Fu Ling*), and the like. To drain the urinary bladder, use Cortex Phellodendri (*Huang Bai*), Rhizoma Anemarrhenae (*Zhi Mu*), and the like. (And) to fortify and dry the spleen, use Rhizoma Atractylodis (*Cang Zhu*), Rhizoma Atractylodis Macrocephalae (*Bai Zhu*), and the like. If these various treatment methods all fail to unblock (urination), then perform ejection since qi conveys and contains water. After ejection, qi will ascend, and when qi ascends, water descends.

Chapter Seventy-two

Bound Stool

(This disease is due to) vacuity, wind, dampness, fire, insufficient fluids and humor, cold, or qi binding. In (all) these cases, a yellow facial complexion can usually be observed. By all means, (one) should not use Nitre (*Xiao*), Sulphur (*Huang*), and the like indiscriminately in all these cases. Semen Crotonis (*Ba Dou*) and Semen Pharbitidis (*Qian Niu*) can also not be used indiscriminately in all cases. It is necessary to observe the great method. Yang formulas rule moistening dryness, while yin formulas rule opening bind. Use Semen Pruni (*Yu Li Ren*), Semen Pruni Persicae (*Tao Ren*), Radix Et Rhizoma Notopterygii (*Qiang*

---

method passing over to the second organ/phase, *i.e.*, lung metal. Passing over both kidneys and lungs to treat the spleen means that one is passing over to the third organ/phase, *i.e.*, spleen earth, away from kidney water, .

Huo), Radix Et Rhizoma Rhei (*Da Huang*), Radix Angelicae Sinensis (*Dang Gui*), and Semen Cannabis Sativae (*Ma Zi Ren*). Powder the above. A small amount of Radix Saussureae Seu Vladimiriae (*Mu Xiang*) and Semen Arecae Catechu (*Bing Lang*) can be added.

For fecal stoppage due to a dry, bound large intestine, (use) *Run Chang Tang* (Moisten the Intestine Decoction), also known as *Dang Gui Run Chang Tang* (*Dang Gui* Moisten the Intestine Decoction).[1] For block of the dark gate[2] with (qi) up-surging into the inhaling gate[3] giving rise to choking and constriction and dry, bound stools, (use) *Tong You Tang* (Free the Dark Decoction).[4] In addition, there may be cases of deep-lying fire in the stomach causing dry, bound stools with no desire for food. Wind bind and blood bind may also cause (fecal) stoppage. Apply dryness-moistening, blood-harmonizing, and wind-coursing in order to achieve natural unblocking. Treat with *Run Chang Wan* (Moisten the Intestine Pills).

---

[1] The decoction consists of Radix Rehmanniae (*Sheng Di*), Radix Glycyrrhizae (*Sheng Gan Cao*), roasted Radix Et Rhizoma Rhei (*Da Huang*), prepared Radix Rehmanniae (*Shu Di*), Apex Radicis Angelicae Sinensis (*Dang Gui Wei*), Rhizoma Cimicifugae (*Sheng Ma*), Semen Pruni Persicae (*Tao Ren*), and Semen Cannabis Sativae (*Ma Zi Ren*), 1 qian for each of the above, and Flos Carthami Tinctorii (*Hong Hua*), 3 fen. The pills mentioned below are composed of Semen Pruni Persicae (*Tao Ren*) and Semen Cannabis Sativae (*Ma Zi Ren*), 1 liang each, Apex Radicis Angelicae Sinensis (*Dang Gui Wei*), roasted Radix Et Rhizoma Rhei (*Da Huang*), and Radix Et Rhizoma Notopterygii (*Qiang Huo*), 1 qian for each of the above.

[2] I.e., the pylorus

[3] I.e., the epiglottis

[4] This consists of smashed Semen Pruni Persicae (*Tao Ren*) and Flos Carthami Tinctorii (*Hong Hua*), 1 fen each, Radix Rehmanniae (*Sheng Di*) and prepared Radix Rehmanniae (*Shu Di Huang*), 5 fen each, Radix Angelicae Sinensis (*Dang Gui*), mix-fried Radix Glycyrrhizae (*Zhi Gan Cao*), and Rhizoma Cimicifugae (*Sheng Ma*), 1 qian for each of the above.

For damp heat causing the disease of dry, bound stools, (use) *Shen Xiong Wan* (Divine Ligusticum Pills).[5] For constipation or fecal blockage with dry, bound stools, blood-quickening and dryness--moistening are the ruling (modalities). For the existence of heat, (use) *Da Cheng Qi Tang* (Major Support the Qi Decoction. But for) cold substances retained and stagnated in the stomach causing constipation and cardiac and abdominal pain, (use) *Bei Ji Wan* (Emergency Pills). For food damaging the *tai yin* and qi stagnation and non-circulation causing the disease, (use) *Mu Xiang Bing Lang Wan* (Saussurea & Areca Pills). For large intestine vacuity constipation with heat, (use) Radix Albus Paeoniae Lactiflorae (*Bai Shao Yao*), 1.5 *liang*, Pericarpium Citri Reticulatae (*Chen Pi*), Radix Rehmanniae (*Sheng Di*), and Radix Angelicae Sinensis (*Dang Gui Shen*), 1 *liang* for each of the above, and Radix Glycyrrhizae (*Gan Cao*), 5 *qian*. Powder the above, make into pills with gruel, and take with boiled water.

In some pertinent discussion, there is a treatment for abdominal distention with (fecal) stoppage. Rub the navel with Semen Pruni Armeniacae (*Xing Ren*), Bulbus Allii Fistulosi (*Cong Bai*), and salt. There is yet another (method): Make Fructus Gleditschiae Sinensis (*Zao Jiao*) and Fructus Immaturus Pruni Mume (*Bai Mei Rou*) into pills with honey and insert (into the anus). Pills can also be made from the juice of these two medicinals which is mixed with honey and boiled down into a paste. Or mix the juice with glutinous rice, stir-fry till dry with their nature preserved, and make into pills with sugar. Or merely use honey-(mixed) Fructus Pruni Mume (*Wu Mei*, as pills). All these kinds of pills can be inserted into the anus. They are all medicinals which open wind heat (and) dry bind.

---

[5] This consists of Radix Et Rhizoma Rhei (*Da Huang*) and Radix Scutellariae Baicalensis (*Huang Qin*), 2 *liang* each, Semen Pharbitidis (*Qian Niu Zi*) and Talcum (*Hua Shi*), 4 *liang* each, and Rhizoma Coptidis Chinensis (*Huang Lian*), Herba Menthae (*Bo He*), and Rhizoma Ligustici Wallichii (*Chuan Xiong*), one half *liang* for each of the above.

Chapter Seventy-three

Block & Repulsion

Block leads to inability to urinate, while repulsion leads to counterflow vomiting. This pattern very often ends in death. Because there is cold above and heat below, it is necessary to use ejection to upraise the transversely barred qi. However, it is alright (even) if no phlegm is ejected. When *Er Chen Tang* is used for ejection, it (nevertheless) implies downbearing (even) while (attempting) to provoke vomiting. In case of central qi vacuity and non-circulation, upbearing and downbearing (medicinals) should be introduced into qi-supplementing ones. (Block and repulsion are characterized by) the *cun* (*kou*) pulse on both hands being four times more exuberant (than normal).

Dai comments: Block and repulsion are spoken of as a sensation of something obstructing at the (level of the) diaphragm, (suspended there) on the verge of ascending but not ascending, on the verge of descending but not descending (with) food unable to go down. This is transversely barred qi.

Chapter Seventy-four

Epileptic Pattern

Epilepsy is not necessarily divided into five types, etc. It is specifically governed by phlegm and (one should) mostly use ejection. (One can) have fright (epilepsy). (One can) have phlegm (epilepsy). (And one can) have fire (epilepsy). Generally speaking, moving phlegm is the rule. The medicinals introduced into the formula are Rhizoma Coptidis Chinensis (*Huang Lian*), Rhizoma Arisaematis (*Nan Xing*), Rhizoma Pinelliae Ternatae

(*Ban Xia*), and Fructus Trichosanthis Kirlowii (*Gua Lou*). Track down phlegm and fire, and treatment, if in accordance with their (relative) quantities, will never not cure. Phlegm should be differentiated from fire. (If) there is heat, use cool medicinals to clear the heart. (If) there is phlegm, it is necessary to use emetics. Afterwards, use (Li) Dong-yuan's *Zhu Sha An Shen Wan* (Cinnabar Calm the Spirit Pills).

In most cases, (the treatment of) this pattern needs the use of ejection. After that, use liver-leveling medicinals such as Pulvis Indigonis (*Qing Dai*), Radix Bupleuri (*Chai Hu*), and Rhizoma Ligustici Wallichii (*Chuan Xiong*). A (variant) version (gives) *Long Hui Wan* (Gentiana & Aloe Pills). Suppose epilepsy is caused by fright. Fright leads the spirit to leave its abode, and, when its abode is left vacant, phlegm may gather there. Qian's *Xie Qing Wan* (Drain the Green-Blue Pills)[1] and *Niu Huang Qing Xin Wan* (Bezoar Clear the Heart Pills)[2] both treat epilepsy.

---

[1] This consists of Radix Angelicae Sinensis (*Dang Gui*), Borneolum (*Bing Pian*), Rhizoma Ligustici Wallichii (*Chuan Xiong*), Fructus Gardeniae Jasminoidis (*Zhi Zi*), Radix Et Rhizoma Rhei (*Da Huang*), Radix Et Rhizoma Notopterygii (*Qiang Huo*), and Radix Ledebouriellae Sesloidis (*Fang Feng*), all in equal amounts.

[2] This consists of Radix Albus Paeoniae Lactiflorae (*Bai Shao Yao*), Tuber Ophiopogonis Japonicae (*Mai Men Dong*), Radix Scutellariae Baicalensis (*Huang Qin*), Radix Angelicae Sinensis (*Dang Gui*), Radix Ledebouriellae Sesloidis (*Fang Feng*), and Rhizoma Atractylodis Macrocephalae (*Bai Zhu*), 1.5 *liang* for each of the above, Radix Bupleuri (*Chai Hu*), Radix Platycodi Grandiflori (*Jie Geng*), Rhizoma Ligustici Wallichii (*Chuan Xiong*), Sclerotium Poriae Cocoris (*Fu Ling*), and Semen Pruni Armeniacae (*Xing Ren*), 1.25 *liang*, Massa Medica Fermentata (*Shen Qu*), stir-fried Pollen Typhae (*Pu Huang*), and Radix Panacis Ginseng (*Ren Shen*), 2.5 *liang* for each of the above, Cornu Antelopis Saigae Tartaricae (*Ling Yang Jiao*), Secretio Moschi Moschiferi (*She Xiang*), and Borneolum (*Bing Pian*), 1 *liang* for each of the above, Cortex Cinnamomi (*Rou Gui*), stir-fried dried blackbean sprouts (*Da Dou Huang Juan*), and stir-fried Gelatinum Corii Asini (*E Jiao*), 1.75 *liang* for each of the above, Radix Ampelopsis Japonicae (*Bai Lian*) and blast-fried Rhizoma Zingiberis (*Pao Jiang*), 7.5 *qian* each, Calculus Bovis (*Niu Huang*), 1.2 *liang*, Cornu Rhinoceroris (*Xi Jiao*), 2 *liang*, Realgar (*Xiong Huang*), 8 *qian*, Radix Dioscoreae Oppositae (*Shan Yao*), 7 *liang*, Radix Glycyrrhizae (*Gan Cao*), 5 *liang*, gold foil (*Jin Bo*), 1,200 (pieces of) foil of which 400 are used as coating, and Fructus Zizyphi Jujubae (*Da Zao*), 100 pieces. Powder the above and make into pills with honey and smashed dates. One pill should weigh 1 *qian*.

Chapter Seventy-five

Impaired Memory

(This is) governed by the heart and the spleen. *Gui Pi Tang* (Return To the Spleen Decoction)[1] and *Ding Zhi Wan* (Settle Orientation Pills) are appropriate (for its treatment). For diminished, meager essence spirit, mostly use *An Shen Wan* (Calm the Spirit Pills) and their like. There are (also) cases of phlegm confounding the cardiac portals.

Dai comments: The name of this disease refers to setting about a matter but failing to carry it through to the end and making neither head nor tail when talking. This should not be compared to being born a stupid idiot, unintelligent of the world.

Chapter Seventy-six

Racing of the Heart

Generally speaking, this is ascribed to blood vacuity. If there is worry and anxiety and (the heart) throbs, this is ascribed to vacuity and scant blood. (However,) in most cases, (if the throbbing) stops and starts,

---

1   This consists of Radix Panacis Ginseng (*Ren Shen*), stir-fried Rhizoma Atractylodis Macrocephalae (*Bai Zhu*), stir-fried Radix Astragali Membranacei (*Huang Qi*), Sclerotium Poriae Cocoris (*Fu Ling*), Arillus Euphoriae Longanae (*Long Yan Rou*), Radix Angelicae Sinensis (*Dang Gui*), Radix Polygalae Tenuifoliae (*Yuan Zhi*), and stir-fried Semen Ziziphi Jujubae (*Suan Zao Ren*), 1 *qian* for each of the above, Radix Saussureae Seu Vladimiriae (*Mu Xiang*) and mix-fried Radix Glycyrrhizae (*Zhi Gan Cao*), 5 *fen* each, all the above boiled together with Rhizoma Zingiberis (*Jiang*) and Fructus Zizyphi Jujubae (*Zao*).

(this is due to) phlegm stirred by fire. In thin people, the cause is usually scant blood, (while) in fat people, (the disease) is ascribed to phlegm. The commonly (seen cases) are usually phlegm. (But) a feeling of a really throbbing heart is scant blood, (In that case, use) *Si Wu Tang* (Four Materials Decoction), *An Shen Wan* (Calm the Spirit Pills), and the like. Racing of the heart is a restless heart with apprehension as if fearing arrest.

Chapter Seventy-seven

Fright Palpitations

For blood vacuity, use *Zhu Sha An Shen Wan* (Cinnabar Calm the Spirit Pills). An(other) formula that treats fright palpitation is *Ding Zhi Wan* (Settle Orientation Pills) plus Succinum (*Hu Po*) and Tuber Curcumae (*Yu Jin*). Phlegm confounding the heart and diaphragm can be treated in every (case) with phlegm(-dispelling) medicinals.

Chapter Seventy-eight

Vexation & Agitation

Roughly speaking, (this is due to) scant blood unable to moisten. This justifies yin-nurturing as the paramount (choice). To treat vexation and agitation with inability to sleep, administer *Liu Yi San* (Six to One Powder) plus Calculus Bovis (*Niu Huang*. In an) internal damage disease like true cold damage (in which case) sweating between the 5-7th days is followed by relapse of fever with vexation and agitation arising with nightfall and calling for water, (use) *Bu Zhong Yi Qi Tang* (Supplement the Center & Boost the Qi Decoction) plus Radix

Praeparatus Aconiti Carmichaeli (*Fu Zi*. However, in an) internal damage disease like cold damage where, after 3 bouts of shivering, there arise taxation fatigue, vexation and agitation, clouding and languor, (use) *Si Jun Zi Tang* (Four Gentlemen Decoction) plus Radix Angelicae Sinensis (*Dang Gui*), Radix Astragali Membranacei (*Huang Qi*), Rhizoma Anemarrhenae (*Zhi Mu*), Tuber Ophiopogonis Japonicae (*Mai Men Dong*), and Fructus Schizandrae Chinensis (*Wu Wei Zi*). In severe cases, the pulse may be thin, rapid, and chaotic, and (the patient) keeps drinking water from the third watch till light. This is original qi vacuity. Boil the (above) formula with Folium Bambusae (*Zhu Ye*) soup. Take a large dose. (But for an) internal damage disease like cold damage with ceaseless groaning, vexation and agitation, fever recurring after sweating, a thin, rapid pulse, and sleeplessness for 5-7 days running, (use) *Bu Zhong Yi Qi Tang* plus 1 *liang* of Radix Panacis Ginseng (*Ren Shen*). Boil together with Folium Bambusae (*Zhu Ye*). (In more) severe cases, add Tuber Ophiopogonis Japonicae (*Mai Men Dong*), Fructus Schizandrae Chinensis (*Wu Wei Zi*), and Rhizoma Anemarrhenae (*Zhi Mu*).

Fire invading the lungs gives rise to vexation, (while fire) invading the kidneys gives rise to agitation. In both cases, (the evil) is located in the upper and is caused by heart fire. When fire is effulgent, metal is wasted away and water becomes deficient. What is left is nothing but fire. Thus, the lungs and kidneys join to cause vexation and agitation.

Chapter Seventy-nine

Heart Disease[1]

In people with heart vacuity and dwindling, there may arise racing of the heart, vexation and restlessness, impaired memory, or confounded

---

[1] Heart disease here does not refer to organic disease of the heart but to mental/emotional disease.

and clouded spirit after disappointment. (In this case, use) *Chen Sha An Shen Wan* (Cinnabar Calm the Spirit Pills). For heart wind[2] with qi heat and exuberant phlegm, (use) *Gun Tan Wan* (Roll Phlegm Pills).[3] For heart disease,, (use) Tuber Curcumae (*Yu Jin*), Fructus Gleditschiae Sinensis (*Zhu Ya Zao Jiao*), Alum (*Bai Fan*), and Scolopendra Subspinipes (*Wu Gong*. But,) strong people with qi repletion, exuberant fire, (and) madness can receive a direct treatment[4] or drink iced slaked lime (*Po Xiao*) solution. For mania with exuberant vacuity fire, administer a soup of Rhizoma Zingiberis (*Jiang*). If iced water is administered instead, instant death results. Urgent and severe fire can be moderated by Radix Glycyrrhizae (*Sheng Gan Cao*). This is able to drain fire. Radix Panacis Ginseng (*Ren Shen*) and Rhizoma Atractylodis Macrocephalae (*Bai Zhu*) can be used instead. Without exception, qi, if superabundant, is fire, and, if insufficient, is qi vacuity.

A person in the prime of his life, corpulent and solid, had heart wind feeble-mindedness. After ejection, he was prescribed the following: Bulbus Fritillariae (*Bei Mu*), Fructus Trichosanthis Kirlowii (*Gua Lou*), Rhizoma Arisaematis (*Nan Xing*), and Rhizoma Coptidis Chinensis (*Huang Lian*), 1 *liang* for each of the above, Tuber Curcumae (*Yu Jin*), Rhizoma Gastrodiae Elatae (*Tian Ma*), Fructus Canari Albi (*Qing Zi*), Radix Glycyrrhizae (*Sheng Gan Cao*), Fructus Immaturus Citri Seu Ponciri (*Zhi Shi*), Fructus Forsythiae Suspensae (*Lian Qiao*), and Radix Sophorae Flavescentis (*Ku Shen*), one half *liang* for each of the above, and Alum (*Bai Fan*) and Fructus Gleditschiae Sinensis (*Zao Jiao*), 2 *qian* each. The above were made into pills. After

---

[2] There are two types of heart wind. Wind intruding into the heart with manifestations of spontaneous sweating, red lips, somnolence, impaired memory, and fright palpitations is a species of external contraction. The other category is internal wind which arises as a result of insufficient heart qi with manifestations of trance, changeable moods, incoherent speech, etc.

[3] This consists of Chlorite Schist (*Meng Shi*), 1 *liang*, wine-steamed Radix Et Rhizoma Rhei (*Da Huang*) and Radix Scutellariae Baicalensis (*Huang Qin*), one half *jin* each, and Lignum Aquilariae Agallochae (*Chen Xiang*), 5 *qian*.

[4] Direct treatment here refers to drainage and precipitation with cool and cold medicinals which are used to directly neutralize the heat causing heart disease.

administration, (he was) prescribed Scolopendra Subspinipes (*Wu Gong*), 2 pieces, one yellow, the other red, fried with sesame oil to yellow, Rhizoma Ligustici Wallichii (*Chuan Xiong*), Radix Ledebouriellae Sesloidis (*Fang Feng*), Rhizoma Arisaematis (*Nan Xing*), Radix Aconiti Coreani (*Bai Fu Zi*), Alum (*Bai Fan*), and Fructus Gleditschiae Sinensis (*Zao Jiao*), 1 *liang* for each of the above, and Tuber Curcumae (*Yu Jin*), one half *liang*. The above were made into pills with Cinnabar (*Zhu Sha*) as coating.

In terms of mania and withdrawal disease, withdrawal is ascribed to yin and mania with frequent excessive joy is ascribed to yang. Frequent anger with a replete pulse (results in) death. A vacuous (pulse indicates) the possibility of a cure. Roughly speaking, this is mostly due to phlegm bound somewhere in the cardiac region of the chest. Treatment normally (consists of) settling the heart spirit and opening bound phlegm. There are also cases of contraction of this disorder due to strike by evils.[5] In that case, it should be treated by a method for treating (ghost) evils. The *Yuan Bing Shi (The Formulated Origin of Disease)*[6] gives a remarkably lucid discussion to this. People who think dual yin is the cause of withdrawal and dual yang is the cause of mania are wrong. Roughly speaking, they both are due to heat.

---

[5]   This refers to possession by supposed ghosts or devils.

[6]   This is the abbreviated name of the *Su Wen Xuan Ji Yuan Bing Shi (The Formulated Origin of Disease Based on the Intricate Mechanism of the Simple Questions)* by Liu Wan-su of the Jin Dynasty (1115-1234CE).

Chapter Eighty

Lumps [Accumulations & Conglomerations in a {variant edition; later editor}]

Lumps (in the abdomen) are phlegm and rheum if located in the middle, accumulated food if located on the right, and dead blood if located on the left. Qi cannot shape into lumps. What gathers to form lumps must be tangible substances (such as) phlegm as well as accumulated food and dead blood. The medicinals to be used are vinegar-cooked Pumice (*Hai Shi*), vinegar-cooked Rhizoma Sparganii (*San Leng*), vinegar-cooked Rhizoma Curcumae Zedoariae (*Peng Zhu*), Semen Pruni Persicae (*Tao Ren*), Flos Carthami Tinctorii (*Hong Hua*), Feces Trogopterori Seu Pteromi (*Wu Ling Zhi*), Rhizoma Cyperi Rotundi (*Xiang Fu*) and Alkaloid (*Shi Jian*). Make into pills and take with Rhizoma Atractylodis Macrocephalae (*Bai Zhu*) soup. In a (variant) edition, there is iron dust (*Zhen Sha*). Concha Arcae Inflatae (*Wa Long Zi*) is able to disperse lumps and phlegm as well. Lumps are always treated by downbearing fire and dispersing food and accumulation. Accumulation refers to phlegm. (However,) to move away lumps of dead blood, great supplementation is necessary. Saltiness treats accumulated phlegm. In case of existence of lumps, it is used to wash away and flush filthy, oily (substances).

One formula that can treat all kinds of gathering and accumulation, concretion and conglomeration (is made by) boiling Radix Althaeae Roseae (*Shu Kui Gen*). After removing the dregs, boil (again) with Radix Panacis Ginseng (*Ren Shen*), Rhizoma Atractylodis Macrocephalae (*Bai Zhu*), Pericarpium Citri Reticulatae (*Chen Pi*), Pericarpium Viridis Citri Reticulatae (*Qing Pi*), Apex Radicis Glycyrrhizae (*Gan Cao Shao*), and Radix Achyranthis Bidentatae (*Niu Xi*). Take hot after putting in a small amount of finely ground Semen Pruni Persicae (*Tao Ren*) and Sodium Sulfate (*Xuan Ming Fen*). Two doses and accumulation lumps will be observed (already) precipitated. (However, for) a heavy (*i.e.*, serious) condition, first supplement and recruit and then carry out (the following) method with additions and subtractions. The great method is to use saltiness to soften and whittling (medicinals) to disperse. The priority is to move qi and open phlegm.

One formula for adhesive ointment to treat gatherings and accumulations (consists of) Radix Et Rhizoma Rhei (*Da Huang*), 2 *liang* [1 *liang* in a {variant} edition {later editor}], and slaked lime (*Po Xiao*), 1 *liang*, powdered separately. Pound with garlic into a paste and apply. When dried, mix with vinegar and re-apply. If lumps are located under the skin but over the membrane, it is necessary to administer qi-supplementing medicinals together with Rhizoma Cyperi Rotundi (*Xiang Fu*) to open these. (Use) in combination with *Er Chen Tang*.

In females, (for) dead blood, food accumulation, and phlegm rheum developing into lumps, possibly located in the lateral costal regions, with abdominal rumbling on movement, a clamoring stomach, and dizziness and body heat which are intermittent, (use) Rhizoma Coptidis Chinensis (*Huang Lian*), 1 *liang*, half stir-fried with Fructus Evodiae Rutecarpae (*Wu Zhu Yu*), half with Fructus Alpiniae Oxyphyllae (*Yi Zhi Ren*), these two medicinals removed afterward, Fructus Gardeniae Jasminoidis (*Shan Zhi*), one half *liang*, stir-fried, Rhizoma Ligustici Wallichii (*Tai Xiong*), one half *liang*, stir-fried, Rhizoma Cyperi Rotundi (*Xiang Fu*), one half to 1 *liang*, soaked in child's urine, Semen Raphani Sativi (*Luo Bo Zi*), 1.5 *liang*, stir-fried, Fructus Crataegi (*Shan Zha Rou*), 1 *liang*, Rhizoma Sparganii (*San Leng*), 5 *qian*, Rhizoma Curcumae Zedoariae (*Peng Zhu*), one half *liang*, boiled in vinegar, Semen Pruni Persicae (*Tao Ren*), one half *liang*, tip preserved, skin removed, and Pericarpium Viridis Citri Reticulatae (*Qing Pi*), one half *liang*, [or Massa Medica Fermentata Cum Exocarpium Semenis Tritici Aestivi {*Mai Pi Qu*}, one half *liang* {later editor}]. Powder the above and make into pills with steamed cake. A (variant) formula includes (in addition) Massa Medica Fermentata (*Shen Qu*), 5 *qian*, Semen Sinapis Albae (*Bai Jie Zi*), 1.5 *liang*, and Concha Arcae Inflatae (*Wa Long Zi*), 1 *liang*, calcined with vinegar. If accumulation disease does not abate in spite of precipitation, this necessitates the administration of accumulation-dispersing medicinals to dissolve (accumulation). Once opened, accumulation will be dispersed.

To treat existence of lumps with flank pain, (use) *Long Hui Wan* (Gentiana & Aloe Pills), 2.5 *qian*, Rhizoma Curcumae (*Pian Jiang Huang*), one half *liang*, and Semen Pruni Persicae (*Tao Ren*), one half *liang*. Powder the above and make into pills with honey. Another formula (consists of) *Long Hui Wan* mixed with white dove droppings. This is able to greatly disperse food accumulation. *Bao He Wan* (Protect & Harmonize Pills) may be used in combination to treat lumps depending on what part (is affected).[1] (But, in treating) various kinds of lumps with central vacuity, lump-attacking (medicinals) may give rise to distention so as to render the situation helpless. (Therefore, one) must avoid using attacking medicinals. *Si Jun Zi Tang* (Four Gentlemen Decoction) plus Rhizoma Pinelliae Ternatae (*Ban Xia*) and Pericarpium Citri Reticulatae (*Chen Pi*) can be taken in a large dose. When the original qi is leveled and restored to normal, attacking medicinals can be used.

To treat glomus lump, (use) Semen Momordicae Cochinensis (*Mu Bie*), [A {variant} edition gives Pericarpium Semenis {Momordicae Cochinensis} instead. {later editor}], 21 pieces. Roast well in a cut up hog's kidney, pound thoroughly, put in 3 *qian* of powdered Rhizoma Coptidis Chinensis (*Huang Lian Mo*), and make into pills the size of mung beans; 30 pills per dose. For pain caused by qi below the navel in the abdomen, (use) Radix Saussureae Seu Vladimiriae (*Mu Xiang*), Semen Arecae Catechu (*Bing Lang*), Rhizoma Sparganii (*San Leng*), Rhizoma Curcumae Zedoariae (*E Zhu*), and Pericarpium Viridis Citri Reticulatae (*Qing Pi*), one half *liang* for each of the above, stir-fried Caulis Akebiae Mutong (*Mu Tong*), one half *liang*, stir-fried Rhizoma Coptidis Chinensis (*Huang Lian*), one half *liang*, Pericarpium Citri Reticulatae (*Chen Pi*), one half *liang*, Fructus Amomi (*Suo Sha*) and Semen Ormosiae Hosiei (*Hong Dou*), 3 *qian* each, and Rhizoma Cyperi Rotundi (*Xiang Fu*), 1 *liang*.

For liver channel blood phase lump pain, the powder form is good but the pill form is especially good: Radix Angelicae Sinensis (*Dang Gui*), one half *liang*, stir-fried Flos Carthami Tinctorii (*Hong Hua*), 1 *qian*, Semen Pruni Persicae (*Tao Ren*), 20 pieces, skinned and tip-nipped, pounded Rhizoma Corydalis Yanhusuo (*Xuan Hu Suo*), one half *liang*, Radix Rubrus Paeoniae

---

[1] The ingredients in this formula are given in the text of Ch. 24, Bk. 2. One should note that *Long Hui Wan* mainly treats problems involving the lateral costal regions, while *Bao He Wan* treats cardiac and abdominal disorders.

Lactiflorae (*Chi Shao Yao*), one half *liang*, Myrrha (*Mo Yao*), 3 *qian*, and Lacca Sinica Exiccata (*Gan Qi*), one half *liang*, stir-fried till no smoke is seen any more. In case of dry stool, add prepared Radix Et Rhizoma Rhei (*Shu Da Huang*).

If people have lumps, whether in the upper, middle, or lower and as long as they are phlegm, (one) should ascertain their favorite food and then use its counteracting medicinals to disperse it. Medication should follow ejection.

A person suffered from phlegm filling up the cardiac region in (their) chest and seemingly coagulating into a whole lump. This obstruction refused to open in spite of attacking. (Therefore, I prescribed) Rhizoma Atractylodis Macrocephalae (*Bai Zhu*), 1 *liang*, Rhizoma Arisaematis (*Nan Xing*), Bulbus Fritillariae (*Bei Mu*), Massa Medica Fermentata (*Shen Qu*), Fructus Crataegi (*Shan Zha*), Rhizoma Curcumae (*Jiang Huang*), Pericarpium Citri Reticulatae (*Chen Pi*), and Sclerotium Poriae Cocoris (*Fu Ling*), 5 *qian* for each of the above, Fructus Gardeniae Jasminoidis (*Shan Zhi*), one half *liang*, Rhizoma Cyperi Rotundi (*Xiang Fu*), 1 *liang*, and Semen Raphani Sativi (*Luo Bo Zi*) and Spina Gleditschiae Sinensis (*Zao Jiao Ci*), 3 *qian* each. All the above were powdered and made into pills with ginger cake.

An(other) person suffered from lumps in the lower abdomen (and was prescribed) Fructus Trichosanthis Kirlowii (*Gua Lou*), Bulbus Fritillariae (*Bei Mu*), Radix Scutellariae Baicalensis (*Huang Qin*), Rhizoma Arisaematis (*Nan Xing*), Rhizoma Atractylodis Macrocephalae (*Bai Zhu*), 1 *liang* for each of above, [one half *liang* in a {variant} edition {later editor}], vinegar-boiled Rhizoma Cyperi Rotundi (*Xiang Fu*), 1 *liang*, prepared Radix Rehmanniae (*Shu Di Huang*), Radix Angelicae Sinensis (*Dang Gui*), Rhizoma Corydalis Yanhusuo (*Xuan Hu Suo*), Semen Pruni Persicae (*Tao Ren*), 5 *qian* for each of the above, and Rhizoma Sparganii (*San Leng*) and Rhizoma Curcumae Zedoariae (*Peng Zhu*), both vinegar-boiled, 5 *qian* each. All the above were powdered and made into pills with Massa Medica Fermentata (*Shen Qu*).

Xiao Shi Wan (Nitre Pills)[2] from the *Qian Jin (Thousand [Pieces of] Gold)*[3] grind lumps, and *San Sheng Gao* (Three Spirits Paste)[4] is (an external remedy) applied over the lumps. [Both of these are efficacious. {later editor}] (I) remember that the master[5] once treated a woman with lumps in the lower abdomen with a choppy pulse. After administering attacking medicinals, the pulse appeared larger. (Later,) *Si Wu Tang* (Four Materials Decoction, was prescribed) with Rhizoma Atractylodis Macrocephalae (*Bai Zhu*), Pericarpium Citri Reticulatae (*Chen Pi*), and Radix Glycyrrhizae (*Gan Cao*) in double amounts as assistants and envoys. Then the pulse became replenished and solid. From time to time, *Xiao Shi Wan* was administered. Two months later, the lumps disappeared completely.

A person, aged 60, who had been fond of wine in the past, contracted a disease as a result of travelling in summerheat. Cold extended up to their knees with a lump in the upper venter like a palm dragging. This caused pain to the lateral costal regions, inability to sleep, reduced food intake, and absence of thirst. (He) had taken by himself 3 raw (*i.e.*, unboiled) doses of *Wu Ji San* (Five Accumulations Powder).[6] The six pulses were all

---

[2] This consists of Nitre (*Xiao Shi*), 6 *liang*, Radix Et Rhizoma Rhei (*Da Huang*), 8 *liang*, and Radix Panacis Ginseng (*Ren Shen*) and Radix Glycyrrhizae (*Gan Cao*), 2 *liang* each.

[3] This is the abbreviated name of the *Bei Ji Qian Jin Fang (Emergency Formulas [Worth] a Thousand [Pieces] of Gold)* written by Sun Si-miao of the Tang Dynasty.

[4] This consists of Pediculus Melonis (*Gua Di*), Radix Ledebouriellae Sesloidis (*Fang Feng*), and Radix Veratri Nigri (*Li Lu*). Powder the above. Take 5 *qian* with boiled water to induce vomit.

[5] The master mentioned here is Zhu Dan-xi. This reiterates that the text was probably written or at least added to by Zhu's students.

[6] This consists of Radix Angelicae (*Bai Zhi*), Rhizoma Ligustici Wallichii (*Chuan Xiong*), mix-fried Radix Glycyrrhizae (*Zhi Gan Cao*), skinned Sclerotium Poriae Cocoris (*Fu Ling*), Radix Angelicae Sinensis (*Dang Gui*), Cortex Cinnamomi (*Rou Gui*), stripped of its outer bark, Radix Paeoniae Lactiflorae (*Shao Yao*), and water-washed Rhizoma Pinelliae Ternatae (*Ban Xia*), 3 *liang* for each of the above, Pericarpium Citri Reticulatae (*Chen Pi*), stripped of its inner white layer, stir-fried Fructus Citri Seu Ponciri (*Zhi Qiao*), and Herba Ephedrae (*Ma Huang*), stripped of its joints and roots,

deep, choppy, and small, but they were not weaker when pressure was applied. (In addition,) they were all rapid, and particularly so on the right hand. Defecation remained normal, but urine was dark-colored. Then *Da Cheng Qi Tang* (Major Support the Qi Decoction) was prescribed with Radix Et Rhizoma Rhei (*Da Huang*) reduced in amount by half but well stir-fried. (Then) Rhizoma Coptidis Chinensis (*Huang Lian*), Radix Paeoniae Lactiflorae (*Shao Yao*), Rhizoma Ligustici Wallichii (*Chuan Xiong*), dry Radix Puerariae Lobatae (*Gan Ge*), and Radix Glycyrrhizae (*Gan Cao*) were added. (The above) were administered in the form of decoction. Fructus Trichosanthis Kirlowii (*Gua Lou Ren*), Rhizoma Pinelliae Ternatae (*Ban Xia*), Rhizoma Coptidis Chinensis (*Huang Lian*), and Bulbus Fritillariae (*Bei Mu*) were (also) administered in the form of pills. After 12 doses had been taken, (the patient's) cold in the feet abated and the lump reduced (in size) by half. Therefore, the medication was stopped. Half a month later, the entire condition was overcome.

Gatherings and accumulations are normally classified as yin and yang. In terms of accumulations, their development has roots, and their pains are located in fixed parts. The pulse is bound and hidden. (While for) gatherings, their development has no roots, and their pains are located in no fixed parts. The pulse (in this case) is floating and bound. (Gatherings and accumulations) are a result of disharmony between yin and yang, vacuity weakness of the viscera and bowels, abnormalities of the four qi[7], and the seven affects.

---

6 *liang* for each of the above, Rhizoma Atractylodis (*Cang Zhu*), soaked with rice water and skinned, 24 *liang*, Radix Platycodi Grandiflori (*Jie Geng*), 12 *liang*, and dry Rhizoma Zingiberis (*Gan Jiang*) and Cortex Magnoliae Officinalis (*Hou Po*), 4 *liang* each. Three *qian* per dose.

7   This refers to the changes of weather characteristic of the four seasons.

Chapter Eighty-one

Tea Mania

Powder Gypsum (*Shi Gao*), Radix Scutellariae Baicalensis (*Huang Qin*), and Rhizoma Cimicifugae (*Sheng Ma*) and take mixed with granulated sugar.

A person was fond of tea. (I prescribed them) Rhizoma Atractylodis Macrocephalae (*Bai Zhu*), soft Gypsum (*Ruan Shi Gao*), Radix Scutellariae Baicalensis (*Pian Qin*), Radix Albus Paeoniae Lactiflorae (*Bai Shao Yao*), Herba Menthae (*Bo He*) with big, round leaves, and bile(-processed) Rhizoma Arisaematis (*Dan Xing*). All the above were powdered, made into a paste with granulated sugar, and, after a meal, were melted in the (patient's) mouth and swallowed with saliva.

Chapter Eighty-two

Shan

(In this condition,) damp heat and accumulated phlegm flow down, (thus) causing pain. Generally speaking, (*shan*) is caused by cold depression, or, in other words, it is phlegm rheum, food accumulation, and dead blood. It specifically governs the liver channel and has nothing to do with the kidney channel. Precipitation is not appropriate.

For *tui shan*[1], which is abundant dampness, moxa at *Da Dun* (Liv 1).[2] For food accumulation and blood stasis causing pain, (use) Fructus Gardeniae Jasminoidis (*Zhi Zi*), Semen Pruni Persicae (*Tao Ren*), Fructus Crataegi (*Shan Zha*), Semen Citri (*Ju He*) [Fructus Immaturus Citri Seu Ponciri {*Zhi Shi*} in a {variant} edition {later editor}], and Fructus Evodiae Rutecarpae (*Zhu Yu*). Take with Succus Zingiberis (*Sheng Jiang Zhi*) soup boiled in water from an eastward running river. For pain which cannot be located by pressing, (*i.e.*, for pain) ascribed to vacuity, use Ramulus Cinnamomi (*Gui Zhi*), stir-fried Fructus Gardeniae Jasminoidis (*Shan Zhi*) and Radix Aconiti (*Wu Tou*). It is necessary to cut (the latter) finely and powder by stir-frying. Make into pills with Succus Zingiberis (*Jiang Zhi*) and take 30-50 pills with ginger soup to thwart the pain.

A formula to treat various kinds of *shan* which is able to settle pain with rapid effect (consists of) Semen Citri (*Ju He*), 50 pieces, stir-fried Fructus Gardeniae Jasminoidis (*Shan Zhi*), and stir-fried Fructus Evodiae Rutecarpae (*Zhu Yu*). If there is overwhelming dampness, add Semen Litchi Chinensis (*Li He*). (Use) all (these medicinals) in equal amounts, taken in the shape of pills.

The medicinals that are important in treating all kinds of *tui* (*shan*) with no pain (are) Rhizoma Atractylodis (*Cang Zhu*), 1 *liang*, Rhizoma Arisaematis (*Nan Xing*), 1 *liang*, Radix Angelicae (*Bai Zhi*), 1 *liang*, ground in water, Fructus Crataegi (*Shan Zha*), 1 *liang*, Rhizoma Ligustici Wallichii (*Chuan Xiong*), 3 *qian*, Semen Immaturus Citri Seu Ponciri (*Zhi Zi*) [Fructus Immaturus Citri Seu Ponciri {*Zhi Shi*} in a {variant} edition {later editor}], 3 *qian*, and Rhizoma Pinelliae Ternatae (*Ban Xia*), 3 *qian*. Powder the above and make into pills with Massa Medica Fermentata (*Shen Qu*) paste. If there is heat, add 1 *liang* of stir-fried Fructus Gardeniae Jasminoidis (*Shan Zhi*). In case of hardened

---

[1] This is a pattern consisting of swollen, hardened testicles with dragging pain, numbness, or insensitivity to pain or touch in males, and lower abdominal distention in females.

[2] Large Pile

(testicles), add one half *liang* of slaked lime (*Po Xiao*). In autumn and winter, add 3.5 *qian* of Fructus Evodiae Rutecarpae (*Zhu Yu*).

To treat *shan*, burn to ash Semen Litchi Chinensis (*Li He*) and Semen Ponciri Trifoliatae (*Gou Ju He*), powder and take with wine. To treat various *shan* by way of attacking, powder two medicinals, Pumice (*Hai Shi*) and Rhizoma Cyperi Rotundi (*Xiang Fu*) and take brewed with Succus Zingiberis (*Sheng Jiang Zhi*). This also treats cardiac pain. (Another method) to treat *shan* (consists of) Semen Citri (*Ju He*), Semen Pruni Persicae (*Tao Ren*), Fructus Gardeniae Jasminoidis (*Zhi Zi*), Fructus Evodiae Rutecarpae (*Zhu Yu*), and Radix Aconiti (*Chuan Wu*). Grind the above into powder, boil, and take. The (above) *Zhi He San* (Orange Seed Powder) merely checks pain. Semen Ponciri Trifoliatae (*Gou Ju He*) is able to treat wooden *shan*.[3]

Shan disease is classified into two types, water qi and damp heat. Swelling may also occur with embraced vacuity. (In that case,) it is necessary to use Radix Panacis Ginseng (*Ren Shen*) and Rhizoma Atractylodis Macrocephalae (*Bai Zhu*) as the sovereigns and coursing and abducting medicinals as assistants. A deep, taut, hollow, and large pulse is its indicator.

(Someone) asked how to treat a person who, following recovery from disease, suffers from pain in the left testicle after drinking water. (I) moxaed at *Da Dun* (Liv 1), applied *Mo Yao Gao* (Rub the Lumbus Paste)[4] which, as it happened, was available, and orally administered Radix Aconiti (*Wu Tou*), Radix Praeparatus Aconiti Carmichaeli (*Fu Zi*), and Secretio Moschi Moschiferi (*She Xiang*. I) Rubbed with (*Mo Yao Gao*) from the scrotum to the ends of the pubic bone and covered (the affected area) with quantities of wet cloth. The pain stopped instantly. After a night, the swelling also disappeared.

---

[3] This refers to swollen, insensitive testicles.

[4] The ingredients in this formula can be found in the text of Ch. 43, Bk. 3.

I used to have orange accumulation in the past. (One day,) while travelling in the mountains, I was extremely hungry when I came across oranges and Chinese yam and ate (some of these). Then the orange eaten stirred the old orange accumulation, and, in addition, the Chinese yam stagnated the qi. In no time, my right testicle became swollen and enlarged with (alternating) cold and heat. I first took 1 or 2 doses of a stomach-balancing formula. The next morning, I concentrated my spirit in order to bring the qi down to the lower burner. Counterflow retching was felt to stir the accumulation. After repeated vomiting, my stomach qi was harmonized, the channels and connecting vessels were coursed and freed, and then recovery followed.

A formula to treat wooden kidney[5] (is made by) collecting the leaves from male Broussonetia Papyrifera (*Chu Shu*), drying (these) in the sun, and powdering (them. Then) make into pills with wine paste and take on an empty stomach with boiled saltwater. As an external (treatment) method, boil down into a thick decoction and fume and wash with Folium Eriobotryae Japonicae (*Pi Ba Ye*), Folium Stachysis Baicalensis (*Ye Zi Su Ye*), Folium Xanthii Sibirici (*Cang Er Ye*), Folium Viticis Viniferae (*Shui Jing Pu Tao Ye*), and Folium Zanthoxyli Bungeani (*Jiao Ye*. However,) to treat painless wooden kidney, (use) Rhizoma Arisaematis (*Nan Xing*), Rhizoma Pinelliae Ternatae (*Ban Xia*), wine-fried Cortex Phellodendri (*Huang Bai*), salt-fried Rhizoma Atractylodis (*Cang Zhu*), Fructus Crataegi (*Shan Zha*), Radix Angelicae (*Bai Zhi*), stir-fried Massa Medica Fermentata (*Shen Qu*), stir-fried Talcum (*Hua Shi*), Fructus Evodiae Rutecarpae (*Zhu Yu*), Herba Laminariae Japonicae (*Kun Bu*), and Fructus Ponciri Trifoliatae (*Gou Ju*. But) enduring shan disease and yellowing disease are suitable for granary-emptying. (And for) pain and inhibited voiding of urine caused by *shan qi*, (use) *Wu Ling San* (Five *Ling* Powder) with finely powdered Fructus Meliae Toosendanis (*Chuan Lian Zi*) added; 2 *qian* (per dose) taken on an empty stomach.

---

[5] The testicles are frequently called the external kidneys in Chinese. Therefore, wooden kidney is another term for wooden *shan*.

Some people have asked about formulas for painless *tui qi* in the lower part, and (I) truly promised an explanation on the spot. (However,) careful thinking (has led me to the conclusion that) no medication should be administered (for this) unless (the patient) is inexorably determined to abstain from thick-flavored (foods) and chamber affairs. Otherwise death is only hastened. For example, Rhizoma Atractylodis (*Cang Zhu*), Massa Medica Fermentata (*Shen Qu*), Radix Angelicae (*Bai Zhi*), Fructus Crataegi (*Shan Zha*), Rhizoma Ligustici Wallichii (*Chuan Xiong*), Semen Immaturus Citri Seu Ponciri (*Zhi Zi*), and Rhizoma Pinelliae Ternatae (*Ban Xia*) are all important medicinals (in treating this), but they are all sordid and abject substances[6] that may stimulate (the patient's) negligence, (thus) making it impossible for them to abstain from sexual desire. In spite of the motive to protect their root, (one) may only obsess them with the disease (more deeply). The disaster of Chen Yan-zheng brought with it much condemnation.[7] What's more, medication (must) vary with the seasons and months, to say nothing of the changeable sovereign, minister, assistant, and envoy. On account of all this, I prefer to be guilty of breaking my promise rather than venturing into what is beyond me. This is a touch of my wandering pen.

An(other) formula to treat *shan* pain (consists of) stir-fried Fructus Crataegi (*Shan Zha*), 4 *liang*, Semen Citri Seu Ponciri (*Zhi He*), Fructus Foeniculi Vulgaris (*Hui Xiang*), and Fructus Gardeniae Jasminoidis (*Shan Zhi*), all the above stir-fried and 2 *liang* each, Radix Bupleuri (*Chai Hu*), 1 *liang*, Cortex Radicis Moutan (*Mu Dan*), 1 *liang*, stir-fried Semen Pruni Persicae (*Tao Ren*), 1 *liang*, stir-fried Fructus Illicii Veri (*Da Hui Xiang*), 1 *liang*, and stir-fried Fructus Evodiae Rutecarpae (*Wu Zhu Yu*), one half *liang*. Make the above into pills and take.

---

[6] These medicinals are spoken of in this way because they are able to boost essence and hence increase sexual desire.

[7] Chen Yan-zheng is probably the name of a person, but the translator has failed to identify him. The sentence seems to say that administration of a formula brought disastrous consequence to this Chen, and, therefore, troubles happened to the attending physician, possibly the author.

A formula to treat *shan* with intermittent acute pain (consists of) salt-fried Rhizoma Atractylodis (*Cang Zhu*), salt-fried Rhizoma Cyperi Rotundi (*Xiang Fu*), and wine-fried Cortex Phellodendri (*Huang Bai*) as the sovereigns, Pericarpium Viridis Citri Reticulatae (*Qing Pi*), Rhizoma Corydalis Yanhusuo (*Xuan Hu Suo*), and Semen Pruni Persicae (*Tao Ren*) as the ministers, Fructus Foeniculi Vulgaris (*Hui Xiang*) as the assistant, and Fructus Alpiniae Oxyphyllae (*Yi Zhi*), salt-fried Radix Praeparatus Aconiti Carmichaeli (*Fu Zi*) and Radix Glycyrrhizae (*Gan Cao*) as the envoys. Powder the above, make a decoction, and take. After a fit of pain is relieved, it will never arise again.

A formula to treat kidney qi[8] (consists of) Fructus Foeniculi Vulgaris (*Hui Xiang*) and Fructus Psoraleae Corylifoliae (*Po Gu Zhi*), 5 *qian* each, Fructus Evodiae Rutecarpae (*Wu Zhu Yu*), stir-fried with salt, 5 *qian*, and Semen Trigonellae Foeni-graeci (*Hu Lu Ba*), 7.5 *qian*. Powder. (Then) extract the juice from Semen Raphani Sativi (*Luo Bo Zi*) by pounding and make (the powder) into pills (with this juice). Take with boiled saltwater.

Swelling *shan* with pain in fat persons (is ascribed to) heat externally and cold internally. (For this, use) *Wu Ling San* plus Fructus Foeniculi Vulgaris (*Hui Xiang*).

A person suffered from *tui shan*. (They were prescribed) Fructus Gardeniae Jasminoidis (*Shan Zhi*), Fructus Crataegi (*Shan Zha*), Fructus Immaturus Citri Seu Ponciri (*Zhi Shi*), Rhizoma Cyperi Rotundi (*Xiang Fu*), Rhizoma Arisaematis (*Nan Xing*), and Fructus Meliae Toosendanis (*Chuan Lian*), 1 *liang* for each of the above, Herba Sargassi (*Hai Zao*) and Semen Pruni Persicae (*Tao Ren*), 7.5 *qian* each, and Fructus Evodiae Rutecarpae (*Wu Zhu Yu*), 2.5 *qian*. The above were powdered and made into pills with ginger cake.

An(other) person had *shan* pain and heart pain. (They were prescribed) stir-fried Fructus Gardeniae Jasminoidis (*Shan Zhi*), 2 *liang*, Rhizoma

---

[8] This is a pattern due to the kidney qi insufficiency manifested by cold, damp genitals, flaccid feet, and low back pain.

Cyperi Rotundi (*Xiang Fu*), 1 *liang*, Rhizoma Atractylodis (*Cang Zhu*), Massa Medica Fermentata (*Shen Qu*), Fructus Germinatus Hordei Vulgaris (*Mai Ya*), 5 *qian* for each of the above, Rhizoma Pinelliae Ternatae (*Ban Xia*), 7 *qian*, Radix Aconiti (*Wu Tou*), and Alkaloid (*Shi Jian*), 3 *qian* each, and Ramulus Cinnamomi (*Gui Zhi*), 1.5 *qian*, which is deleted in the spring. Powder the above, make into pills with cake, the size of mung beans; 100 pills per dose taken with boiled saltwater.

(Yet) an(other) person suffered from *shan* which, when pain arose, formed in the abdomen into a lump that would disappear when the pain ceased. (They were prescribed) vinegar-boiled Rhizoma Sparganii (*San Leng*), 1 *liang*, vinegar-boiled Rhizoma Curcumae Zedoariae (*Peng Zhu*), 1 *liang*, Massa Medica Fermentata (*Shen Qu*) and Fructus Germinatus Hordei Vulgaris (*Mai Ya*), both stir-fried, 1 *liang* each, Tuber Curcumae (*Jiang Huang*), 1 *liang*, ginger-processed Rhizoma Arisaematis (*Nan Xing*), 1 *liang*, Rhizoma Atractylodis Macrocephalae (*Bai Zhu*), 2 *liang*, Radix Saussureae Seu Vladimiriae (*Mu Xiang*) and Lignum Aquilariae Agallochae (*Chen Xiang*), 3 *qian* each, and Fructus Gardeniae Jasminoidis (*Shan Zhi*) and Semen Citri Seu Ponciri (*Zhi He*), 5 *qian* each, both stir-fried. Powder the above and make into pills with ginger cake.

A thwarting formula which is divinely remarkable (consists of) finely-sliced, stir-fried Radix Aconiti (*Wu Tou*) and stir-fried Fructus Gardeniae Jasminoidis (*Zhi Zi Ren*. This formula) should be used, however, with additions and subtractions. This (disease) is due to damp heat which results from cold depression. Fructus Gardeniae Jasminoidis is used to dispel dampness and Radix Aconiti to break cold depression. In addition, these two are medicinals for the lower burner and, when led by Fructus Gardeniae Jasminoidis, Radix Aconiti becomes too swift to stay in the stomach.

Chapter Eighty-three

The Ears

Deafness and ringing in the ears (are due to) the existence of phlegm, fire, and qi vacuity. Deafness with abundant heat in the *shao yang* and *jue yin* is ascribed to fire in every case. (In this case,) it is appropriate to open phlegm and dissipate wind heat with *Tong Sheng San* (Communicate with the Divinity Powder), *Gun Tan Wan* (Roll Phlegm Pills), and the like. (But) deafness following a great disease requires supplementing yin and downbearing fire. Deafness may also be due to yin fire stirring. (These two conditions) should be treated in the same way (by using) *Si Wu Tang* (Four Materials Decoction) plus medicinals such as Cortex Phellodendri (*Huang Bai*). (Another) method is to drip the bile of a male rat into the ears. The disease of deafness invariably requires *Long Hui* (Gentiana & Aloe [Pills]) and *Si Wu (Tang)* to nurture yin. There are also cases with damp hot phlegm, (requiring) *Bing Lang Shen Xiong* (Areca Divine Ligusticum [Pills]). Booming in the ears is also (due to) absence of yin. (While) deafness of the ears due to (heat) depression is treated with *Tong Sheng San* with Radix Et Rhizoma Rhei (*Da Huang*) roasted in wine and stir-fried thrice with wine before being mixed with the other ingredients which should (also) be stir-fried with wine.

For ringing in the ears in people addicted to wine, (use) *Mu Xiang Bing Lang Wan* (Saussurea & Areca Pills). For ringing in the ears due to excessive drinking of wine, (use) large doses of *Tong Sheng San* plus Fructus Citri Seu Ponciri (*Zhi Qiao*), Radix Bupleuri (*Chai Hu*), Radix Et Rhizoma Rhei (*Da Huang*), Radix Glycyrrhizae (*Gan Cao*), Rhizoma Arisaematis (*Nan Xing*), Radix Platycodi Grandiflori (*Jie Geng*), Pericarpium Viridis Citri Reticulatae (*Qing Pi*), and Herba Seu Flos Schizonepetae Tenuifoliae (*Jing Jie*. In case of) no improvement, (administer) *Si Wu Tang*. Ringing in the ears invariably requires *Dang Gui Long Hui Wan* (*Dang Gui* Gentiana & Aloe Pills) which should be taken after a meal. For people with replete qi, administer *Bing Lang Shen Xiong (Wan)*.

For dampness of the ears with swelling and pain, (use) *Liang Ge* (Cool the Diaphragm [Powder]) plus wine-fried Radix Et Rhizoma Rhei (*Da Huang*), one half *liang*, wine-soaked Radix Scutellariae Baicalensis (*Huang Qin*), Radix Ledebouriellae Sesloidis (*Fang Feng*), Herba Seu Flos Schizonepetae Tenuifoliae (*Jing Jie*), and Radix Et Rhizoma Notopterygii (*Qiang Huo*. In addition, a mixture consisting of) more Borneolum (*Nao*) than Secretio Moschi Moschiferi (*She Xiang*) can be blown into (the ears). In case of dampness, add Alumen (*Bai Ku Fan*). For pus in the ears which will not dry, (a mixture of) Calomelas (*Qing Fen*), powdered Cortex Phellodendri (*Huang Bai Mo*), and Os Sepiae Seu Sepiellae (*Hai Piao Xiao*) can be blown in (the ears). For ear ulceration, apply powdered, dry Bulbus Fritillariae (*Bei Mu*. For) discharge of pus from the ears, (use) *Tao Hua San* (Peach Blossom Powder). The formula is comprised of Alum (*Bai Fan*) and Radix Mirabilis Jalapae (*Yan Zhi*), 1 *qian* each, and Secretio Moschi Moschiferi (*She Xiang*), 1 character. Powder the above. (Then) dab this powder onto a cloth swab and roll the swab to dry (the pus. And in case of) heat in the ears with acute pain, blow Alum (*Ku Bai Fan*) into the ears. It is still better to blow in ash-burnt Folium Indocalami Tessellati (*Qing Ruo*).

Chapter Eighty-four

The Nose

Drinker's nose is (due to) blood heat entering the lungs. (For this,) boil *Si Wu Tang* (Four Materials Decoction) plus Pericarpium Citri Reticulatae (*Chen Pi*), wine-processed Flos Carthami Tinctorii (*Hong Hua*), and wine-fried Radix Scutellariae Baicalensis (*Huang Qin*. After decoction,) mix in several drops of good wine and then take with stir-fried, powdered Feces Trogopterori Seu Pteromi (*Wu Ling Zhi*). This is effective. Another formula (is made by) mixing Rhizoma Coptidis Chinensis (*Huang Lian*) with tung oil. Heat with a fire (made with) Ramulus Aristolochiae (*Tian Diao Teng*) and apply hot (as a dressing).

Some people may ask, does the name, drinker's nose, suggest that it is certainly a result of drinking hot wine? The answer is no. Those not drinking wine may also become diseased with this. The nose is the portal of the lungs and the foot *yang ming* passes up towards the inner canthi on either side of it. It is located in the center of the face and the center is ascribed to earth. It serves as a gate for the entrance and exit of the breath in the process of respiration. Moreover, the essence and brightness of qi and blood all go up and pour into the face, entering the portals there. On account of all this, damp heat in the stomach together with the blood transformed in the middle burner may be transported up into the lungs and, following the breath of respiration, may fume and steam the tip of the nose. (Finally, this becomes) congealed and bound in the skin, dying (the nose) red. In extreme (cases, this redness) is not limited to the nose but spreads all over the face. (To treat this,) I often use powdered Flos Campsis Grandiflorae (*Ling Xiao Hua*) and Lithargyum (*Mi Tuo Seng*). These are mixed with saliva and applied. (This is) extremely effective. Another formula (consists of) Folium Xanthii Sibirici (*Cang Er Ye*). Steam with wine, powder, and apply. (It) resolves heat toxin best of all.

To treat nasal sink[1], (use) Rhizoma Arisaematis (*Nan Xing*), Rhizoma Pinelliae Ternatae (*Ban Xia*), Rhizoma Atractylodis (*Cang Zhu*), Radix Angelicae (*Bai Zhi*), Massa Medica Fermentata (*Shen Qu*), wine-proc-essed Radix Scutellariae Baicalensis (*Huang Qin*), Flos Magnoliae Liliflorae (*Xin Yi*), and Herba Seu Flos Schizonepetae Tenuifoliae (*Jing Jie*, (whereas,) nasal polyp is (ascribed to) streaming food accumulation and hot phlegm in the stomach. To treat the root, it is necessary to disperse food accumulation. Externally, insert into the nose each time a small amount of (a mixture of) 2 *qian* of Alumen (*Hu Die Fan*), 1 *qian*

---

[1]   Wiseman *et al.* render *bi yuan* as deep source nasal congestion. This is a disorder of the nose manifested by copious purulent mucus from the nose with obstruction, and, in extreme cases, vertigo and dizziness.

of Herba Cum Radice Asari Sieboldi (*Xi Xin*), and one half *qian* of Radix Angelicae (*Bai Zhi*).

The face and nose turning black on exposure to cold requires the use of clearing heat and transforming stasis and enriching and engendering new blood. Not till blood is able to move itself will the color change (to normal). Process *Si Wu Tang* with wine and then add wine-processed Radix Scutellariae Baicalensis (*Pian Qin*), Pericarpium Citri Reticulatae (*Chen Pi*), Radix Glycyrrhizae (*Sheng Gan Cao*), and wine-processed Flos Carthami Tinctorii (*Hong Hua*). Boil with fresh Rhizoma Zingiberis (*Sheng Jiang*) and drink with powdered Feces Trogopterori Seu Pteromi (*Wu Ling Zhi*). For those of fat form with weak qi, the addition of wine-processed Radix Astragali Membranacei (*Huang Qi*) is also effective.

Chapter Eighty-five

Foot Qi[1]

This requires the use of medicinals able to upraise dampness from below used in combination with qi and blood (medicinals). Those introduced into the formula include Radix Rehmanniae (*Sheng Di Huang*), wine-washed Cortex Phellodendri (*Huang Bai*), wine-fried Rhizoma Atractylodis (*Cang Zhu*), salt-fried Rhizoma Coptidis Chinensis (*Huang Lian*), Rhizoma Atractylodis Macrocephalae (*Bai Zhu*), Radix Stephaniae Tetrandrae (*Fang Ji*), Semen Arecae Catechu (*Bing Lang*), Rhizoma Ligustici Wallichii (*Chuan Xiong*), Caulis Akebiae Mutong (*Mu Tong*), Pericarpium Citri Reticulatae (*Chen Pi*), Apex Radicis Glycyrrhi-

---

[1] This is a pattern mainly manifested in the initial stage by numbness and water swelling of the feet and legs and mental and cardiac disorders in the advanced stage. It should be noted that this is not athlete's foot which is also called foot qi in Chinese.

zae (*Gan Cao Shao*), and powdered Cornu Rhonoceroris (*Xi Jiao Xiao*). If there is heat, add Radix Scutellariae Baicalensis (*Huang Qin*) and Rhizoma Coptidis Chinensis (*Huang Lian*). If there is phlegm, add Succus Bambusae (*Zhu Li*) and Succus Zingiberis (*Jiang Zhi*). In case of great fever or in summerheat weather, add Gypsum (*Shi Gao*). In case of difficult evacuation of solid stools, add Semen Pruni Persicae (*Tao Ren*). In case of inhibited voiding of urine, add wild Radix Achyranthis Bidentatae (*Du Niu Xi*. However,) in case of streaming food accumulation, use Rhizoma Atractylodis (*Cang Zhu*), Cortex Phellodendri (*Huang Bai*), Radix Stephaniae Tetrandrae (*Han Fang Ji*), Rhizoma Arisaematis (*Nan Xing*), Rhizoma Ligustici Wallichii (*Chuan Xiong*), Radix Angelicae (*Bai Zhi*), Cornu Rhinoceroris (*Xi Jiao*), and Semen Arcae Catechu (*Bing Lang*). Powder the above and make into pills. In case of blood vacuity, add Radix Achyranthis Bidentatae (*Niu Xi*) and vanquished (*i.e.,* processed) Plastrum Testudinis (*Bai Gui Ban*) and make into pills with Massa Medica Fermentata (*Shen Qu*) paste. Constant swelling (of the feet) is specifically governed by damp heat. Master Zhu[2] has (specific) formulas for this.

There are cases of foot qi surging up into the heart.[3] This is blood vacuity with fire qi ascending. It is appropriate (to use) *Si Wu Tang* (Four Materials Decoction) plus stir-fried Cortex Phellodendri (*Huang Bai*). In addition, stick some powdered Radix Praeparatus Aconiti Carmichaeli (*Fu Zi*) the size of a coin mixed with saliva onto the point *Yong Quan* (Ki 1)[4] and then moxa at it to drain and attract the heat. Spasms are ascribed to blood heat in every case. (In this case,) *Zuo Jin Wan* (Left Gold Pills) can downbear liver fire.

---

[2]   *I.e.,* Zhu Dan-xi. This is another piece of evidence that this book was not entirely written by Zhu himself.

[3]   This refers to a later stage of foot qi in which there appear cardiac problems, such as asthma, abdominal swelling, and heart failure.

[4]   Gushing Spring

For foot qi swelling, (use) Fructus Immaturus Citri Seu Ponciri (*Zhi Shi*), Radix Et Rhizoma Rhei (*Da Huang*), Radix Angelicae Sinensis (*Dang Gui*), and Radix Et Rhizoma Notopterygii (*Qiang Huo*. But for) distressed aching in the limb joints, heavy shoulders and upper back, inhibited chest and diaphragm, aching pain all over the body, and (dampness) streaming down into the lower legs and feet causing swelling and pain, (use) *Dang Gui Nian Tong Tang* (*Dang Gui* Stifle Pain Decoction. And for) various (cases of) dampness intruding into the low back and knees causing heaviness and pain and puffy swelling of the feet and lower legs, (use) *Chu Shi Dan* (Eliminate Dampness Elixir): Gummum Olibani (*Ru Xiang*) and Myrrha (*Mo Yao*), 1 *liang* each, (both) ground, Semen Pharbitidis (*Qian Niu*), ground and sifted, one half *liang*, Semen Arcae Catechu (*Bing Lang*), Radix Clematidis Chinensis (*Wei Ling Xian*), Radix Rubrus Paeoniae Lactiflorae (*Chi Shao Yao*), Rhizoma Alismatis (*Ze Xie*), Semen Tinglizi (*Ting Li*), and Radix Euphorbiae Kansui (*Gan Sui*), 2 *liang* for each of the above, Herba Cirsii Japonicae (*Da Ji*), 3 *liang*, and Pericarpium Citri Reticulatae (*Chen Pi*), 6 *liang*, stripped of its white inner layer. Powder the above and make into pills with paste.

In case of foot qi developing from dampness and from below, treat the dampness and the qi (with) Fructus Perillae Frutescentis (*Zi Su*), stir-fried Cortex Phellodendri (*Huang Bai*), Radix Paeoniae Lactiflorae (*Shao Yao*), Fructus Chaenomelis Lagenariae (*Mu Gua*), Rhizoma Alismatis (*Ze Xie*), Caulis Akebiae Mutong (*Mu Tong*), Radix Stephaniae Tetrandrae (*Fang Ji*), Semen Arecae Catechu (*Bing Lang*), Rhizoma Atractylodis (*Cang Zhu*), Fructus Citri Seu Ponciri (*Zhi Qiao*), Radix Glycyrrhizae (*Gan Cao*), Rhizoma Cyperi Rotundi (*Xiang Fu*), and Radix Et Rhizoma Notopterygii (*Qiang Huo*). In case of more pain, add Radix Saussureae Seu Vladimiriae (*Mu Xiang*). In case of more swelling, add Pericarpium Arecae (*Da Fu Pi*). In case of fever, add Rhizoma Coptidis Chinensis (*Huang Lian*).

For weak feet with sinew pain, (use) Radix Achyranthis Bidentatae (*Niu Xi*), 2 *liang*, Radix Albus Paeoniae Lactiflorae (*Bai Shao*), 1.5 *liang*, and wine-processed Cortex Phellodendri (*Huang Bai*), Rhizoma Anemarrhenae (*Zhi Mu*), and stir-fried Radix Glycyrrhizae (*Gan Cao*), 5 *qian* for each of the above. Make into pills with wine paste and take.

For damp phlegm foot qi with efflux diarrhea, (use) Rhizoma Atractylodis (*Cang Zhu*), 2 *liang*, Radix Ledebouriellae Sesloidis (*Fang Feng*), Semen Arecae Catechu (*Bing Lang*), and Talcum (*Hua Shi*), 1 *liang* for each of the above, Rhizoma Cyperi Rotundi (*Xiang Fu*), 8 *qian*, Rhizoma Ligustici Wallichii (*Chuan Xiong*), 6 *qian*, Radix Scutellariae Baicalensis (*Tiao Qin*) and Caulis Akebiae Mutong (*Mu Tong*), 4 *qian* each, and Radix Glycyrrhizae (*Gan Cao*), 3 *qian*. (Take) either in the shape of pills or powder.

Jian Bu Wan (Nimble Steps Pills) are composed of Radix Rehmanniae (*Sheng Di*), 1.5 *liang*, Apex Radicis Angelicae Sinensis (*Gui Wei*), Pericarpium Citri Reticulatae (*Chen Pi*), Radix Paeoniae Lactiflorae (*Shao Yao*), Radix Achyranthis Bidentatae (*Niu Xi*), Rhizoma Atractylodis (*Cang Zhu*), and Rhizoma Atractylodis Macrocephalae (*Bai Zhu*), 1 *liang* for each of the above, Fructus Evodiae Rutecarpae (*Zhu Yu*) and Radix Scutellariae Baicalensis (*Tiao Qin*), 5 *qian* each, Semen Arecae Catechu (*Da Fu Zi*), 3 *qian*, and Ramulus Cinnamomi (*Gui Zhi*), 2 *qian*. Powder and make into pills; 100 pills per dose taken with Medulla Tetrapanacis Papyriferi (*Tong Cao*) soup before a meal.

A female with pain and swelling in the feet (was prescribed) Radix Rehmanniae (*Sheng Di Huang*), stir-fried Cortex Phellodendri (*Huang Bai*), Rhizoma Arisaematis (*Nan Xing*), Rhizoma Ligustici Wallichii (*Chuan Xiong*), Rhizoma Atractylodis (*Cang Zhu*), Radix Achyranthis Bidentatae (*Niu Xi*), Radix Gentianae Scabrae (*Long Dan*), and wine-washed Flos Carthami Tinctorii (*Hong Hua*).

A person with twitching sinews in the big toes, gradually up [3 characters missing] near to the lumbus and terminating there. (He) used to enjoy abundant supplies (of clothing and rich food). As a result of drinking [3 characters missing] damp heat damaging blood. *Si Wu Tang* plus Radix Scutellariae Baicalensis (*Huang Qin*), Flos Carthami Tinctorii (*Hong Hua*) [2 characters missing].[5]

---

[5] In relationship to this next to the last paragraph, there is a paragraph in Ch. 19, Bk. 2 where the author gives a similar description of a case aged nearly 30. This paragraph is, practically speaking, illegible because of too many characters having

A male, nearly 30 years of age, who was used to having (a diet) of thick flavor and was irascible, [3 characters missing], a point painful in the hip joints on both sides, [1 character missing] relieved [3 characters missing] averse to cold with thirst at one time but absence of thirst at another. Diaphragm [3 characters missing] wind medicinals, absence of blood supplementing medicinals. The next spring, his knees [3 characters missing] severely, his food intake decreased, his form was thin. Towards the end of the spring, his knees became so swollen [3 characters missing] contract or stretch, his pulse was bowstring, large, rather replete, and choppy/astringent in the *cun* section, all rapid and short, (with) frequent voiding of scant urine. Then (I treated him) as [3 characters missing] accumulated in the *tai yin* and *yang ming*. The treatment [3 characters missing] in the chapter in detail.

---

been lost in the long course of this book's hand-copied circulation. To help the reader get something from the reading of this paragraph, the translator, though aware of the risk of wild guesses, has taken the liberty of trying to fill in as many blanks as possible. The following is his best guess as to how this paragraph might have originally read:

A person had twitching of sinews in (his) big toes gradually extending to the knees and finally near to the lower back where the twitching ended. Because he used to enjoy abundant supplies of clothing and food and (indulged in) dietary irregularities, damp heat damaged his blood. He was treated with *Si Wu Tang* plus Radix Scutellariae Baicalensis (*Huang Qin*), Flos Carthami Tinctorii (*Hong Hua*), and an unidentifiable ingredient.

The last paragraph in this chapter has too may missing characters to even try to fill in the blanks.

Book Six

Chapter Eighty-six

Atony

(This disease) is classified into heat, damp phlegm, blood vacuity, and qi vacuity (types). The specific ruling (method) is to nurture lung qi, nurture the blood, and clear metal. It should not be treated as wind. (In terms of) damp heat, (Li) Dong-yuan's *Jian Bu Wan* (Nimble Steps Pills) plus Radix Scutellariae Baicalensis (*Huang Qin*), Cortex Phellodendri (*Huang Bai*), and Rhizoma Atractylodis (*Cang Zhu*, are effective). The formula of *Jian Bu Wan* includes Radix Et Rhizoma Notopterygii (*Qiang Huo*) and Radix Bupleuri (*Chai Hu*) 5 *qian* each, stir-fried Talcum (*Hua Shi*), 5 *qian*, mix-fried Radix Glycyrrhizae (*Zhi Gan Cao*), 5 *qian*, wine-washed Radix Trichosanthis Kirlowii (*Tian Hua Fen*), 5 *qian*, Radix Ledebouriellae Sesloidis (*Fang Feng*), 2 *liang*, Rhizoma Alismatis (*Ze Xie*), 3 *qian*, wine-washed Radix Stephaniae Tetrandrae (*Fang Ji*), 1 *qian*, Radix Aconiti (*Chuan Wu*), 1 *qian*, wine stir-fried Radix Sophorae Flavescentis (*Ku Shen*), 1 *qian*, and Cortex Cinnamomi (*Rou Gui*), one half *qian*. Powder the above and make into pills with wine paste; 70 pills per dose taken on an empty stomach with a decoction of *Yu Feng Tang* (Overcome Wind Decoction).[1]

For damp phlegm, (use) *Er Chen Tang* (Two Aged Decoction) plus Rhizoma Atractylodis (*Cang Zhu*), Rhizoma Atractylodis Macrocephalae (*Bai Zhu*), Radix Scutellariae Baicalensis (*Huang Qin*), Cortex Phelloden-

---

[1] This consists of Radix Paeoniae Lactiflorae (*Shao Yao*), Rhizoma Ligustici Wallichii (*Chuan Xiong*), stir-fried Bombyx Batryticatus (*Jiang Can*), Radix Platycodi Grandiflori (*Jie Geng*), Herba Cum Radice Asari Sieboldi (*Xi Xin*), Rhizoma Arisaematis (*Nan Xing*), Cinnabar (*Zhu Sha*), and Radix Et Rhizoma Notopterygii (*Qiang Huo*), one half *liang* for each of the above, Herba Ephedrae (*Ma Huang*), Radix Ledebouriellae Sesloidis (*Fang Feng*), Radix Angelicae (*Bai Zhi*), Rhizoma Gastrodiae Elatae (*Tian Ma*), and processed Buthus Martensi (*Zhi Quan Xie*), 1 *liang* for each of the above, and Radix Glycyrrhizae (*Gan Cao*), 3 *qian*. Note that this formula is usually taken in the form of pills, and it is also called *Yu Feng Dan* (Overcome Wind Elixir).

dri (*Huang Bai*), Succus Zingiberis (*Jiang Zhi*), and Succus Bambusae (*Zhu Li*. For) blood vacuity, (use) *Si Wu Tang* (Four Materials Decoction) plus Radix Scutellariae Baicalensis (*Huang Qin*), Cortex Phellodendri (*Huang Bai*), and Rhizoma Atractylodis (*Cang Zhu*). Take with *Bu Yin Wan* (Supplement Yin Pills). For qi vacuity, (use) *Si Jun Zi Tang* (Four Gentlemen Decoction) plus Radix Scutellariae Baicalensis (*Huang Qin*), Cortex Phellodendri (*Huang Bai*), Rhizoma Atractylodis (*Cang Zhu*), etc.

There are also cases of dead blood and cases of food accumulation obstructed and unable to descend. Roughly speaking, all these are ascribed to heat and require Radix Panacis Ginseng (*Ren Shen*), Rhizoma Atractylodis Macrocephalae (*Bai Zhu*), *Si Wu*[2], Cortex Phellodendri (*Huang Bai*), etc. For atony in strong people, (use) *Liang Ge San* (Cool the Diaphragm Powder). For atony in old or empty people, (use) *Ba Wei Wan* (Eight Flavors Pills).[3] A farmer was hunch backed with hypertonicity of the feet, [for which, see the *Yi Yao* {*Essentials of Medicine*; later editor}].

The *Su Wen (Simple Questions)* classifies atony into five kinds. (However,) all these various kinds of atony start from the lungs. When heat (in the lungs) enters the five viscera, it develops into different patterns (of atony). Generally speaking, the only appropriate (method) is to supplement and nurture (yin. If patients with atony) are treated as

---

[2]   This refers to the ingredients in *Si Wu Tang, i.e.,* Radix Angelicae Sinensis (*Dang Gui*), Rhizoma Ligustici Wallichii (*Chuan Xiong*), Radix Albus Paeoniae Lactiflorae (*Bai Shao Yao*), and prepared Radix Rehmanniae (*Shu Di Huang*). A formula name is often used to refer to the medicinals it contains, and in that case, it should be regarded as a collective name of certain medicinals rather than indicating the final form of preparation, a decoction for instance.

[3]   This consists of Radix Rehmanniae (*Di Huang*), 8 *liang*, Radix Dioscoreae Oppositae (*Shan Yao*), and Fructus Corni Officinalis (*Shan Zhu Yu*), 4 *liang* each, Rhizoma Alismatis (*Ze Xie*), Sclerotium Poriae Cocoris (*Fu Ling*), and Cortex Radicis Moutan (*Mu Dan Pi*), 3 *liang* each, and Ramulus Cinnamomi (*Gui Zhi*) and blast-fried Radix Praeparatus Aconiti Carmichaeli (*Fu Zi*), 1 *liang* each. Powder these ingredients and make into pills the size of Chinese parasol tree seeds with honey; 15-25 pills per dose.

external contraction of wind evils, how can the disaster of evacuating vacuity and replenishing repletion be avoided? Some may ask, why is atony treated only through the single channel of the *yang ming*? The master said: All the various kinds of atony are generated by lung heat. This one sentence brings out the essential (point) of the method of treating (this condition). The classic (*i.e., Nei Jing [Inner Classic]*) states: The east is replete and the west is empty. The south should be drained and the north supplemented. Here, supplementation and drainage are spoken of in terms of mutual engendering and mutual restraining relationships (of the five phases). The great classic and the great method never go beyond this. The east, wood, is the liver. The west, metal, is the lungs. The south, fire, is the heart. The north, water, is the kidneys. Among the five phases, fire alone is dual. The kidneys have two phases, but water occupies (only) one of them. (On account of all this,) yang is constantly superabundant, while yin is constantly insufficient. Therefore, the classic states: One water is no match for two fires. This is the only logical conclusion. Metal, a dry substance, is located above. It governs qi and is in awe of fire. Earth, damp by nature, is located in the center and is in awe of wood. Fire upflames by nature. In case of sexual desire beyond measure, water loses that which nourishes it, and fire, now daunted by nothing, bullies its restrained (phase). Subjected to fire evils, lung metal becomes hot. Wood has an unyielding, quick temper. When the lungs are subjected to evil heat, metal loses that which nourishes it, and wood, now daunted by nothing, bullies spleen earth. Affected by wood evils, (spleen earth) is damaged. When the lungs are hot, they lose control over (the qi of) the whole body, and when the spleen is hot, the four limbs are no longer capable of use. Thus various kinds of atony arise.

When the south is drained, lung metal is cleared and the east is no longer replete. Then what can damage the spleen? When the north is supplemented, heart fire is downborne and the west is no longer vacuous. Then what can damage the lungs? It follows that when the *yang ming* is replenished, the gathering sinews are moistened and enabled to bundle the bones and disinhibit the joints. There is no better treatment method for atony than this. Master Luo[4] also states: When wind and fire are mutually flaming, it is necessary to enrich the kidneys. (Li) Dong-yuan chose Cortex Phellodendri (*Huang Bai*) as the sovereign and supplementing medicinals like Radix Astragali Membranacei (*Huang Qi*) as assistants, stipulating no fixed formulas. (Among those he treated,) there were cases complicated by phlegm accumulation, excessive dampness, excessive heat, half dampness and half heat, or complicated by cold [qi in a {variant} edition {later editor}]. (He) designed (various) formulas in accordance with particular diseases. How good (he) was at treating atony! However, even though the medicinals are particularly appropriate and efficacious, if (the patient) is negligent in appropriate nurturing and care, a divine doctor cannot achieve a cure. (Eating) abundant produce (*i.e.*, fresh vegetables and fruits) gives rise to yang (disease) and thick flavors generate heat. This is a maxim left by the past sages. I am certain that persons suffering from atony can be sure of no safety unless they remain indifferent to the flavor of food.

Da Bu Wan (Great Supplement Pills) remove kidney channel fire, dry dampness in the lower burner, and treat flaccid sinews and bones. In case of qi vacuity, take with qi-supplementing medicinals. In case of blood vacuity, take with blood-supplementing medicinals. These are never used by themselves.

Bu Shen Wan (Supplement the Kidneys Pills) and *Hu Qian Wan* (Tiger in Hiding Pills) both can treat atony and their method of administration is the same as with *Da Bu Wan*. Cortex Phellodendri (*Huang Bai*) and Rhizoma Atractylodis (*Cang Zhu*) are essential ingredients in treating atony.

---

[4] Luo Long-ji, Song Dynasty, author of the *Nei Jing Shi Yi Fang Lun* (*The Treatise on Making Good the Omissions in the Inner Classic Formulas*). Little is known of this author's life.

A person suffered from yang atony.[5] (They were prescribed) Rhizoma Anemarrhenae (*Zhi Mu*), Cortex Phellodendri (*Huang Bai*), both stir-fried, 1 *liang* each, Fructus Lycii Chinensis (*Gou Qi*), 1 *liang*, wine-soaked Radix Achyranthis Bidentatae (*Niu Xi*), 1 *liang*, ginger stir-fried Cortex Eucommiae Ulmoidis (*Du Zhong*), 1 *liang*, Radix Panacis Ginseng (*Ren Shen*), 1 *liang*, Radix Dioscoreae Oppositae (*Shan Yao*), 1 *liang*, Plastrum Testudinis (*Gui Ban*) and Os Tigridis (*Hu Gu*), both processed, 1 *liang* each, wine-washed Radix Dipsaci (*Xu Duan*), 1 *liang*, Herba Cynomorii Songarici (*Suo Yang*), 2 *liang*, Radix Angelicae Sinensis (*Dang Gui*), 2 *liang*, Semen Cuscutae (*Tu Si Zi*), Fructus Schizandrae Chinensis (*Wu Wei Zi*), and Pericarpium Citri Reticulatae (*Chen Pi*), 5 *qian* for each of the above, and Rhizoma Atractylodis Macrocephalae (*Bai Zhu*), 1 *liang*. In a (variant) formula, there is 2 *liang* of Herba Cistanchis (*Cong Rong*) and Rhizoma Atractylodis Macrocephalae and Pericarpium Citri Reticulatae are deleted. The above were powdered and made into pills with paste.

A person more than 20 years of age suffered from a persistently erect, swollen, and atonic (*i.e.*, impotent) penis. Its skin was sunken, constantly wet, and rubbed against his thighs, (thus) causing inability to walk. (This was accompanied by) ascending qi from the lateral costal regions and weak, feeble hands and feet. First, a large dose of *Xiao Chai Hu Tang* (Minor Bupleurum Decoction) was prescribed with Rhizoma Coptidis Chinensis (*Huang Lian*) added to move damp heat and Cortex Phellodendri (*Huang Bai*) added in small amount to downbear upwardly counterflowing qi. The swelling reduced by half but there was a hardened place still undispersed on the penis. Then the single ingredient, Pericarpium Viridis Citri Reticulatae (*Qing Pi*) as the sovereign, plus small amounts of qi-dissipating [wind-dissipating {in a variant edition; later editor}] medicinals were administered in the form of powder. Externally, Succus Fructi Luffae Cylindricae (*Si Gua Zhi*) mixed with powdered Galla Rhi Chinensis (*Wu Bei*) was applied and a cure was obtained.

---

[5] Here, yang atony means impotence.

Chapter Eighty-seven

Tetany

Roughly speaking, (this condition) is similar to epilepsy. (However,) compared with epilepsy, it is vacuous (in nature. Therefore,) it is appropriate to combine a (specific) treatment with supplementation. For qi vacuity accompanied by fire and phlegm, (use) Radix Panacis Ginseng (*Ren Shen*), Succus Bambusae (*Zhu Li*), and the like. It is absolutely not permitted to treat this as wind with the addition of wind(-dispelling) medicinals. To treat wine tuggings with abundant wind, (use) Rhizoma Atractylodis Macrocephalae (*Bai Zhu*), 5 *qian*, Radix Panacis Ginseng (*Ren Shen*), 2.5 *qian*, Radix Glycyrrhizae (*Gan Cao*), 3 *qian*, Pericarpium Citri Reticulatae (*Chen Pi*) and Rhizoma Atractylodis (*Cang Zhu*), 1 *qian* for each of the above, Rhizoma Gastrodiae Elatae (*Tian Ma*), finely sliced and soaked in wine, 1 *qian*, wine-soaked Radix Albus Paeoniae Lactiflorae (*Bai Shao Yao*), 1 *qian*, Radix Ledebouriellae Sesloidis (*Fang Feng*), 5 *fen*, and Rhizoma Ligustici Wallichii (*Chuan Xiong*), 5 *fen*. Powder the above and make into pills. In case of copious urine, add Fructus Schizandrae Chinensis (*Wu Wei Zi*).

Chapter Eighty-eight

Heat in the Palms of the Hands
& Soles of the Feet

(This) is ascribed to heat depression. Use *Huo Yu Tang* (Fire Depression Decoction): Radix Puerariae Lobatae (*Ge Gen*), Radix Bupleuri (*Chai Hu*), and Radix Albus Paeoniae Lactiflorae (*Bai Shao Yao*), 1 *liang* for each of the above, mix-fried Radix Glycyrrhizae (*Zhi Gan Cao*), 1 *liang*, Radix Ledebouriellae Sesloidis (*Fang Feng*), 5 *qian*, and Rhizoma

Cimicifugae (*Sheng Ma*), 1 *liang*; 3 *qian* per dose. Put in 3 *cun* of Bulbus Allii Fistulosi (*Cong Bai*), boil, and take moderately hot. Another formula (consists of) Fructus Gardeniae Jasminoidis (*Zhi Zi*), Rhizoma Cyperi Rotundi (*Xiang Fu*), Radix Angelicae (*Bai Zhi*), Rhizoma Atractylodis (*Cang Zhu*), Rhizoma Pinelliae Ternatae (*Ban Xia*), and Rhizoma Ligustici Wallichii (*Chuan Xiong*). Powder the above and make into pills with flour paste. For fire depression with steaming bones in the palms of the hands and soles of the feet, (use) *Cao Huan Dan* (Grass Return Elixir).[1]

Chapter Eighty-nine

Numbness & Insensitivity of the Hands & Feet

Numbness is ascribed to qi vacuity, and insensitivity is ascribed to damp phlegm and dead blood. (Li) Dong-yuan explains that numbness and insensitivity are due to non-circulation of qi, and that it is necessary to supplement the qi in the lungs.

A fat female with qi depression suffered from a numb tongue, dizziness, numb hands and feet, qi obstruction with phlegm, and constipation. (She was prescribed) *Liang Ge San* (Cool the Diaphragm Powder) with Rhizoma Arisaematis (*Nan Xing*), Rhizoma Cyperi Rotundi (*Xiang Fu*), and Rhizoma Ligustici Wallichii (*Chuan Xiong*) added to open (depression).

---

[1] A.k.a. Zhang Tian Shi's *Cao Huan Dan* in full. This consists of Cortex Radicis Lycii (*Di Gu Pi*), Radix Rehmanniae (*Sheng Di Huang*), Rhizoma Acori Graminei (*Shi Chang Pu*), Radix Achyranthis Bidentatae (*Niu Xi*), Radix Polygalae Tenuifoliae (*Yuan Zhi*), Semen Cuscutae (*Tu Si Zi*), all in equal amounts. Zhang Tian Shi or Zhang the Heavenly Scholar, also named Ling or Dao-ling, was the founder of the Five *Dou* of Grain School of Taoism.

Chapter Ninety

Inversion

There is yang inversion and yin inversion. When yang becomes decrepit below, this is cold (inversion). When yin becomes decrepit below, this is heat (inversion). There is a detailed discussion in the *Yuan Bing Shi (The Formulation of the Origin of Disease)*. (This condition) is (also) commonly due to qi and blood vacuity (and also to) phlegm and heat. To treat phlegm, (use) Rhizoma Atractylodis Macrocephalae (*Bai Zhu*) and Succus Bambusae (*Zhu Li*). To treat heat, (use) *Cheng Qi Tang* (Support the Qi Decoction). And in case of external contraction (of wind cold), add Succus Zingiberis (*Jiang Zhi*) and wine to resolve and dissipate this. (With) qi vacuity, the pulse is fine. (With) blood vacuity, the pulse is hollow. (With) heat inversion, the pulse is rapid. (With) external contraction, the pulse is floating. (With) repletion phlegm, the pulse is wiry.

A female more than 30 years of age with a white facial complexion and a long form constantly bore grudges and indignation in her heart. One night, she unexpectedly gave birth to a child and immediately postpartum, had clouding inversion, falling unconscious of people. She was promptly moxaed at *Qi Hai* (CV 6)[1] with 15 cones. After resurrection, (she) was administered Radix Panacis Ginseng (*Ren Shen*), Rhizoma Atractylodis Macrocephalae (*Bai Zhu*), and other medicinals, and she recovered 2 months later.

An(other) female, aged 19, bore but kept suppressing her angry qi. One day, she broke into a great fit (of fury), shouting and on the verge of inversion. This was phlegm obstructing above and fire starting below and surging up. (The medicinals) prescribed first were Rhizoma Cyperi Rotundi (*Xiang Fu*), 5 qian, Radix Glycyrrhizae (*Sheng Gan Cao*),

---

[1] Sea of Qi

3 *qian*, and Rhizoma Ligustici Wallichii (*Chuan Xiong*), 7 *qian*. These were boiled with child's urine and Succus Zingiberis (*Jiang Zhi*) and taken. Later Pulvis Indigonis (*Qing Dai*), Radix Panacis Ginseng (*Ren Shen*), and Radix Aconiti Coreani (*Bai Fu Zi*) were administered in the form of pills. A small degree of improvement was achieved but (the disease) was not exterminated. Then great (*i.e.*, drastic) ejection was applied, and relief followed. After that, *Dao Tan Tang* (Conduct Phlegm Decoction) plus ginger-fried Rhizoma Coptidis Chinensis (*Huang Lian*), Rhizoma Cyperi Rotundi (*Xiang Fu*), and fresh Rhizoma Zingiberis (*Sheng Jiang*) were prescribed and taken with *Long Hui Wan* (Gentiana & Aloe Pills).

Chapter Ninety-one

Various Eye Diseases (With Throat Disorders Appended [trans.])

Zhi Bao Gao (Consummately Precious Paste) treats fulminant breaking out of heat congestion with screen (in the eye) with remarkable efficacy. It consists of de-oiled Semen Prinsepiae Uniflorae (*Rui Ren*) and Borax (*Peng Sha*), 1 *qian* each, Cinnabar (*Chen Sha*), 3 *fen*, and Borneolum (*Bing Pian*), 1 *fen*. Powder extremely finely together, mix with honey, and drop (in the eye).

To treat ulcers on the rims of the eyelid, use Herba Menthae (*Bo He*), Herba Seu Flos Schizonepetae Tenuifoliae (*Jing Jie*) and Herba Cum Radicis Asari Sieboldi (*Xi Xin*), all in equal amounts. Powder coarsely, burn till smoke is seen no more, and drop into the eye. The (processing) method is like burning incense. Place a celadon bowl smeared with a small amount of honey over the smoke till the smoke is seen no more. Then collect (the honey) and preserve it in a ceramic container. All cases of copious tearing (due to) wind heat in the eyes (can be treated by) dropping (this in them).

Concerning *Ping Feng Zhi Lei San* (Level Wind to Check Tearing Powder) there is a rhyme:

> Wind heat tearing complicated by pain,
> *Cang Fu Xiong Xin He Zhi*[1] restrain.
> *Xia Ku Fang Guo Lao Mu Zei*[2],
> Boil and take, and everything will be okay.

Another formula for (eye) drops (is made by) breaking Calcareous Spar (*Han Shui Shi*) into pieces. Soak in child's urine for 7 days (and) dry in the sun for 7 days. Soak again for another 7 days, grind, put in 5 *fen* of Calomelas (*Qing Fen*) per *liang*, grind again extremely finely, expose to night dew for 7 nights, and dry in the sun for 7 days. Before use, add a tiny amount of Borneolum (*Bing Pian*) and then drop (in the eye).

To treat blood vacuity eyes, use *Sheng Shu Di Huang Wan* (Raw & Prepared Rehmannia Pills. These consists of) Radix Rehmanniae (*Sheng Di Huang*) and prepared Radix Rehmanniae (*Shu Di Huang*), 2 *liang* each, and Herba Dendrobii (*Shi Hu*) and Radix Scrophulariae Ningpo-ensis (*Xuan Shen*), 1 *liang* each. Powder and make into pills with honey. In winter months, sudden pain in the eye also requires resolving and dissipating (wind heat. In this case,) the use of cool medicinals is not allowed. (But) for screen growing over the dark of the eye, use Cortex Phellodendri (*Huang Bai*) and Rhizoma Anemarrhe-nae (*Zhi Mu*) in every case. For pain in the eye, (use) Rhizoma Anemarrhenae (*Zhi Mu*) and Cortex Phellodendri (*Huang Bai*) to drain kidney fire, Radix Angelicae Sinensis (*Dang Gui*) to nurture yin, and Radix Et Rhizoma Notopterygii (*Qiang Huo*) to lead these to the (*tai yang*) channel. (And) for wind tearing in the eye, take a number of

---

[1] This consists of Rhizoma Atractylodis (*Cang Zhu*), Radix Praeparatus Aconiti Carmichaeli (*Fu Zi*), Rhizoma Ligustici Wallichii (*Chuan Xiong*), Flos Magnoliae Liliflorae (*Xin Yi*), Herba Menthae (*Bo He*), and Radix Angelicae (*Bai Zhi*).

[2] This consists of Spica Prunellae Vulgaris (*Xia Gu Cao*), Radix Ledebouriellae Sesloidis (*Fang Feng*), Radix Glycyrrhizae (*Guo Lao*), and Herba Equiseti Hiemalis (*Mu Zei*).

pills of *Long Hui Wan* (Gentiana & Aloe Pills) 3 times per day after meals.

A person suffered from eye disease which never failed to arise in spring and summer. This should be treated as (heat) depression. (In this case, use) wine-soaked Radix Scutellariae Baicalensis (*Huang Qin*), 2 *liang*, ginger-processed Rhizoma Arisaematis (*Nan Xing*), 2 *liang*, Rhizoma Cyperi Rotundi (*Xiang Fu*) and Rhizoma Atractylodis (*Cang Zhu*), both soaked in urine, 2 *liang* each, Fructus Forsythiae Suspensae (*Lian Qiao*), 2 *liang*, stir-fried Fructus Gardeniae Jasminoidis (*Shan Zhi*), 1 *liang*, urine-soaked Rhizoma Ligustici Wallichii (*Dao Xiong*), 1.5 *liang*, wine-soaked Pericarpium Citri Reticulatae (*Chen Pi*), one half *liang*, wine-steamed Radix Gentianae Scabrae (*Long Dan Cao*), one half *liang*, Rhizoma Raphani Sativi (*Luo Bo*), one half *liang*, Pulvis Indigonis (*Qing Dai*), one half *liang*, and Radix Bupleuri (*Chai Hu*), 3 *qian*. Powder the above and make into pills with Massa Medica Fermentata (*Shen Qu*) paste.

A person with sunken eyes (was prescribed) Radix Rehmanniae (*Sheng Di*) and prepared Radix Rehmanniae (*Shu Di*), 1 *jin* each, Semen Pruni Armeniacae (*Xing Ren*), 4 *liang*, Herba Dendrobii (*Shi Hu*), and Radix Achyranthis Bidentatae (*Niu Xi*), one half *jin* each, Radix Ledebouriellae Sesloidis (*Fang Feng*), 6 *liang*, and Fructus Citri Seu Ponciri (*Zhi Qiao*), 5 *liang*, taken in the shape of honey pills.

To treat sudden breaking out of heat congestion and swelling causing pain (in the eyes, use) *Si Wu Tang* plus Radix Gentianae Scabrae (*Long Dan Cao*), Radix Stephaniae Tetrandrae (*Fang Ji*), Radix Ledebouriellae Sesloidis (*Fang Feng*), and Radix Et Rhizoma Notopterygii (*Qiang Huo*). Dry, ulcerated eyelid rims due to wind require a wind formula to dry them, (such as) *Chai Hu San* (Bupleurum Powder): Radix Bupleuri (*Chai Hu*), Radix Et Rhizoma Notopterygii (*Qiang Huo*), Radix Ledebouriellae Sesloidis (*Fang Feng*), Radix Rehmanniae (*Sheng Di Huang*), Radix Rubrus Paeoniae Lactiflorae (*Chi Shao Yao*), Radix Glycyrrhizae (*Gan Cao*), Radix Platycodi Grandiflori (*Jie Geng*), and Herba Seu Flos Schizonepetae Tenuifoliae (*Jing Jie*).

For internal obstruction of the eyes with dim and clouding vision due to taxation and toil and dietary irregularity, (use) *Man Jing Zi Tang* (Turnip Seed Decoction).[3] To treat internal obstruction, (use) *Si Wu Tang* plus wine-fried Radix Scutellariae Baicalensis (*Huang Qin*), Rhizoma Coptidis Chinensis (*Huang Lian*), and Cortex Phellodendri (*Huang Bai*). A sucking agent (*i.e.*, a medicinal to melt in the mouth, which consists of) Fructus Immaturus Pruni Mume (*Shuang Mei*), Bombyx Batryticatus (*Jiang Can*), and Alum (*Bai Fan*). Mix into pills, wrap in silk cloth, and melt in the mouth.

A formula for throat *bi* (is made by) putting common house centipedes (*You Yan*) into Fructus Immaturus Pruni Mume (*Bai Mei*), mix well and melt in the mouth. To treat wind heat throat *bi*, first administer *Qian Min Tang* (Thousand Strings of Coins Decoction) and afterwards *Si Wu Tang* plus Cortex Phellodendri (*Huang Bai*) and Rhizoma Anemarrhenae (*Zhi Mu*). When yin is nurtured, fire will be downborne. Another formula (consists of) making pills of powdered Fructus Gleditschiae Sinensis (*Zhu Ya Zao Jiao*) and Fructus Immaturus Pruni Mume (*Bai Mei*). Melt in the mouth. (Again) another formula (consists of) 1 *liang* of Radix Rubiae Cordifoliae (*Qian Cao*) as 1 dose. (This) downbears fire in the blood. (Yet) another formula (is composed of) Nitre (*Yan Xiao*), one half *qian*, Alumen (*Ku Fan*), 1 *qian*, and Borax (*Peng Sha*), 1 *qian*. Powder together, brew with Succus Radicis Achyranthis Bidentatae (*Du Niu Xi Zhi*) obtained by pounding, and take.

Run Hou San (Moisten the Throat Powder) treats qi depression night heat with a dry throat and choking and obstruction. (It consists of) Radix Platycodi Grandiflori (*Jie Geng*), 2.5 *qian*, debarked Radix Glycyrrhizae (*Fen Cao*), 1 *qian*, Placenta Hominis (*Zi He Che*), 4 *qian*, Rhizoma Cyperi Rotundi (*Xiang Fu Zi*), 3 *qian*, and Massa Medica Fermentata made with Galla Rhi Chinensis and Folium Camelliae Sinensis (*Bai Yao Jian*), 1.5 *qian*. Powder the above finely and apply

---

[3] This consists of Radix Astragali Membranacei (*Huang Qi*) and Radix Panacis Ginseng (*Ren Shen*), 1 *liang* each, mix-fried Radix Glycyrrhizae (*Zhi Gan Cao*), 8 *qian*, Fructus Viticis (*Man Jing Zi*), 2.5 *qian*, Cortex Phellodendri (*Huang Bai*), 3 *qian*, and Radix Albus Paeoniae Lactiflorae (*Bai Shao Yao*), 3 *qian*.

inside the mouth. (However,) in case of sores growing in and damaging the throat, do not use fresh Rhizoma Zingiberis (*Sheng Jiang*), since it causes hot pain. Moreover, it is capable of dispersing without contracting. (While) sore throat necessarily requires Herba Seu Flos Schizonepetae Tenuifoliae (*Jing Jie,* and) upflaming yin fire necessarily requires Radix Scrophulariae Ningpoensis (*Xuan Shen*). For sore throat, powder Borax (*Peng Sha,*) alone or together with Chalcanthitum (*Dan Fan*), Bombyx Batryticatus (*Jiang Can*), and Alumen (*Bai Fan*). Pound together with Fructus Immaturus Pruni Mume (*Shuang Mei*) and melt in the mouth. To treat all kinds of sore throat, obtain Radix Rosae Multiflorae (*Dao Zhai Ci Gen*), wash clean, grind with a tiny amount of good vinegar, and drop into the throat and ear. Itching foretells healing.

Sores growing in the throat with pain are ascribed to heat. In most cases, this is vacuity fire wandering out of control, intruding into the throat. In case of repletion fire, use Radix Panacis Ginseng (*Ren Shen*), honey-fried Cortex Phellodendri (*Huang Bai*), and Herba Seu Flos Schizonepetae Tenuifoliae (*Jing Jie*). In case of vacuity fire, use Radix Panacis Ginseng (*Ren Shen*) and Succus Bambusae (*Zhu Li*). In case of heat, use Rhizoma Coptidis Chinensis (*Huang Lian*), Herba Seu Flos Schizonepetae Tenuifoliae (*Jing Jie*), Herba Menthae (*Bo He*), and Nitre (*Xiao Shi*). Mix with honey and melt in the mouth. In case of blood vacuity, use *Si Wu Tang* with Succus Bambusae (*Zhu Li*) added.

To treat throat *bi* or blood threads running from the nose which coagulate and form a hanging ball of blood in the throat, pound and smash Radix Achyranthis Bidentatae (*Du Niu Xi, i.e.*), the erect, single stemmed *Gu Chui Cao*, mix with a small amount of good vinegar, grind, collect 3-5 drops of the juice, and drop into the nose. (The ball) will break instantly.

A fat person who used to have fat meat and fine grains frequently suffered from sore throat, nasal congestion, and coughing of phlegm when taxed and overworked. (They were prescribed) *Liang Ge San* (Cool the Diaphragm Powder) plus Radix Platycodi Grandiflori (*Jie Geng*), Herba Seu Flos Schizonepetae Tenuifoliae (*Jing Jie*), Rhizoma Arisaematis (*Nan Xing*), and Fructus Immaturus Citri Seu Ponciri (*Zhi Shi*).

Du Qing-bi's *Tong Shen San* (Free the Spirit Powder) is a very effective formula for the treatment of throat *bi* via ejecting wind phlegm. The formula is seen in the chapter on wind (*i.e.*, Ch. 1). An ejecting agent for throat wind[4] (consists of) Bombyx Batryticatus (*Jiang Can*), Fructus Gleditschiae Sinensis (*Ya Zao*), and Alum (*Bai Fan*). Powder, brew with pickle solution, pour down (the throat), and then operate mechanical emesis. The needling method is to prick *Shao Shang* (Lu 11)[5] with a three-edged needle. Recuperation follows bleeding instantly.

Chapter Ninety-two

Mouth Sores

If administration of cool medicinals does not achieve recovery, the qi is insufficient in the middle burner and vacuity fire is floating above out of control. (To treat this, use) *Li Zhong Tang* (Rectify the Center Decoction). In severe cases, add Radix Praeparatus Aconiti Carmichaeli (*Fu Zi*. But for) mouth sores due to replete heat, (use) *Liang Ge San* (Cool the Diaphragm Powder), *Gan Ju Tang* (Licorice & Platycodon Decoction)[1], and *Fu Yan San* (Going to the Banquet Powder).[2] For erosion in the mouth, boil Radix Rosae Multiflorae (*Ye Qiang Wei Gen*) and rinse the mouth with the decoction. For excessive dissipation in

---

[4] This refers to acute inflammation of the throat with distressed rapid dyspneic breathing, difficulty speaking and swallowing, etc.

[5] Lesser *Shang*. *Shang* refers to the note associated with the metal phase.

[1] This is composed of 2 *liang* of Radix Platycodi Grandiflori (*Jie Geng*) and 1 *liang* of Radix Glycyrrhizae (*Gan Cao*); 2 *qian* per dose.

[2] This consists of Rhizoma Alpiniae Officinalis (*Gao Liang Jiang*), Radix Aconiti (*Cao Wu Tou*), Herba Cum Radicis Asari Sieboldi (*Xi Xin*), and Herba Seu Flos Schizonepetae Tenuifoliae (*Jing Jie*), 2 *liang* for each of the above.

wine, indulgence in sex, taxation fatigue, and sleeplessness with a smooth, glossy, skinless (*i.e.*, furless) tongue or insomnia and taxation fatigue as a result of central qi damaged by worry and thought, (also use) *Li Zhong Tang* plus Radix Praeparatus Aconiti Carmichaeli (*Fu Zi*). Drink cool. If mouth sores are caused by earth vacuity of the middle burner with inability to take in food and (hence) ministerial fire surging upward without obstacle, use *Li Zhong Tang* since Radix Panacis Ginseng (*Ren Shen*), Rhizoma Atractylodis Macrocephalae (*Bai Zhu*), and Radix Glycyrrhizae (*Gan Cao*) supplement earth vacuity and dry Rhizoma Zingiberis (*Gan Jiang*) dissipates blazing fire. In severe cases, add Radix Praeparatus Aconiti Carmichaeli (*Fu Zi*). Another formula (consists of) Rhizoma Coptidis Chinensis (*Huang Lian*), Pulvis Indigonis (*Qing Dai*), and Cortex Phellodendri (*Huang Bai*). Powder and melt in the mouth. To treat white erosions covering the entire mouth, (use) Fructus Piperis Longi (*Bi Ba*), 1 *liang*, and Cortex Phellodendri (*Hou Huang Bai*), 1 *liang*, roasted by fire. Powder the above, boil in millet vinegar, mix with the preceding formula after boiling for a while, and rinse the mouth with it. Afterwards, rinse the mouth with boiled water and recovery will be achieved. In severe cases, rinsing twice (suffices).

A person had a sore growing on their lip. (In this case,) petals of Flos Albus Nelumbinis Nuciferae (*Bai He Hua Ban*) were stuck (to the sore).

To treat double tongue[3], grind finely good Chalcanthitum (*Dan Fan*) and apply (to the affected part. In addition, take) *Man Jing Zi Tang* (Turnip Seed Decoction). For blood weakness, yin water vacuity, and yang fire exuberance with the pupils (of the eyes) scattered and injured, and blurred, flowery vision, (use) *Shu Di Huang Wan* (Prepared Rehmannia Pills)[4], also known as *Zi Yin Di Huang Wan* (Enrich

---

[3] This refers to inflammation under the tongue which forms a tangible protrusion.

[4] This consists of prepared Radix Rehmanniae (*Shu Di Huang*), 1.6 *qian*, Radix Dioscoreae Oppositae (*Shan Yao*), Fructus Corni Officinalis (*Shan Zhu Yu*), wine-processed Radix Angelicae Sinensis (*Dang Gui*), Radix Albus Paeoniae Lactiflorae (*Bai Shao Yao*), and Rhizoma Ligustici Wallichii (*Chuan Xiong*), 8 *fen* for each of the above, Cortex Radicis Moutan (*Mu Dan Pi*), Rhizoma Alismatis (*Ze Xie*), Sclerotium Poriae

Yin Rehmannia Pills. But) for sudden reddening and swelling (of the eye), use (Liu) Shou-zhen's *San Re Yin Zi* (Dissipate Heat Drink).[5] In case of constipation, add Radix Et Rhizoma Rhei (*Da Huang*). In case of pain, add Radix Angelicae Sinensis (*Dang Gui*) and Radix Rehmanniae (*Di Huang*. And) in case of vexation and insomnia, add Fructus Gardeniae Jasminoidis (*Zhi Zi*).

For years long eye disorders, moxa the end of the crease at the base joint lateral to the nail of the thumb till seven cones are burned up. (In addition,) drink loess and honey solution.

Chapter Ninety-three

Bone Stuck in the Throat

Dry Ootheca Mantidis (*Sang Piao Xiao*) by hanging, powder, and blow in (the throat). A formula to resolve stuck fish bones (consists of) powdered, charred, granulated sugar, powdered Folium Perillae Frutescentis (*Zi Su Ye*), and powdered Talcum (*Hua Shi*). Mix into a pill, wrap in cloth, and retain in the mouth. Swallow the saliva and the bone will go down.

Cocoris (*Fu Ling*), Radix Polygalae Tenuifoliae (*Yuan Zhi*), Rhizoma Acori Graminei (*Shi Chang Pu*), wine-processed Rhizoma Anemarrhenae (*Zhi Mu*), and wine-processed Cortex Phellodendri (*Huang Bai*).

[5] This consists of Radix Ledebouriellae Sesloidis (*Fang Feng*), Radix Et Rhizoma Notopterygii (*Qiang Huo*), Radix Scutellariae Baicalensis (*Huang Qin*), and Rhizoma Coptidis Chinensis (*Huang Lian*), 1 *liang* for each of the above; 5 *qian* per dose. Boil and take.

Chapter Ninety-four

Throat

Roughly speaking, throat *bi* is usually ascribed to phlegm heat and is treated by retaining a slice of Radix Pruni Salicinae (*Li Shi Gen*) in the mouth and, in addition, applying water-ground Radix Pruni Salicinae around the neck. This offers an instant cure. Radix Pruni Salicinae must be freshly dug out in the garden. In severe cases, perform mechanical emesis with tung oil. A (variant) method is to use Rhizoma Belamcandae (*She Gan*) and the water from a whirlpool as an emetic.

Circling the throat wind[1] is ascribed to phlegm heat. (For this,) it is appropriate to use mechanical emesis with a goose quill dabbed with tung oil. To treat sore throat, (use) Herba Seu Flos Schizonepetae Tenuifoliae (*Jing Jie*), Radix Angelicae Sinensis (*Dang Gui*), Radix Platycodi Grandiflori (*Jie Geng*), and Radix Glycyrrhizae (*Gan Cao*). Boil, rinse (the mouth) with (this decoction), and take. (But) for dry, painful throat, (use) *Si Wu Tang* (Four Materials Decoction) plus Radix Platycodi Grandiflori (*Jie Geng*), Herba Seu Flos Schizonepetae Tenuifoliae (*Jing Jie*), Cortex Phellodendri (*Huang Bai*), and Rhizoma Anemarrhenae (*Zhi Mu*). This offers an instant cure.

For heat and pain in the throat, (use) *Gan Jie Tang* (Licorice & Platycodon Decoction) plus Herba Seu Flos Schizonepetae Tenuifoliae (*Jing Jie*). If there is fever, add Radix Scutellariae Baicalensis (*Huang Qin*) and Fructus Citri Seu Ponciri (*Zhi Qiao*). For hemilateral headache with incessant running nose and sore throat, (use) *Gan Jie Tang* plus Herba Seu Flos Schizonepetae Tenuifoliae (*Jing Jie*), Herba Menthae (*Bo He*), Fructus Citri Seu Ponciri (*Zhi Qiao*), and Herba Ephedrae (*Ma Huang*). Perspiration after administration leads to resolution. In case of

---

[1]   This refers to an acute, deep-seated inflammation involving the throat manifested by inability to swallow, dyspnea, rales, clenched jaw, and even suffocation.

hemilateral swelling (of the throat), add Fructus Perillae Frutescentis (*Zi Su*). In winter months, (such swelling may be caused by) wind cold depressed hemilaterally.

Chapter Ninety-five

Vesicular Sore[1]

(For this,) obtain *Tong Sheng San* (Communicate with the Divinity Powder) and smashed Lumbricus (*Qui Yin*). Stir-fry for a short while and mix with honey. This is remarkable when applied to the affected area. If (the lesion) develops upwards from the belly, this is internal heat effusing outward. (In that case,) still take *Tong Sheng San.*

Chapter Ninety-six

Toothache

For toothache, use powdered Rhizoma Arisaematis (*Nan Xing*) seasoned with Fructus Immaturus Pruni Mume (*Bai Mei*) to attract drool, Herba Seu Flos Schizonepetae Tenuifoliae (*Jing Jie*) and Herba Menthae (*Bo He*) to dissipate wind heat, and Halitum (*Qing Yan*), which enters the kidneys and bones. Frequently rub (the teeth) with and melt these in the mouth. (To treat) tooth decay, powder and fill in the holes with Resina Alois (*Lu Hui*) and Resina Liquidambaris

---

[1] This refers to a lesion or rash consisting of a great many thin-walled, transparent vesicles of various sizes, the largest of which may possibly be as big as a hen's egg. These fester easily.

Taiwanianae (*Bai Jiao Xiang*. To treat) *yang ming* wind heat toothache, burn equal amounts of Radix Et Rhizoma Rhei (*Da Huang*) and Rhizoma Cyperi Rotundi (*Xiang Fu*) separately with their natures preserved, put in a small amount of Halitum (*Qing Yan*), powder finely, and constantly rub the teeth with these. (To treat) loose teeth with wide spaces in between, burn 1 *liang* of the leg bone of a white goat to ash with nature preserved, powder together with 1 *qian* of Rhizoma Cimicifugae (*Sheng Ma*) and one half *qian* of Rhizoma Coptidis Chinensis (*Huang Lian*), and rub (the teeth with this powder. To treat) clenched jaw and teeth, dab powdered Alum (*Bai Fan*) and Bombyx Batryticatus (*Jiang Can*) onto Fructus Immaturus Pruni Mume (*Bai Mei*). Rub (the teeth) and the jaw will open instantly.

For toothache with cold and heat and swelling, (use) *Tiao Wei Cheng Qi Tang* (Regulate the Stomach & Support the Qi Decoction) plus Rhizoma Coptidis Chinensis (*Huang Lian*. To treat) worm-bitten teeth (*i.e.*, tooth decay), use Venum Bufonis Bufonis (*Chan Su*. Also to treat) toothache, rub (the teeth) with powdered Semen Firmianae Simplicis (*Wu Tong Lu*) mixed with a small amount of Secretio Moschi Moschiferi (*She Xiang*. While) great toothache necessarily requires Fructus Piperis Nigri (*Hu Jiao*) and Fructus Piperis Longi (*Bi Ba*) which are able to dissipate floating heat in the teeth, Rhizoma Cimicifugae (*Sheng Ma*) and Calcareous Spar (*Han Shui Shi*) as supervisors, and acrid, cool medicinals as assistants, such as Herba Menthae (*Bo He*), Herba Seu Flos Schizonepetae Tenuifoliae (*Jing Jie*), and Herba Cum Radicis Asari Sieboldi (*Xi Xin*) to restrain wood.[1] Another formula (consists of) using cool medicinals to prevent the ache. This entails a similar treatment: Fructus Piperis Longi (*Bi Ba*), Fructus Zanthoxyli Bungeani (*Chuan Jiao*), Herba Menthae (*Bo He*), Herba Seu Flos Schizonepetae Tenuifoliae (*Jing Jie*), Herba Cum Radicis Asari Sieboldi (*Xi Xin*), Camphora (*Zhang Nao*), and Halitum (*Qing Yan*). For severe toothache, (use) Radix Ledebouriellae Sesloidis (*Fang Feng*), Radix Et Rhizoma Notopterygii (*Qiang Huo*), and Halitum (*Qing Yan*) to penetrate internally and Herba Cum Radicis Asari Sieboldi (*Xi Xin*), Fructus Piperis Longi (*Bi Ba*), and

---

[1] Wood, *i.e.*, the liver, should be restrained because bad toothache is usually ascribed in Chinese medicine to effulgent liver fire.

Fructus Zanthoxyli Bungeani (*Chuan Jiao*) to settle pain. Another formula (consists of) ash-burnt Herba Cum Radicis Taraxaci Mongolici (*Pu Gong Ying*), Rhizoma Cyperi Rotundi (*Xiang Fu*), Radix Angelicae (*Bai Zhi*), and Halitum (*Qing Yan*).

For yin vacuity with fresh blood exiting from the teeth and qi depression, add Radix Achyranthis Bidentatae (*Niu Xi*), Rhizoma Cyperi Rotundi (*Xiang Fu*), Nodus Radicis Glycyrrhizae (*Sheng Gan Cao Jie*), and Cacumen Biotae Orientalis (*Ce Bai Ye*) to *Si Wu Tang* (Four Materials Decoction). For toothache with swelling, (use) Rhizoma Cimicifugae (*Sheng Ma*), Radix Angelicae (*Bai Zhi*), Radix Ledebouriellae Sesloidis (*Fang Feng*), Herba Seu Flos Schizonepetae Tenuifoliae (*Jing Jie*), Herba Menthae (*Bo He*), Radix Glycyrrhizae (*Gan Cao*), Radix Platycodi Grandiflori (*Jie Geng*), and the like.

For upper toothache, moxa *San Li* (LI 10).[2] For lower toothache, moxa *San Jian* (LI 3).[3] (To treat) worm-eaten teeth, fumigate (the teeth) with Semen Crotonis (*Ba Dou*). In case of no avail, use one half *liang* of powdered Semen Phaseoli Radiati (*Lu Dou Fen*), 1 *qian* of Arsenolitum (*Ren Yan*), and one half *qian* of Secretio Moschi Moschiferi (*She Xiang*). A formula to secure the teeth (consists of) goat's leg bone (*Yang Jing Gu*) burnt to ash with nature preserved, 3 *qian*, Radix Angelicae Sinensis (*Dang Gui*), 2 *qian*, and Radix Angelicae (*Bai Zhi*), Fructus Gleditschiae Sinensis (*Zhu Ya Zao Jiao*), and Halitum (*Qing Yan*), 1 *qian* for each of the above. Powder and rub (the teeth with these).

---

[2] (Arm) Three *Li*

[3] Third Space

Chapter Ninety-seven

Prolapse of the Rectum

(This may be due to) qi heat, qi vacuity, blood heat, or blood vacuity. For qi heat, (use) Radix Scutellariae Baicalensis (*Huang Qin*), fresh desirable, 6 *liang*, and Rhizoma Cimicifugae (*Sheng Ma*), 1 *liang*. Powder and make into pills with Massa Medica Fermentata (*Shen Qu*). For qi vacuity, supplement the qi with Radix Panacis Ginseng (*Ren Shen*), Radix Astragali Membranacei (*Huang Qi*), Rhizoma Ligustici Wallichii (*Chuan Xiong*), Radix Angelicae Sinensis (*Dang Gui*), Rhizoma Cimicifugae (*Sheng Ma*), and the like. For blood vacuity, (use) *Si Wu Tang* (Four Materials Decoction). For blood heat, cool the blood with *Si Wu Tang* plus stir-fried Cortex Phellodendri (*Huang Bai*).

One method to treat prolapse of the rectum (consists of) supporting and sending (the rectum) in with powdered Galla Rhi Chinensis (*Wu Bei Zi, i.e.*, with the powder applied on the prolapsed rectum, hold and send in the rectum by hand). If one operation fails to contract (the rectum), do this over again. Five to seven operations will surely succeed.

Chapter Ninety-eight

Goiter Qi

(In order to treat this,) it is first necessary to abstain from thick flavored (food). Powder 1.2 *liang* of Herba Sargassi (*Hai Zao*) and 1 *liang* of Rhizoma Coptidis Chinensis (*Huang Lian*), put a small amount in the palm, lap from time to time, and swallow with saliva. When (the goiter) reduces to 2/3 its size, it is necessary to stop administration (of these medicinals).

Chapter Ninety-nine

Vomiting of Worms

Stir-fry Galenitum (*Hei Xi*) to ash, mix with powdered Semen Arecae Catechu (*Bing Lang*), and take with thin gruel.

Chapter One Hundred

Lung *Yong*[1]

(If lung *yong*) is already broken and intruded by wind, it is incurable. (Otherwise, it can be treated by) *Sou Feng Tang* (Track Wind Decoction)[2] as an emetic. This comes from the *Yi Lei Yuan Rong (Commander in Chief of the Medical Realm)*.[3] In terms of a specific formula, there is only one decoction for tracking down pus. To contract and close the openings of the sores, administer Cortex Albizziae Julibrissinis (*He Huan Pi*) with a thick soup of Radix Ampelopsis Japonicae (*Bai Lian*).

---

[1]   This is a pattern of suppuration from the lungs accompanied by coughing, dyspnea, and expectoration of foul smelling phlegm, pus, and blood.

[2]   This consists of Radix Ledebouriellae Sesloidis (*Fang Feng*), 6 *qian*, Radix Panacis Ginseng (*Ren Shen*), boiled separately, 4 *qian*, Rhizoma Pinelliae Ternatae (*Ban Xia*), 3 *qian*, Gypsum (*Shi Gao*), 8 *qian*, Bombyx Batryticatus (*Jiang Can*), 2 *qian*, powder collected from the surface of dried persimmon (*Shi Shuang*), 5 *qian*, brewed in afterwards, and Secretio Moschi Moschiferi (*She Xiang*), 1 *fen*.

[3]   This is a book written in 1291 CE by Wang Hao-gu, pupil of Liu Wan-su and Li Dong-yuan. It is so named because it mainly treats cold damage based on the methods of the founder of that theory, Zhang Zhong-jing.

For lung atony, administer *Ren Shen Ping Fei San* (Ginseng Level the Lungs Powder). The treatment of lung atony focuses on nurturing the lung, nurturing the qi, nurturing the blood, and clearing metal.

I once treated a woman who was more than 20 years of age. She suffered from a festering hole in the chest. Expectoration of pus and blood from the mouth occurred at the same time as discharge from the hole. A formula for supplementing qi and blood composed of Radix Panacis Ginseng (*Ren Shen*), Radix Astragali Membranacei (*Huang Qi*), and Radix Angelicae Sinensis (*Dang Gui*) was prescribed, to which were added certain heat-abating and pus-dispelling medicinals.

Chapter One Hundred One

Intestinal *Yong*

(This) is treated as damp heat (and) food accumulation. If there is phlegm accumulation and streaming dead blood in the large intestine, use *Tao Ren Cheng Qi Tang* (Persica Support the Qi Decoction) plus Fructus Forsythiae Suspensae (*Lian Qiao*) and Radix Gentianae Macrophyllae (*Qin Jiao*). Breaks close to the anus with intrusion of wind are difficult to treat. Use Radix Ledebouriellae Sesloidis (*Fang Feng*) and the like.

Chapter One Hundred Two

Breast *Yong*

(The medicinals) to be introduced into the formula (for this condition) include Pericarpium Viridis Citri Reticulatae (*Qing Pi*), Fructus

Trichosanthis Kirlowii (*Gua Lou*), Folium Citri (*Ju Ye*), Fructus Forsythiae Suspensae (*Lian Qiao*), tip-preserved Semen Pruni Persicae (*Tao Ren*), Spina Gleditschiae Sinensis (*Zao Jiao Ci*), and Nodus Radicis Glycyrrhizae (*Gan Cao Jie*). In case of breaks, (add) large quantities of Radix Panacis Ginseng (*Ren Shen*) and Radix Astragali Membranacei (*Huang Qi*).

Once broken, breast nodes seldom end in survival. The only choice is to greatly supplement (with) Radix Panacis Ginseng (*Ren Shen*), Radix Astragali Membranacei (*Huang Qi*), Rhizoma Ligustici Wallichii (*Chuan Xiong*), Radix Angelicae Sinensis (*Dang Gui*), Pericarpium Viridis Citri Reticulatae (*Qing Pi*), Rhizoma Atractylodis Macrocephalae (*Bai Zhu*), Fructus Forsythiae Suspensae (*Lian Qiao*), Radix Albus Paeoniae Lactiflorae (*Bai Shao Yao*), and Radix Glycyrrhizae (*Gan Cao*). A (variant) formula includes Fructus Trichosanthis Kirlowii (*Gua Lou*, in addition). In case of breast rocks before breaking, add Radix Bupleuri (*Chai Hu*) and Rhizoma Ligustici Wallichii (*Xiong*) from the Tian Tai Mountains.

To treat small nodes in the breast, (use) Rhizoma Arisaematis (*Nan Xing*), Bulbus Fritillariae (*Bei Mu*), Nodus Radicis Glycyrrhizae (*Gan Cao Jie*), and Fructus Trichosanthis Kirlowii (*Gua Lou*), 1 *liang* for each of the above, and Fructus Forsythiae Suspensae (*Lian Qiao*) and Pericarpium Viridis Citri Reticulatae (*Qing Pi*), each 5 *qian*. For breast *yong*, suckling taxation, and hot swelling, (use) calcined Gypsum (*Shi Gao*), burnt Cortex Betulae Platyphyllae (*Hua Pi*), Semen Trichosanthis Kirlowii (*Gua Lou Zi*), Nodus Radicis Glycyrrhizae (*Gan Cao Jie*), and Pericarpium Viridis Citri Reticulatae (*Qing Pi*). To treat suckling breast *yong*, (use) Flos Lonicerae Japonicae (*Jin Yin Hua*), Radix Fagopyri Cymosi (*Tian Qiao Mai*), and Ramulus Cayratiae Japonicae (*Zi Ge Teng*), all in equal amounts. Boil with vinegar and wash (with the decoction. In this case,) one single ingredient, Flos Lonicerae Japonicae (*Jin Yin Hua*), will also do.

(To treat) breast *yong*, apply Succus Radicis Rehmanniae (*Sheng Di Huang Zhi*) and change it when it becomes hot. This never fails to be effective. Another formula (is made by) pounding 1 old piece of Fructus Trichosanthis Kirlowii (*Gua Lou*), boil in 1 *dou* of wine down to 6 *sheng*, and take 3 times per day. (Yet) another formula is given in a rhyme:

What matters suckling breast *yong* in women?
Burn Fructus Gleditschiae Sinensis (*Zao Jiao*) and mix with Concha Mactrae
    Quadrangularis (*He Fen*)!
Once a character of this ash is brewed with heated wine,
The patient claps her hands, laughing happy and gay.

Another formula (is made by) pounding and spreading Herba Leonuri Heterophylli (*Yi Mu Cao*, over the sore) or mix its dry powder with water and apply. (Still) another formula (consists of) rubbing Cornu Cervi (*Lu Jiao*) in water to make a thick fluid and apply. (And still) another formula: stir-fry and powder Fructus Trichosanthis Kirlowii (*Gua Lou Zi*) and take 2 *qian* with wine before sleep.

For cracked nipples, apply powdered Flos Caryophylli (*Ding Xiang*). If (the nipple is dry), mix with saliva (before applying). For postpartum breast *yong* in women, (use) Radix Angelicae (*Bai Zhi*), Radix Angelicae Sinensis hairs (*Dang Gui Xu*), Fructus Forsythiae Suspensae (*Lian Qiao*), Radix Rubrus Paeoniae Lactiflorae (*Chi Shao Yao*), Herba Seu Flos Schizonepetae Tenuifoliae (*Jing Jie Sui*), and Pericarpium Viridis Citri Reticulatae (*Qing Pi*), 5 *fen* for each of the above, Bulbus Fritillariae (*Bei Mu*), Radix Trichosanthis Kirlowii (*Tian Hua Fen*), and Radix Platycodi Grandiflori (*Jie Geng*), 1 *qian* for each of the above, Fructus Trichosanthis Kirlowii (*Gua Lou*), half a piece, and Nodus Radicis Glycyrrhizae (*Gan Cao Jie*), 1.5 *qian*. Boil the above in water, take when half hungry/half full (*i.e.*, between meals), and sip by sip. If there is heat, add Radix Bupleuri (*Chai Hu*) and Radix Scutellariae Baicalensis (*Huang Qin*). Wine, meat, and acrid spices are prohibited. The dressing is composed of Rhizoma Arisaematis (*Nan Xing*), Calcareous Spar (*Han Shui Shi*), Fructus Gleditschiae Sinensis (*Zao Jiao*), Bulbus Fritillariae (*Bei Mu*), Radix Angelicae (*Bai Zhi*), Radix Aconiti (*Cao Wu*), and Radix Et Rhizoma Rhei (*Da Huang*). Powder, mix with vinegar, and then apply.

The breasts are where the *yang ming* passes, and the nipples are ascribed to the *jue yin*. If the breast-feeding mother has thick flavored (food) or bears indignation or grudges, qi will, therefore, stop circulating and the portals will become blocked. (Because) milk is no longer able to come out, the blood of the *yang ming* becomes hot and transforms into pus. There are, however, cases where the breath of the baby is burning hot and, when it is blown (upon the mother's breast), gives rise to nodes (in the mother's nipples). Right at the onset, in defiance of the pain, (one) must soften (the nodes) by rubbing. Then the qi is freed and (the nodes) are dispersed and dissipated. If one misses the chance to treat (in this way), *yong* and boils are bound to develop. If stagnation of the *jue yin* is to be coursed, use Pericarpium Viridis Citri Reticulatae (*Qing Pi*) to clear heat from the *yang ming*, Gypsum (*Shi Gao*) to move away foul blood, and Nodus Radicis Glycyrrhizae (*Sheng Gan Cao Jie*) to disperse swelling toxins. Semen Trichosanthis Kirlowii (*Gua Lou Zi*, alone) or together with fresh Folium Citri (*Qing Ju He*), Myrrha (*Mo Yao*), Spina Gleditschiae Sinensis (*Zao Jiao Ci*), Flos Lonicerae Japonicae (*Jin Yin Hua*), and Radix Angelicae Sinensis (*Dang Gui*) can be added. (This formula) can be taken either as a powder or a decoction with additions and subtractions with a small amount of wine as the assistant. At the same time, moxa at the swollen parts, 2-3 cones. This is very effective. Do not unscrupulously needle or lance (or this will) incur intricate diseases.

In addition, as a cumulative result of worry, a dormant node may develop, (hard) like a turtle's shell (but) with no pain or itching. This takes more than 10 years to develop into a sunken sore, called suckling breast rock because it forms a depression like a rock cave. It is incurable. If, at the initial stage of its generation, (one) eliminates the root of the disease by keeping the heart tranquil and the spirit calm and administers certain treatment, recovery is possible.

My nephew's wife contracted this pattern at the age of 18. She was quick tempered and her pulse was replete. It was her worries over the future which presented difficulty. I administered her a decoction made of one single ingredient, Pericarpium Viridis Citri Reticulatae (*Qing Pi*), and, from time to time, *Si Wu Tang* with additions and subtractions. Two months later, she recovered.

Chapter One Hundred Three

Cavalier's *Yong*[1]

Obtain 4 *liang* of debarked Radix Glycyrrhizae (*Da Fen Cao*) with nodules. Roast. Then quench and soak in 1 bowl of river water. When the water is out, powder Radix Glycyrrhizae and mix with a small amount of carbonized Fructus Gleditschiae Sinensis (*Zao Jiao Hui*). Divide into 4 doses and take brewed with boiled water. This offers great effect. Another formula (consists of) Nodus Radicis Glycyrrhizae (*Gan Cao Jie*), Radix Angelicae (*Bai Zhi*), and Rhizoma Coptidis Chinensis (*Huang Lian*), all in equal amounts. Slice and boil in water. For broken (*yong*), apply Os Draconis (*Long Gu*), Alumen (*Ku Bai Fan*), and Hallyositum Rubrum (*Chi Shi Zhi*, as a dressing).

A person suffered from cough above and breaking kidney *yong*[2] below. (They were prescribed) Radix Scrophulariae Ningpoensis (*Xuan Shen*), stir-fried Cortex Phellodendri (*Huang Bai*), Pulvis Indigonis (*Qing Dai*), Cornu Rhinoceroris (*Xi Jiao*), Fructus Crataegi (*Shan Zha*), Nodus Radicis Glycyrrhizae (*Gan Cao Jie*), Massa Medica Fermentata (*Shen Qu*), Fructus Germinatus Hordei Vulgaris (*Mai Ya*), Semen Pruni Persicae (*Tao Ren*), and Fructus Forsythiae Suspensae (*Lian Qiao*), all the above powdered and made into pills.

A formula to treat genital toxin[3] (consists of) Fructus Gardeniae Jasminoidis (*Shan Zhi*), Radix Et Rhizoma Rhei (*Da Huang*), Gummum

---

[1]   This is a suppurative inflammation of the perineum. It is also known as pendent or suspended *yong*.

[2]   Here kidney refers to the external kidneys, *i.e.*, the testicles.

[3]   This is also known as transverse bowstring mass, bubo sore, or the initial stage of venereal disease affecting the groins.

Olibani (*Ru Xiang*), Myrrha (*Mo Yao*), and Radix Angelicae Sinensis (*Dang Gui*), 5 *fen* for each of the above, Semen Trichosanthis Kirlowii (*Gua Lou Ren*), 2 *liang*, and Hematitum (*Dai Zhe Shi*), 1 *qian*, all as one dose. Boil. Another formula (consists of) Semen Momordicae Cochinensis (*Mu Bie Zi*), Radix Et Rhizoma Rhei (*Da Huang*), Semen Trichosanthis Kirlowii (*Gua Lou Ren*), Radix Gentianae Scabrae (*Long Dan Cao*), and Semen Pruni Persicae (*Tao Ren*). Boil the above down to a thick decoction, settle overnight, and take warm early the next morning.

(Yet) another formula (is composed of) Bombyx Batryticatus (*Bai Jiang Can*) and Flos Immaturus Sophorae Japonicae (*Huai Hua*). Powder together and take brewed with wine. A (variant) formula includes wine-processed Radix Et Rhizoma Rhei (*Da Huang*. Still) another formula (consists of) 3 *cun* of Radix Pruni Salicinae (*Li Shi Gen*). Grind finely with equal amount of fresh Rhizoma Zingiberis (*Sheng Jiang*), brew in hot boiled water, and take on an empty stomach. (And still) another formula (is composed of) Radix Et Rhizoma Rhei (*Da Huang*) and Concha Ostreae (*Mu Li*), 2.5 *qian* each, skinned Fructus Trichosanthis Kirlowii (*Gua Lou*), 1 piece, and debarked Radix Glycyrrhizae (*Gan Cao*, no amount given). Grate the above as 1 dose. Boil in water and take on an empty stomach.

Chapter One Hundred Four

Fixed to the Bone *Yong*[1]

(This is due to) extreme heat in the blood phase. As soon as it is perceived, administer Pericarpium Viridis Citri Reticulatae (*Qing Pi*) and Nodus Radicis Glycyrrhizae (*Gan Cao Jie*). Later, it is necessary to nurture the blood. At the initial stage of leg swelling, use Radix Panacis Ginseng (*Ren Shen*), Radix Astragali Membranacei (*Huang Qi*),

---

[1]   This is a deep-lying, usually suppurative sore that can reach and affects the bone.

and Sclerotium Poriae Cocoris (*Fu Ling*), 2 *qian* for each of the above, and Semen Trichosanthis Kirlowii (*Gua Lou Ren*), 48 pieces. Divide into 2 doses, put in Succus Bambusae (*Zhu Li*), heat, and take. If there is incessant pain at point *Huan Tiao* (GB 30)[2], (one) should take measure to prevent fixed to the bone *yong* from growing. [For details, see the *Yi Yao* {*Essentials of Medicine;* later editor}].

Chapter One Hundred Five

Swelling Toxins

Tie Quan San (Iron Ring Powder) treats *yong* and *ju* swelling toxins. (It consists of) Gummum Olibani (*Ru Xiang*) and Myrrha (*Mo Yao*), one half *liang* each, Radix Et Rhizoma Rhei (*Da Huang*), Rhizoma Coptidis Chinensis (*Huang Lian*), Cortex Phellodendri (*Huang Bai*), Rhizoma Arisaematis (*Nan Xing*), Rhizoma Pinelliae Ternatae (*Ban Xia*), Radix Ledebouriellae Sesloidis (*Fang Feng*), Radix Et Rhizoma Notopterygii (*Qiang Huo*), Fructus Gleditschiae Sinensis (*Zao Jiao*), Nodus Radicis Glycyrrhizae (*Gan Cao Jie*), Radix Aconiti (*Cao Wu*), and Gelatinum Corii Asini (*E Jiao*), put in afterwards, 1 *liang* for each of the above. Powder the above, mix into a paste with vinegar, heat in an earthenware or stone vessel till black, and then apply to the affected part with a goose's quill. It is applied hot in case of cold and cold in case of heat.

Clove sore with a deep root requires cutting open with a needle or a knife. Then apply Venum Bufonis Bufonis (*Can Su*) on the tip (of the sore) and later administer (the following) medication. Powder Flos Chrysanthemi Indici (*Ye Ju*), mix in wine, and drink till tipsy. When one falls asleep, the pain will be settled and heat eliminated. There is no need to remove the clove sore. It will heal by itself.

---

[2] Jumping Round

A method for removing pus without separating (*i.e.*, breaking) the skin is a treatment for various swelling toxins. (It consists of) stir-fried and finely cut donkey hoof (*Lu Ti*), 1 *liang*, stir-fried, powdered Fructus Fagopyri Esculenti (*Qiao Mai Mian*), 1 *liang*, salt (*Bai Yan*), one half *liang*, and Radix Aconiti (*Cao Wu*), 4 *qian*, stripped of its skin. Powder the above, mix with water and roll into cakes. Bake over a small fire till slightly yellow, (cool) to discharge fire toxins and grind. (Then) mix into a paste with vinegar, spread on a piece of paper, and stick to the affected part. Water will exit from the hair pores and the swelling will disappear by itself.

To treat celestial snake head[1], (use) Herba Melastomae Dodecandri (*Ye Luo Su*), also called *Huang Si Cao*, Lignum Lonicerae Japonicae (*Jin Yin Hua Teng*), also called *Yang Er Teng*, Herba Seu Radix Cayratiae Japonicae (*Wu Ye Zi*), Lignum Argyreiae Sanguinii (*Ge Teng*), and Radix Fagopyri Cymosi (*Tian Qiao Mai*), all cut finely, 10 *fen* each. Boil with good millet vinegar down to a thick decoction. Wash after steaming (the affected part with it). Another formula (is made by) pounding human feces together with clay and spreading this over the affected part. It will heal. To treat celestial fire cinnabar sore[2], (use) stir-fried Lumbricus (*Qu Shan*) with clay, grind finely, mix with sesame oil, and apply. Another formula which is also good (is made by) burning pheasant or goose feather to ash, mix with sesame oil, and apply.

To treat all kinds of clove sores, (use) Kalimeris Indicae (*Zi Geng Ju*), either the root, stem, leaves, or flowers will do. Extract the juice by grinding and then drop in the mouth and drink. White beeswax (*Bai La*) promotes contraction by nature. [This has already been discussed in the *Yi Yao* {*Essentials of Medicine;* later editor}]. To treat *yong* and *ju*, collect the wax from one layer of comb, put in Alum (*Bai Fan*), place on a stone and melt with a fire. (Then) grind with water, mix with oil,

---

[1]   Also called snake head cinnabar sore, this is a suppurative sore on the palmar side of the tip of the finger shaped like a snake head.

[2]   This is called celestial fire sore because this lesion develops astonishingly rapidly like a fire. It is called cinnabar sore because of its red color.

and apply. Another formula (consists of) Radix Glycyrrhizae (*Gan Cao*) soaked in human feces. It greatly treats swelling toxins. This is (discussed) in detail in the chapter on warm spring (*i.e.*, Ch. 16, Bk. 1.)

In treating *yong* and *ju*, it is necessary to identify the channels and connecting vessels (involved). Of the six yang channels and six yin channels, some are abundant in qi but scanty in blood, while others are abundant in blood but scanty in qi. (Thus) they should not be treated indiscriminately. The *shao yang* is abundant in qi but scanty in blood, and (therefore,) muscles and flesh (related to it) grow with difficulty. The logical treatment for it is to prevent and expel toxins. Even disinhibitors cannot be used indiscreetly.

My uncle was liable to worry and taxed his spirit. At about 50, he had a red swelling, the size of a chestnut kernel on the lateral side of his left upper arm. I warned him not to take this lightly and (I) first administered him a thick soup made of Radix Panacis Ginseng (*Ren Shen*). He was better after a moderate perspiration was induced. After administration of scores of doses, (the swelling) was healed. A little more than 10 days later, a violent wind that could pull up trees broke out, and a red thread grew over his (old) sore, wrapping the upper back and reaching the right ribs. I said that there was no other choice but to administer large doses of *Ren Shen Tang* (Ginseng Decoction)[3] plus supplementing medicinals such as Rhizoma Ligustici Wallichii (*Chuan Xiong*) and Rhizoma Atractylodis Macrocephalae (*Bai Zhu*). After 2 months' administration, he recovered.

The son of a Mr. Li, aged 30, had mishaps in succession. In addition, he was lustful and (suffered from) taxation. There was a red swelling

---

[3] The formula, *Ren Shen Tang* (Ginseng Decoction) consists of Radix Panacis Ginseng (*Ren Shen*), Rhizoma Polygonati Odorati (*Wei Rei*), Radix Scutellariae Baicalensis (*Huang Qin*), Rhizoma Anemarrhenae (*Zhi Mu*), and Sclerotium Poriae Cocoris (*Fu Ling*), 3 *liang* for each of the above, Rhizoma Atractylodis Macrocephalae (*Bai Zhu*), Pericarpium Citri Reticulatae (*Ju Pi*), Rhizoma Phragmitis Communis (*Lu Gen*), and Fructus Gardeniae Jasminoidis (*Zhi Zi Ren*), 4 *liang* for each of the above, and Gypsum (*Shi Gao*), 8 *liang*. The translator suspects, however, that the author is here simply referring to a soup made from Radix Panacis Ginseng (*Ren Shen*).

the size of a chestnut kernel on the lateral side of his left leg. A physician administered 2 doses of *Cheng Qi Tang* (Support the Qi Decoction) to him to precipitate (toxins), and another physician bid him to take *Jie Du Tang* (Resolve Toxins Decoction)[4] to (also) precipitate (toxins). On examination, I found his pulse replete (thus prognosticating death). It turned out (later) that he died.

The buttocks are located behind the lower abdomen, and moreover, in the lower (part of the body. Thus) they are consummate yin within the yin. It is a long way there and they are located in a remote place. Although the (foot) *tai yang* is abundant in blood, it is difficult for qi to travel over (there), and scarcely is blood able to reach there either. (A sore) growing (on the buttocks) after middle age, requires supplementation (and this) takes precedence (over other treatment methods). Without the cumulative virtue of supplementation, in most cases, a disastrous consequence will present itself after the sore has formed a scab. Or a (serious) disease will develop half a year or so later. A poor physician is ignorant of this and may commit grave blunders. Be careful and cautious.

In treating *yong* swelling, it is necessary to distinguish swellings from open sores and to treat accordingly. It is not permitted to recklessly administer *Wu Xiang Lian Qiao Tang* (Five Fragrances Forsythia Decoction)[5] and the like. Before the opening (of the swelling, one)

---

[4] This consists of Radix Et Rhizoma Rhei (*Da Huang*), Fructus Citri Seu Ponciri (*Zhi Qiao*), Radix Glycyrrhizae (*Gan Cao*), Rhizoma Coptidis Chinensis (*Huang Lian*), Radix Scutellariae Baicalensis (*Huang Qin*), Fructus Gardeniae Jasminoidis (*Zhi Zi Ren*), Radix Ledebouriellae Sesloidis (*Fang Feng*), Cortex Phellodendri (*Huang Bai*), and Radix Rubrus Paeoniae Lactiflorae (*Chi Shao Yao*).

[5] This consists of Lignum Aquilariae Agallochae (*Chen Xiang*), Fructus Forsythiae Suspensae (*Lian Qiao*), Ramus Loranthi Seu Visci (*Sang Ji Sheng*), Flos Caryophylli (*Ding Xiang*), Rhizoma Belamcandae (*She Gan*), Radix Angelicae Duhuo (*Du Huo*), Gummum Olibani (*Ru Xiang*), Rhizoma Cimicifugae (*Sheng Ma*), Radix Et Rhizoma Rhei (*Da Huang*), Caulis Akebiae Mutong (*Mu Tong*), Radix Et Rhizoma Notopterygii (*Qiang Huo*), Radix Glycyrrhizae (*Gan Cao*), Secretio Moschi Moschiferi (*She Xiang*), and fresh Radix Saussureae Seu Vladimiriae (*Qing Mu Xiang*), all in equal amount, 4 *qian* per dose.

should perform expulsion from within in combination with dispersal. After opening, supplement the qi and blood. Upon palpation, if the swelling feels hot, there is pus. If it does not feel hot, there is no pus.

Chapter One Hundred Six

Nodulations

To treat (nodulations) in adults and children, whether located in the nape of the neck, (the front of) the neck, on the legs, or the arms, if there is swelling toxins, it is usually located under the skin but over the membrane. (Since such) nodulations are usually produced by non-dissipating streaming phlegm, (one) should ascertain what food (the patient) favors and then administer, after ejection and precipitation, medicinals (counteracting that food) to dissipate bind.

(For a node) on the head or the nape, (use) Bombyx Batryticatus (*Jiang Can*), stir-fried Radix Et Rhizoma Rhei (*Da Huang*), wine-soaked Pulvis Indigonis (*Qing Dai*), and bile(-processed) Rhizoma Arisaematis (*Dan Xing*). Powder, make into pills with honey, and melt in the mouth. For phlegm nodes growing on the chin and in the region below the cheeks, (use) *Er Chen Tang* plus Fructus Forsythiae Suspensae (*Lian Qiao*), Radix Ledebouriellae Sesloidis (*Fang Fen*), Rhizoma Ligustici Wallichii (*Chuan Xiong*), Spina Gleditschiae Sinensis (*Zao Jiao Ci*), wine-processed Radix Scutellariae Baicalensis (*Huang Qin*), Rhizoma Atractylodis (*Cang Zhu*), and Bombyx Batryticatus (*Jiang Can*).

A female who was more than 40 years of age and had a white facial complexion, a thin form, and quick temper had had an overwhelming disappointment. Three month later, (she developed) a mass over the ribs in the flank below the breast which grew steadily to screen the heart. (This was accompanied by) a moderate pain, oppression of the diaphragm, food intake reduced by 3/4, a bitter taste in the mouth in the morning, and a faint, short, choppy pulse on both hands. [For details, see the chapter on qi and blood causing disease in Book 4 (*i.e.*, Ch. 51). {later editor}].

Chapter One Hundred Seven

Small & Large Scrofulous Lumps

(These are due to) heat of the qi, blood, and phlegm. Mash blackish, ripe Fructus Mori Albi (*Sang Ren*), simmer down into a paste, brew with boiled water, and take. If dried in the sun, powdered, and taken, the red (fruit) is also effective. Another formula (is made by) burning large Cipangopaludina Chinensis (*Tian Luo*) with its meat to ash with nature preserved, powder, put in a small amount of Secretio Moschi Moschiferi (*She Xiang*), and then apply. If (the lump is) wet, apply dry. If it is dry, apply after mixing with oil. Another formula (consists of) using Spica Prunellae Vulgaris (*Xia Ku Cao*. This) is especially able to dissipate bound qi and accomplish the feat of supplementing and nurturing the blood vessel of the *jue yin* with the ability to abate cold and heat. A vacuity case can entirely rely on it. For a repletion case, add moving and dissipating medicinals to assist it. Externally, moxa can also achieve steady effect.

Chapter One Hundred Eight

Open Wound Wind (*i.e.*, Tetanus)

Open wound wind, blood congealed in the heart, and needle wandering in the flesh, these three patterns all can be treated by the following miraculous formula. Burn to ash 1 *qian* of duck's plume, grind finely, and take with wine. Radix Ledebouriellae Sesloidis (*Fang*

Feng), dried Buthus Martensi (*Quan Xie*), and the like are all (also) important medicinals for open wound wind. More often than not, this ends in death, and nothing but Buthus Martensi can open (this wind). Powder 10 scorpions and take with wine, 3 times a day. For open wound wind with fever, (use) Fructus Trichosanthis Kirlowii (*Gua Lou Ren*), 9 *qian*, Talcum (*Hua Shi*), 1.5 *qian*, Rhizoma Arisaematis (*Nan Xing*), Rhizoma Atractylodis (*Cang Zhu*), stir-fried Cortex Phellodendri (*Huang Bai*), Radix Rubrus Paeoniae Lactiflorae (*Chi Shao Yao*), and Pericarpium Citri Reticulatae (*Chen Pi*), 1 *qian* for each of the above, Rhizoma Coptidis Chinensis (*Huang Lian*), Radix Scutellariae Baicalensis (*Huang Qin*), and Radix Angelicae (*Bai Zhi*), 5 *qian* for each of the above, and Radix Glycyrrhizae (*Sheng Gan Cao*), a small amount. Slice the above, boil with 3 slices of fresh ginger, and take.

Chapter One Hundred Nine

Shank Sores

A formula for a plaster (for this problem consists of) Gummum Olibani (*Ru Xiang*), Myrrha (*Mo Yao*), Mercurius (*Shui Yin*), and Radix Angelicae Sinensis (*Dang Gui*), 5 *qian* for each of the above, Rhizoma Ligustici Wallichii (*Chuan Xiong*) and Bulbus Fritillariae (*Bei Mu*), 1 *liang* each, Minium (*Huang Dan*), 2.5 *liang*, and sesame oil (*Ma You*), 6 *liang*. Slice the above and fry all except the Minium and Mercurius with the sesame oil till black. After removing the dregs, put in the Minium and Mercurius and again fry till black. Stir into a paste with a peach (or) willow twig.

Another formula includes Os Draconis (*Sheng Long Gu*), Sanguis Draconis (*Xue Jie*), and Hallyositum Rubrum (*Chi Shi Zhi*), 1 *liang* together for (all) 3 ingredients, Crinis Carbonisatus (*Xue Yu*), a fingerful, yellow beeswax (*Huang La*), 1 *liang*, and Resina Liquidambaris Taiwanianae (*Bai Jiao Xiang*), 1 *liang*. (Obtain) an appropriate amount of sesame oil. First fry the hair with the oil. After boiling for a short while, remove the hair. (Then) put in the wax and Resina Liquidambaris Taiwanianae first and the Os Draconis, Sanguis Draconis, and Hallyositum Rubrum (second). Stir evenly and then put (the container with the processed medicinals) over a basin of water to cool. Collect after they are cooled and preserve in a ceramic vessel. Before treating a sore, roll some (of this paste) into a thin layer, apply over the sore, and cover with a bamboo shoot leaf. Three days later, turn the layer over and apply once again. At the same time, take blood-quickening medicinals (internally).

Another formula (is made by) boiling Folium Ilicis Chinensis (*Dong Qing Ye*) in granulated sugar solution. After boiling for a short while, take out, dry by pressing with a rock, and then apply on the sore. Change (the leaf) 2 times per day. (Yet) another formula (is made by) burning dandruff (*Tou Gou*) to ash. Pound with Fructus Zizyphi Jujubae (*Zao Rou*) into a paste. Beforehand, wash (the affected area) clean with a soup of Herba Allii Fistulosi (*Cong*) and Fructus Sophorae Japonicae (*Jiao*) and dab Calomelas (*Qing Fen*) onto the sore to dry it. Then apply the above paste and cover with tung oil paper. (Still) another formula (consists of) Concha Mactrae Quadrangularis (*He Fen*), Folium Camelliae Sinensis (*La Cha*), Radix Sophorae Flavescentis (*Ku Shen*), Pulvis Indigonis (*Qing Dai*), and Lithargyum (*Mi Tuo Seng*). Beforehand, wash the sore with river water. Mix the above with lard from a pig killed in the last month and apply (on the sore).

Another formula (consists of) Cortex Radicis Lycii (*Di Gu Pi*), 1 *liang*, Nodus Radicis Glycyrrhizae (*Gan Cao Jie*), one half *liang*, and white beeswax (*Bai La*), one half *liang*. Fry Cortex Radicis Lycii and Radix Glycyrrhizae well in 4 *liang* of sesame oil over (neither) a slow (nor) fierce fire. Remove the dregs, put 1.5 *liang* of Minium (*Huang Dan*) and the white wax in, heat over a vigorous fire till black, spread over a piece of paper, and then apply. (Again) another formula (consists of) Folium Ilicis Chinensis (*Dong Qing Ye*). Boil in vinegar and apply. Shank sores in females are usually ascribed to blood congelation. (For these,) administer *Bu Sun Huang Qi Tang* (Mend Detriment Astragalus

Decoction)[1] in the *Ju Fang (Collected Formulas)*. A formula for shank sores (consists of) Calomelas (*Qing Fen*), carbonate of lead (*Ding Fen*), another form of carbonate of lead (*Wa Fen*), and Sodium Sulphate (*Xuan Ming Fen*), all in equal amounts. Powder, mix with rainwater, and spread on the bottom of a bowl. Smoke with 5 *liang* of Folium Artemisiae Argyii (*Ai*) till all is burned up. (Collect), powder finely, mix with marrow from the long leg bone of a goat, spread onto a piece of oil paper, and apply after washing (the affected area) with a soup of Herba Allii Fistulosi (*Cong*) and Fructus Sophorae Japonicae (*Jiao*). Band with a soft cloth. (Yet) another formula (is composed of) 1 *liang* of Rhizoma Coptidis Chinensis (*Huang Lian*). Cut, boil in 2 cups of water down to 1 cupful, remove the dregs, and put in a piece of oil paper. Continue boiling till all (the liquid) is dried up, take out the paper, rub yellow wax onto it, and bind the sore with it.

Chapter One Hundred Ten

Injuries & Wounds from Slips & Falls

Brew 4 *liang* each of Succus Zingiberis (*Jiang Zhi*) and sesame oil in wine and take. Use Lignum Sappanis (*Su Mu*) to quicken the blood, Rhizoma Coptidis Chinensis (*Huang Lian*) to downbear fire, and Rhizoma Atractylodis Macrocephalae (*Bai Zhu*) to harmonize the center. Boil in child's urine and take. This is remarkable.

If blood stasis is located below, it can be precipitated. However, it is necessary to first supplement and prop up (the qi) before precipitating.

---

[1]   This consists of Radix Astragali Membranacei (*Huang Qi*), Semen Astragali Complanati (*Bai Ji Li*), Fructus Meliae Toosendanis (*Chuan Lian Zi*), Radix Aconiti (*Chuan Wu Tou*), Semen Phaseoli Calcarati (*Chi Xiao Dou*), stir-fried Lumbricus (*Di Long*), and Radix Ledebouriellae Sesloidis (*Fang Feng*), 1 *liang* for each of the above, and Radix Linderae Strychnifoliae (*Wu Yao*), 2 *liang*. Powder and make into pills the size of Chinese parasol tree seeds with wine paste; 15 pills per dose.

If blood stasis is located above, it is appropriate to drink Succus Allii Tuberosi (*Jiu Zhi*, alone) or together with urine. Drinking cold water is absolutely prohibited, (since) blood becomes congealed once it meets with cold water. Even if a thread of blood should enter the heart, death follows instantly.

Jie Gu San (Join the Bone Powder, consists of) Myrrha (*Mo Yao*), 5 *qian*, Pyritum (*Zi Ran Tong*), 5 *liang*, calcined with vinegar, Talcum (*Hua Shi*), 2 *liang*, Os Draconis (*Long Gu*), 3 *qian*, Hallyositum Rubrum (*Chi Shi Zhi*), 3 *qian*, and Secretio Moschi Moschiferi (*She Xiang*), 1 character, ground separately. Powder the above and, (except for the musk,) boil in as much good vinegar (as necessary) to submerge all the ingredients, the more (vinegar) the better. (Continue boiling) till all (the vinegar) is out and stir-fry till completely dry. Before taking, put in the Secretio Moschi Moschiferi. Place on the tongue and take with warmed wine. The disease may be located above or below and, accordingly, (these medicinals) should be taken (either) before or after a meal. If the bone is joined but pain persists, delete Os Draconis and Hallyositum Rubrum. The more taken, the better. This is particularly effective. Another formula (consists of) Pericarpium Benincasae Hispidae (*Dong Gua Pi*) and Gelatinum Corii Asini (*E Jiao*) in equal amounts. Stir-fry dry, powder, brew with wine, and take. Intoxication is the measure (of the dosage).

To treat a broken bone thrust inward with darkened blood (as a result of) accidentally slipping, (use) Talcum (*Hua Shi*), 6 *fen*, and Radix Glycyrrhizae (*Gan Cao*), 1 *fen*. Powder and take with Radix Panacis Ginseng (*Ren Shen*) soup. Then obtain 1 cupful each of undiluted Succus Zingiberis (*Jiang Zhi*) and good millet vinegar and 4 pieces of Fructus Gymnocladi Chinensis (*Fei Zao*) with solitary seeds. Break and crumble Fructus Gymnocladi Chinensis, put into the mixture of Succus Zingiberis and vinegar, filter out the dregs with a cloth. Boil down into a paste and apply as a plaster. (It is) applicable even if (there are wounds) all over the body.

Chapter One Hundred Eleven

Flogging Wounds

Cortex Phellodendri (*Huang Bai*), Radix Rehmanniae (*Sheng Di Huang*), and Cortex Cercis Chinensis (*Zi Jing Pi*) are all important medicinals in treating blood heat causing pain. Cool formulas remove blood stasis and should be used first, such as *Ji Ming San* (Cock Crow Powder).[1] Powder Radix Rehmanniae (*Sheng Di Huang*) and Cortex Phellodendri (*Huang Bai*), mix with child's urine, and apply or (use) with Succus Allii Tuberosi (*Jiu Zhi*) added. If (the wound is) not open, smash Herba Allii Tuberosi (*Jiu Cai*) and Bulbus Allii Fistulosi (*Cong Tou*), stir-fry, and apply while hot. When (these become) cool, change them. A plaster is composed of Cortex Cercis Chinensis (*Zi Jing Pi*), Gummum Olibani (*Ru Xiang*), Myrrha (*Mo Yao*), Radix Rehmanniae (*Sheng Di Huang*), Cortex Phellodendri (*Huang Bai*) Radix Et Rhizoma Rhei (*Da Huang*), and others. Another formula (is made by) holding Auricula Juda (*Mu Er*) in a wooden ladle, make into a pap by soaking with boiling water, and stir till the water is no more seen. (Then) pound in an earthenware basin and apply on the wound. (Yet) another formula (is made by) pounding any amount of tender Radix Boehmeriae Niveae (*Zhu Ma Gen*) with salt after washing clean. Then apply on the wound. (This is) miraculously effective. In severe cases, salt should be used in great quantities. (And yet) another formula (is made by) powdering Radix Et Rhizoma Rhei (*Da Huang*) and Cortex Phellodendri (*Huang Bai*), mix with Succus Radicis Rehmanniae (*Sheng Di Huang Zhi*), and apply. When (it becomes) dry, change, and (re-)apply. (This is also) remarkably effective.

---

[1] This consists of Semen Arecae Catechu (*Bing Lang*), 7 pieces, Pericarpium Citri Reticulatae (*Chen Pi*), and Fructus Chaenomelis Lagenariae (*Mu Gua*), 1 *liang* each, Fructus Evodiae Rutecarpae (*Wu Zhu Yu*), 2 *qian*, Radix Platycodi Grandiflori (*Jie Geng*) and fresh Rhizoma Zingiberis (*Sheng Jiang*), one half *liang* each, and Fructus Perillae Frutescentis (*Zi Su*), 3 *qian*. Powder the above and divide into 8 doses. Boil and take on an empty stomach.

Chapter One Hundred Twelve

Short Ears[1]

Make Spora Lygodii Japonici (*Hai Jin Sha*), Talcum (*Hua Shi*), and Radix Glycyrrhizae (*Gan Cao*) into pills with gruel and take. Do not administer decoctions. Just swallow 50 pills of *Jiang Gong Wan* (Deep-Red Palace Pills). [The treatment is the same as for small and large scrofulous lumps. {later editor}]

The formula, *Jiang Gong Wan*, (consists of) Fructus Forsythiae Suspensae (*Lian Qiao*), 1 *liang*, Rhizoma Ligustici Wallichii (*Chuan Xiong*), 1 *liang*, wine-washed Radix Angelicae Sinensis (*Dang Gui*), 1 *liang*, Fructus Germinatus Hordei Vulgaris (*Mai Ya*), and Fructus Crataegi (*Shan Zha*), 1 *liang* each, Semen Pruni Persicae (*Tao Ren*), 1 *liang*, Resina Alois (*Lu Hui*), 1 *liang*, Nodus Radicis Glycyrrhizae (*Gan Cao Jie*), 1 *liang*, Semen Brassicae Campestris (*Yun Tai Zi*), 1 *liang*, Rhizoma Coptidis Chinensis (*Huang Lian*), 1.5 *liang*, stir-fried with wine, Rhizoma Arisaematis (*Nan Xing*), 1.5 *liang*, Radix Scutellariae Baicalensis (*Pian Qin*), 1.5 *liang*, Rhizoma Cimicifugae (*Sheng Ma*), 1.5 *liang*, wine-washed Herba Sargassi (*Hai Zao*), 1.5 *liang*, Radix Et Rhizoma Notopterygii (*Qiang Huo*), 5 *qian*, Radix Platycodi Grandiflori (*Jie Geng*), 5 *qian*, Radix Ledebouriellae Sesloidis (*Fang Feng*), one half *liang*, Rhizoma Atractylodis Macrocephalae (*Bai Zhu*), 2 *liang*, and Radix Et Rhizoma Rhei (*Da Huang*), 1 *liang*, steamed with wine thrice. Powder the above and make into pills with Massa Medica Fermentata (*Shen Qu*) paste. (If the sore) is already open, add 1 *liang* of Radix Panacis Ginseng (*Ren Shen*). The plaster (to be used) is made by boiling Nodus Radicis Glycyrrhizae (*Gan Cao Jie*) and Bombyx Batryticatus (*Jiang Can*).

---

[1] This is also known as auricular piles or polyp in the ear.

Chapter One Hundred Thirteen

Frostbite

Mix powdered Lithargyum (*Mi Tuo Seng*) with well-heated tung oil and apply.

Chapter One Hundred Fourteen

Lower Body *Gan* Sores[1]

Use Concha Mactrae Quadrangularis (*He Fen*), Folium Camelliae Sinensis (*La Cha*), Radix Sophorae Flavescentis (*Ku Shen*), Pulvis Indigonis (*Qing Dai*), and Lithargyum (*Mi Tou Seng*). Beforehand, wash the sore clean with river water. Then mix the above medicinals with lard from a pig killed in the last month and apply. Another formula (is made by) de-oiling Crinis (*Tou Fa*) by washing with salt water and then washing with boiled water. Dry in the sun and burn to ash. Beforehand, wash the sore clean with clear rice water. Grind the hair ash finely and apply and (the sore) will soon scab (over).

Early in the summer, a person who had previously been suffering from lower body *gan* sore contracted loose bowels with a slightly oppressed diaphragm. After having been administered *Zhi Zhong Tang*

---

[1] In fact, this is the modern disease syphilis. It consists of round, clearly outlined ulcerations with a hardened base on the external genitals.

(Treat the Center Decoction)[2], (he) suffered from (such severe) clouding and oppression as if (he were) dying. The pulse on both (hands) was choppy and heavy (*i.e.*, soggy or sodden), a little wiry, and seemingly rapid. This was a severe case of lower body *gan* sore. He was administered 5 doses of *Dang Gui Long Hui Wan* (*Dang Gui*, Gentiana & Aloe Pills) and the loose bowels improved. Then (he) was administered *Xiao Chai Hu* (Minor Bupleurum [Decoction]) with Rhizoma Pinelliae Ternatae (*Ban Xia*) deleted and Rhizoma Coptidis Chinensis (*Huang Lian*), Radix Paeoniae Lactiflorae (*Shao Yao*), and Rhizoma Ligustici Wallichii (*Chuan Xiong*) added. After 5-6 doses were administered, (he) recovered.

---

[2] This consists of Radix Panacis Ginseng (*Ren Shen*), blast-fried Rhizoma Zingiberis (*Pao Jiang*), Rhizoma Atractylodis Macrocephalae (*Bai Zhu*), mix-fried Radix Glycyrrhizae (*Zhi Gan Cao*), Pericarpium Citri Reticulatae (*Chen Pi*), and Pericarpium Viridis Citri Reticulatae (*Qing Pi*), all in equal amounts; 3 *qian* per dose.

Chapter One Hundred Fifteen

Burns & Scalds

Make a plaster with Cortex Phellodendri (*Huang Bai*) and the lard of a pig killed in the last month. Dry by stir-frying, powder, and apply. Another formula (is made by) powdering Rhizoma Polygoni Cuspidati (*Ku Zhang*), mix with water, and apply. (And) another formula (is made by) dabbing Succus Fructi Immaturi Diospyroris (*Shi Qi Shui*)[1] with a goose quill (onto the wound).

---

[1] This succus or juice is made by mashing unripe persimmons, mixing with water, and allowing this mixture to settle. The clear fluid without the dregs is collected for use.

Chapter One Hundred Sixteen

Open Incised Wounds

One method for treating open incised wounds and also dog bites (is performed as follows). At the *wu* watch[1] of the 5th day of the 5th lunar month, pound and grind 1 *jin* of lime (*Shi Hui*) together with 1 *jin* of Herba Allii Tuberosi (*Jiu*). Extract the juice, make into cake, powder, and apply. Another formula that treats open incised wounds (consists of) Galla Rhi Chinensis (*Wu Bei Zi*) and Fructus Perillae Frutescentis (*Zi Su*) in equal amounts. Powder and apply. (Yet) another formula (consists of) Resina Liquidambaris Taiwanianae (*Bai Jiao Xiang*), 3 *qian*, and Os Draconis (*Long Gu*), 1 *qian*. Powder and apply. (Still) another formula (is composed of) Galla Rhi Chinensis (*Wu Bei Zi*) and Medulla Junci Effuci (*Deng Xin Cao*). Burn separately equal amounts with their nature preserved, powder, and apply. (And still) another method (is performed by) finely slicing debarked Radix Glycyrrhizae (*Da Fen Cao*). Put this into a fresh bamboo (tube) and preserve in the manure pit (for some time). Then dry, powder, and apply. [For details (about the processing method), see the chapter on warm spring (*i.e.*, Ch. 16, Bk. 1). {later editor}].

---

[1] *I.e.*, 11 AM-1 PM. Note that the *wu* meaning the seventh terrestrial branch is pronounced the same as *wu* meaning five in Chinese.

Chapter One Hundred Seventeen

Rabid Dog Bite

To treat rabid dog bite, obtain hair from the head of a child, stir-fry with fresh Rhizoma Cyperi Rotundi (*Xin Xiang Fu*) and Flos Chrysanthemi Indici (*Ye Ju*), grind finely, and brew in wine. Drink this till (one becomes) intoxicated. An(other) method for treating dog bite (consists of) applying Fructus Perillae Frutescentis (*Zi Su*) after chewing in the mouth. (And) another method (consists of) applying charcoal after breaking it up and powdering it.

Chapter One Hundred Eighteen

Sores & *Xian*

For the treatment *xian* sores (commonly associated with various types of tinea, a) formula (one can) use (includes) Calomelas (*Qing Fen*), Realgar (*Xiong Huang*), Fructus Cnidii Monnieri (*She Chuang Zi*), and Cortex Hibisci Syricaci (*Chuan Jin Pi*). Powder together. (Then) scrape the *xian* and rub Radix Rumicis Crispi (*Yang Ti Gen*) with vinegar. Mix the fluid (so obtained with the above powder), and then apply. Another formula to treat *xian* sores (is made by) powdering Resina Alois (*Lu Hui*) and Radix Et Rhizoma Rhei (*Da Huang*) and apply. (Yet) another formula (consists of) rubbing Radix Rumicis Japonici (*Yang Ti Tu Cai Gen*) in good vinegar and apply. (And still) another formula (consists of) Semen Crotonis (*Ba Dou*), Semen Ricini Communis (*Cao Ma Zi*), both husked, 14 pieces each, and Mylabris Phalerata (*Ban Mao*), 7 pieces. Fry till black with 2 *liang* of sesame oil. Remove the dregs, put in 3 *qian* of powdered Resina Alois (*Lu Hui Mo*) and 5 *qian* of white wax (*Bai La*), and continue frying over a small fire down to a paste.

Collect and preserve in a ceramic vessel. Before using, scrape the *xian* gently and then apply the medicine. Overnight, a moderate swelling will appear. Healing will follow.

To treat *jie* (*i.e.*, scabious) sores in adults and children, (use) Fructus Gleditschiae Sinensis (*Zhu Ya Zao Jiao*) with pods removed, calcined Alum (*Bai Fan*), Calomelas (*Qing Fen*), and Fructus Piperis Nigri (*Hu Jiao*), each a small amount. Powder together, put in Camphora (*Zhang Nao*) and Petroleum (*Zhu You*), and pound evenly. Apply (before going to bed) in the evening. For plum sore[1] and purulent nest sore, Fructus Piperis Nigri should be deleted.

There are three kinds of sores. In case of purulent vesicle sore, the ruling (method) is to treat heat (with) Radix Scutellariae Baicalensis (*Huang Qin*), Rhizoma Coptidis Chinensis (*Huang Lian*), Radix Et Rhizoma Rhei (*Da Huang*), Calcareous Spar (*Han Shui Shi*), and Fructus Cnidii Monnieri (*She Chuang*), 3 *qian* for each of the above, Sulphur (*Liu Huang*) and Minium (*Huang Dan*), 5 *fen* each, Alumen (*Ku Fan*), 1 *qian*, Pyrolusite (*Wu Ming Yi*), and Radix Angelicae (*Bai Zhi*), 7 *fen* each, Semen Arecae Catechu (*Bing Lang*), 1 piece; Calomelas (*Qing Fen*), 1.2 *qian*, a small amount of Radix Saussureae Seu Vladimiriae (*Mu Xiang*), used only in the presence of pain. Powder the above, mix with sesame oil, and apply (as a dressing).

In case of sand sores[2], the ruling (method) is to kill worms (*i.e.*, parasites, with) Semen Praeparatus Ulmi Macrocarpae (*Wu Yi*), 2 *qian*, Herba Clinopodi Confineae (*Jian Cao*), 1 *qian*, Fructus Cnidii Monnieri (*She Chuang Zi*), 2 *qian*, Alum (*Bai Fan*), 1 *qian*, Alumen (*Ku Fan*), 1 *qian*, Fructus Evodiae Rutecarpae (*Wu Zhu Yu*), 1 *qian*, Rhizoma Atractylodis (*Cang Zhu*), one half *liang*, Cortex Magnoliae Officinalis (*Hou Po Pi*), 5

---

[1] This refers to ringworm shaped like a plum.

[2] This condition is acquired by walking in wet sand along river banks or sea beaches as a result of a small, red, poisonous worm bite. It manifests as small red spots on the legs and feet. There is usually itching and sometimes there is pain, often with fever.

fen, Realgar (*Xiong Huang*), 5 *fen*, Calcareous Spar (*Han Shui Shi*), 2 *qian*, Cortex Phellodendri (*Huang Bai*), 1 *qian*, and Calomelas (*Qing Fen*), 10 small cupfuls. Powder the above, mix with oil, and apply.

Lai[3] *jie* sores break out in spring. The ruling (method) is to promote scabbing and open depression. After scratching, it is appropriate to dress with Alum (*Bai Fan*), 2 *qian*, Fructus Evodiae Rutecarpae (*Wu Zhu Yu*), 2 *qian*, Camphora (*Zhang Nao*), 5 *fen*, Calomelas (*Qing Fen*), 10 small cupfuls, Calcareous Spar (*Han Shui Shi*), 3.5 *qian*, Fructus Cnidii Monnieri (*She Chuang Zi*), 3 *qian*, Cortex Phellodendri (*Huang Bai*), 1 *qian*, Radix Et Rhizoma Rhei (*Da Huang*), 1 *qian*, Sulphur (*Liu Huang*), 1 *qian*, and Semen Arecae Catechu (*Bing Lang*), 1 piece. Powder the above and plaster (the sore).

For *jie* sores, (use) Semen Praeparatus Ulmi Macrocarpae (*Wu Yi*), one half *liang*, Rhizoma Dryopteris (*Guan Zhong*), 1 *liang*, Alumen (*Ku Bai Fan*), 5 *qian*, soft Gypsum (*Ruan Shi Gao*), 5 *qian*, Radix Et Rhizoma Rhei (*Da Huang*), 5 *qian*, Sulphur (*Liu Huang*), 2.5 *qian*, Realgar (*Xiong Huang*), 2.5 *qian*, and Camphora (*Zhang Nao*), one half *liang*, put in afterwards. Powder the above, mix with sesame oil, and apply. It is necessary to wash the scabs off the sore before dressing.

Related to the medication for sores, in case of purulent nest sore, the rule is to treat heat and dry dampness using Pyrolusite (*Wu Ming Yi*). In case of dry, itching (sores), the rule is to open depression using Fructus Evodiae Rutecarpae (*Wu Zhu Yu*). In case of *xian*-like worm sores[4], the rule is to abate heat and kill worms using Semen Praeparatus Ulmi Macrocarpae (*Wu Yi*), Rhizoma Dryopteris Crassirhizomae (*Hei Gou Ji*), Realgar (*Xiong Huang*), Sulphur (*Liu Huang*), and Mercurius (*Shui Yin*) to kill worms, Alum (*Bai Fan*) to stop itching, Camphora (*Zhang Nao*) to penetrate flesh, 1 *fen* (in amount), Resina Pini (*Song Xiang*), and (in case of sores) on the head, adding a large amount of Radix Et Rhizoma Rhei (*Da Huang*) and 1 *fen* of Calcitum (*Fang Jie Shi*).

---

[3] This refers to favus or any kind of cutaneous disease causing large scale loss of hair.

[4] This refers to sores where tiny mites can be observed.

Rhizoma Coptidis Chinensis (*Huang Lian*) and Fructus Cnidii Monnieri (*She Chuang Zi*) are able to settle itching and kill worms.

Related to purulent swelling, if there is much dampness, add carbonized Cortex Pini (*Song Pi Hui*). If there is much swelling, add Radix Angelicae (*Bai Zhi*) to open depression. If there is much pain, add Radix Angelicae and Calcitum (*Fang Jie Shi*). If there are many worms, add Radix Veratri Nigri (*Li Lu*) and Mylabris Phalerata (*Ban Mao*). If there is much itching, add water-ground Alum (*Bai Fan*. And) if there is much dampness, add sesame oil mixed (sic).

In case of scrotal sores, usually introduce Fructus Evodiae Rutecarpae (*Wu Zhu Yu*). In case of dry *jie* with bleeding, usually introduce Radix Et Rhizoma Rhei (*Da Huang*) and Rhizoma Coptidis Chinensis (*Huang Lian*) mixed with pig's lard (*Zhu Zhi*). In case of worms, usually introduce any amount of carbonate of lead (*Xi Hui*), Semen Praeparatus Ulmi Macrocarpae (*Wu Yi*), and Semen Arecae Catechu (*Bing Lang*) which can kill worms. In case of red (sores), introduce Minium (*Huang Dan*. And) in case of green-blue (sores), introduce Pulvis Indigonis (*Qing Dai*).

A sore, if located above, usually (requires) administering *Tong Shen San* (Free the Spirit Powder). A sore, if located below, is usually (rooted) in the viscera and (thus) requires precipitation. For swollen foot, prescribe damp heat (removing) medicinals in connection with the blood phase.

One formula to treat sores with abundant dampness (consists of) Concha Ostreae (*Mu Li*), 2 *liang*, Fructus Cnidii Monnieri (*She Chuang*), 1 *liang*, Radix Angelicae (*Bai Zhi*), 1 *liang*, Fructus Zanthoxyli Bungeani (*Chuan Jiao*), 3 *qian*, Calcareous Spar (*Han Shui Shi*), 5 *qian*, Calomelas (*Qing Fen*), 20 small cupfuls, Realgar (*Xiong Huang*), 5 *qian*, and Fructus Evodiae Rutecarpae (*Wu Zhu Yu*), 2.5 *qian*. Powder the above finely, mix with sesame oil, and apply (as a dressing).

For an ointment for moxibustion sores which refuse to close their opening, (use) Rhizoma Coptidis Chinensis (*Huang Lian*), Nodus Radicis Glycyrrhizae (*Gan Cao Jie*), Radix Angelicae (*Bai Zhi*), Minium

(*Dan*), and oil. A formula for scabies (consists of) Fructus Cnidii Monnieri (*She Chuang*), 1 *liang*, Sulphur (*Liu Huang*), 1.5 *qian*, Calomelas (*Qing Fen*, in amounts) for 20 packets, Melanteritum (*Qing Fan*), 1.5 *qian*, Alum (*Ming Fan*), 1 *qian*, Minium (*Huang Dan*), 1.5 *qian*, and Galla Rhi Chinensis (*Wu Bei Zi*), 1.5 *qian*, stir-fried for a short time till yellow. Powder the above finely, mix with sesame oil, and apply (as a dressing). It is prohibited to expose (the sore) to lamplight and fire. (This dressing) is remarkably efficacious.

A formula for *jie* sores (is made by) powdering Minium (*Huang Dan*) and Semen Myristicae Fragrantis (*Rou Dou Kou*), mix with sesame oil, and apply. To treat wounds on horseback developing into sores (*i.e.*, saddle sores), spread the whites of a hen's egg as an ointment and (allow) to adhere (to the sore). Leave in place till it comes off by itself at which time (the sore) will be healed. A formula to treat *xian* (consists of) Cortex Hibisci Syricaci (*Chuan Jin Pi*) and Semen Arecae Catechu (*Bing Lang*). First scratch (the affected part) and then smear with (these medicinals) rubbed with good vinegar. Another formula which treats a damp, itching scrotum (is made by) powdering Lithargyum (*Mi Tuo Seng*), dry Rhizoma Zingiberis (*Gan Jiang*), and Talcum (*Hua Shi*). Apply dry. (Yet) another formula (is made by) first boiling Fructus Evodiae Rutecarpae (*Wu Zhu Yu*) and washing with the decoction. Then use the following medicinals: Fructus Evodiae Rutecarpae (*Wu Zhu Yu*), 5 *qian*, Calcareous Spar (*Han Shui Shi*), 3 *qian*, Cortex Phellodendri (*Huang Bai*), 1.5 *qian*, Radix Et Rhizoma Rhei (*Da Huang*), 2.5 *qian*, Camphora (*Zhang Nao*), 3 *qian*, Fructus Cnidii Monnieri (*She Chuang Zi*), 3 *qian*, Calomelas (*Qing Fen*), 1 small cupful, Alumen (*Ku Fan*), 3 *qian*, Sulphur (*Liu Huang*), 2 *qian*, Semen Arecae Catechu (*Bing Lang*), 3 *qian*, and Radix Angelicae (*Bai Zhi*), 3 *qian*. Powder the above and apply.

A formula to treat sores on the head (consists of) pig's fat (*Zhu You*), 2.5 *qian*, half raw, half cooked, Realgar (*Xiong Huang*), 2.5 *qian*, and Mercurius (*Shui Yin*), 2.5 *qian*. Grind the above evenly and apply on the sore. Another formula (consists of) Rhizoma Ligustici Wallichii (*Chuan Xiong*) and wine-processed Radix Scutellariae Baicalensis (*Huang Qin*), 5 *qian* (each), wine-processed Radix Paeoniae Lactiflorae (*Shao Yao*), 5 *qian*, Pericarpium Citri Reticulatae (*Chen Pi*), 5 *qian*, wine-processed Rhizoma Atractylodis Macrocephalae (*Bai Zhu*), 5 *qian*, wine-processed Radix Angelicae Sinensis (*Dang Gui*), 1.5 *liang*, wine-processed Rhizoma Gastrodiae Elatae (*Tian Ma*), 7.5 *qian*, Herba Xanthii Sibirici (*Cang Er*), 7.5 *qian*, wine-processed Cortex Phellodendri (*Huang Bai*), 4 *qian*, wine-processed, debarked Radix Glycyrrhizae (*Fen Cao*), 4 *qian*, and Radix Ledebouriellae Sesloidis (*Fang Feng*), 3 *qian*. Powder the above, heat in water to a boil, and take 4-5 times a day. After taking, have a short nap.

Chapter One Hundred Nineteen

Worm Toxins (*i.e.*, Toxins from Insects, Parasites, Snakes & Vermin)

To treat nine *li* flyer, *i.e.*, wasp, toxins, bore a hole in Fructus Gleditschiae Sinensis (*Zao Jiao*), place this hole directly over the point stung by the wasp, and then moxa 3 cones in the hole. (The sting) will heal. To treat centipede bite, moxa with dried Buthus Martensi (*Quan Xie*) in the same way as for the nine *li* flyer (sting). To treat (the bite of) all kinds of snake, rub a small amount of Radix Paridis Petiolatae (*Jin Xian Chong Lou*) in water and apply (the fluid) to the bitten place. At the same time, drink wine brewed with powdered Radix Paridis Petiolatae. Another formula (is made by) finely grinding Folium Sapii Sebiferi (*Wu Jiu Shu Ye*), Herba Houttuyniae Cordatae (*Yu Xing Cao*), Herba Saginae Japonicae (*Di Song*), Herba Teucrii Viscidi (*Zhou Mian Cao*), or Semen Cassiae Torae (*Cao Jue Ming*), any of them alone will also do, and apply on the bitten place. To treat centipede bite toxins, smear Radix Panacis Ginseng (*Ren Shen*, on the bite). Another formula (consists of) setting a spider over the wound. It offers a rapid effect. Choose a spider that survives after it is put into water.

Chapter One Hundred Twenty

Poisoning

To resolve poisonous mushroom toxins, drink a decoction made from Radix Saussureae Seu Vladimiriae (*Mu Xiang*) and Pericarpium Viridis Citri Reticulatae (*Qing Pi*) in equal amounts. To resolve the toxins of various medicinals, obtain 2 *liang* of Galla Rhi Chinensis (*Wu Bie Zi*), grind finely, brew in warm, limeless wine, and take. If the toxins are located above, vomiting will occur. If they are located below, diarrhea will occur. In case of food toxins from horse and cow meat, grind 4 *liang* of Radix Glycyrrhizae (*Da Gan Cao*), brew in limeless wine, and drink. In a short while the patient will have violent vomiting and violent diarrhea. In case of thirst, do not drink water. Otherwise death is bound (to occur). Another formula to treat poisonous mushroom toxins (consists of) eating the heads of stone-head fish, *i.e.*, the yellow croaker (Pseudosciaena crocea/polyactis).

Chapter One Hundred Twenty-one

Barbarian Qi[1]

A formula to treat barbarian qi (consists of) iron dust (*Gang Sha*), Lithargyum (*Mi Tuo Seng*), Alum (*Ming Fan*), Aerugo (*Tong Qing*), Radix Aconiti Coreani (*Bai Fu Zi*), and Cinnabar (*Chen Sha*). Beforehand, wash (the affected area) 2-3 times with a soup of Fructus

---

[1] *I.e.*, body odor or bromhidrosis. In ancient times, the races, usually nomads, living north and west of China were collectively called *hu ren* (barbarians or foreigners). These people smelled of mutton and beef because these were their main foods. Therefore, bromhidrosis was called barbarian qi or *hu qi*.

Gleditschiae Sinensis (*Zao Jiao*) and then apply (the above powdered medicinals). Not [5 characters missing]. Another formula (is made by) adding Minium (*Huang Dan*) and Mercurius (*Shui Yin*) to the above formula. Dab the powder with Fructus Immaturus Pruni Mume (*Bai Mei Rou*) and rub (the affected area with it. Yet) another formula (is made by) grinding Minium (*Huang Dan*), Lithargyum (*Mi Tuo Seng*), and Alumen (*Ku Bai Fan*) very finely, dab the powder onto steamed cake, and rub.

Book Seven

Women's Disorders

Chapter One

Menstrual Disease

The menstrual water is yin blood. Since yin must necessarily comply with yang, (the menses) is red agreeing with the color of fire. It corresponds to the moon above and flows in a regular way. Thus it acquires (its) name.[1] The menses is the spouse of qi and flows by the strength of qi. (Therefore,) lump formation is congelation of qi. Pain prior to menstruation is (due to) stagnation of qi. (But) pain following (menstruation) is (due to) vacuity of both qi and blood. A light colored (flow) is also (due to) vacuity of blood which is diminished and blended with water. (While) menstrual hemafecia with (blood) running frenetically is (due to) chaos of qi. A purple colored (flow) is (due to) heat qi. (And) a blackish colored (flow) is (due to) extreme heat.

Whenever observing purple or blackish (blood) with pain or clots, people nowadays declare without justification these to be (due to) invasion of wind cold and (thus) prescribe warm and hot formulas. This is erroneous. Occasionally, there is indeed such a case, but it is one out of a hundred or a thousand. Blackish menstrual flow is the color of water, and the purple color turning to black is a result of increasing heat and invariably the complication of water transformation. Thus it is that hyperactivity never fails to do harm but can be brought under control when restrained.[2]

---

[1] Menstruation, *jing*, also means channel in Chinese. Therefore, the menstrual flow can be regarded as a display of the circuit of the channels in females.

[2] This is a famous set phrase in TCM, *kang hai cheng zhi* in shortened form. In most cases, it means treating hyperactivity by a counter-balancing method. But in this context, it seems to the translator also to imply that hyperactivity, in the extreme, may turn to its opposite or acquire part of the nature of its opposite. Thus, blackish-purple blood clots are mainly produced by heat but partly also by water vacuity, the opposite to heat or fire. Therefore, treatment should focus on draining

Pain on the verge of menstruation is (ascribed to) blood repletion [qi stagnation in a {variant} edition {later editor}], requiring Semen Pruni Persicae (*Tao Ren*), Rhizoma Cyperi Rotundi (*Xiang Fu*), Rhizoma Coptidis Chinensis (*Huang Lian*), and the like. Pain before menstruation is also (ascribed to) qi stagnation. (While) pain after menstruation is (due to) vacuity containing within it heat. (For this, use) *Si Wu* (Four Materials [Decoction]) plus Radix Scutellariae Baicalensis (*Huang Qin*) and Rhizoma Coptidis Chinensis (*Huang Lian*). A (variant) version says (it is due to) vacuity of qi and blood, (requiring) *Ba Wu Tang* (Eight Materials Decoction) with additions and subtractions.

Delayed menstruation with pain is (due to) vacuity in addition to the existence of heat. Early menstruation is (due to) blood heat. A (variant) version says (it is due to) dual vacuity of qi and blood, (requiring) *Si Wu (Tang)* plus such (medicinals) as Radix Scutellariae Baicalensis (*Huang Qin*) and Rhizoma Coptidis Chinensis (*Huang Lian*). In a fat person, additionally treat phlegm. For delayed menstruation (due to) scant blood, (use) Rhizoma Ligustici Wallichii (*Chuan Xiong*), Radix Angelicae Sinensis (*Dang Gui*), Radix Panacis Ginseng (*Ren Shen*), Rhizoma Atractylodis Macrocephalae (*Bai Zhu*), and phlegm(-expelling) medicinals.

For irregular menstruation with thin and pale blood water, it is appropriate to supplement qi and blood (with) Radix Panacis Ginseng (*Ren Shen*), Rhizoma Atractylodis Macrocephalae (*Bai Zhu*), Rhizoma Ligustici Wallichii (*Chuan Xiong*), Radix Angelicae Sinensis (*Dang Gui*), Radix Astragali Membranacei (*Huang Qi*), Rhizoma Cyperi Rotundi (*Xiang Fu*), and Radix Paeoniae Lactiflorae (*Shao Yao*). In case of low back pain, add Gelatinum Corii Bovis Tauri (*Jiao Zhu*), Folium Artemisiae Argyii (*Ai Ye*), and Rhizoma Corydalis Yanhusuo (*Xuan Hu Suo*).

Delayed menstruation with purple, black clots is (due to) blood heat and is invariably accompanied by pain. (For this, use) *Si Wu Tang* plus Rhizoma Cyperi Rotundi (*Xiang Fu*), Rhizoma Coptidis Chinensis

---

fire and, at the same time, at supplementing yin blood.

(*Huang Lian*), and the like. (But) delayed menstruation with pale colored (blood) is (due to) abundant phlegm. (For this,) use *Er Chen Tang* (Two Aged Decoction) plus Rhizoma Ligustici Wallichii (*Chuan Xiong*) and Radix Angelicae Sinensis (*Dang Gui*).

Menstruation with purple clots is (due to) extreme heat. (For this, use) *Si Wu Tang* plus Rhizoma Coptidis Chinensis (*Huang Lian*), etc. In case of menses failing to come after due time, extract more than half cupful of juice by pounding Radix Achyranthis Bidentatae (*Du Niu Xi*). Mix with 1 *qian* of powdered Rhizoma Corydalis Yanhusuo (*Xuan Hu Suo*) and one half *qian* each of powdered Rhizoma Cyperi Rotundi (*Xiang Fu*) and powdered Fructus Citri Seu Ponciri (*Zhi Qiao*). Take in the morning.

For abdominal pain on the verge of menstruation, use *Yi Qi San* (Depressed Qi Powder) which is composed of *Si Wu Tang* plus Pericarpium Citri Reticulatae (*Chen Pi*), Rhizoma Corydalis Yanhusuo (*Xuan Hu Suo*), Cortex Radicis Moutan (*Mu Dan Pi*), and Radix Glycyrrhizae (*Gan Cao*). In case of severe pain, (add) spraying-onbean wine. In case of slight pain only, boil Herba Cyperi Rotundi (*Suo Cao*) in child's urine, mix with a small amount of Radix Scutellariae Baicalensis (*Huang Qin*), and take in the shape of pills.

For blackish menstrual flow with thirst, fatigue, a weakened form, a black complexion, and an arrhythmic, somewhat rapid pulse, use stir-fried Radix Scutellariae Baicalensis (*Huang Qin*), 3 *qian*, Radix Glycyrrhizae (*Gan Cao*), 2 *qian*, and Radix Rubrus Paeoniae Lactiflorae (*Chi Shao Yao*) and Rhizoma Cyperi Rotundi (*Xiang Fu*), 5 *qian* each. Make into pills and take. Another formula (is made by) powdering Terra Flava Usta (*Fu Long Gan*) and Pulvis Fumi Carbonisati (*Bai Cao Shuang*). Make into pills with paste.

If abundant phlegm occupying the sea of blood[3] results in abundant flow, the eyes invariably become gradually clouded. Such (a condition) is seen in fat persons. Use Rhizoma Arisaematis (*Nan Xing*), Rhizoma

---

[3]   *I.e.*, the penetrating vessel, which is closely connected with menstruation in females

Cyperi Rotundi (*Xiang Fu*), Rhizoma Ligustici Wallichii (*Chuan Xiong*), and Rhizoma Atractylodis (*Cang Zhu*). Make into pills and take. Advanced and abundant (menstrual flow) in fat persons (is due to) abundant phlegm with blood vacuity and the existence of heat. (For this, use) Rhizoma Arisaematis (*Nan Xing*), Rhizoma Atractylodis Macrocephalae (*Bai Zhu*), Rhizoma Atractylodis (*Cang Zhu*), Rhizoma Coptidis Chinensis (*Huang Lian*), Rhizoma Cyperi Rotundi (*Xiang Fu*), and Rhizoma Ligustici Wallichii (*Chuan Xiong*). Powder and make into pills.

For desiccated blood amenorrhea, (use) *Si Wu Tang* plus Semen Pruni Persicae (*Tao Ren*) and Flos Carthami Tinctorii (*Hong Hua*). For amenorrhea (due to) fat filling up the body in corpulent persons, (use) *Dao Tan Tang* (Conduct Phlegm Decoction) plus Rhizoma Ligustici Wallichii (*Chuan Xiong*) and Rhizoma Coptidis Chinensis (*Huang Lian*). Do not use Radix Rehmanniae (*Di Huang*) since it obstructs the diaphragm, unless fried with Succus Zingiberis (*Sheng Jiang Zhi*).

Jiao Jia Di Huang Wan (Cross-processed Rehmannia Pills) in females treat menstrual irregularities, blood clots, qi glomus, and abdominal pain. (They consists of) Radix Rehmanniae (*Sheng Di Huang*), 1 *jin*, old fresh Rhizoma Zingiberis (*Sheng Jiang*), 1 *jin*, Rhizoma Corydalis Yanhusuo (*Xuan Hu Suo*), Radix Angelicae Sinensis (*Dang Gui*), Rhizoma Ligustici Wallichii (*Chuan Xiong*), and Radix Albus Paeoniae Lactiflorae (*Bai Shao Yao*), 2 *liang* for each of the above, Myrrha (*Mo Yao*) and Radix Saussureae Seu Vladimiriae (*Mu Xiang*), 1 *liang* each, Semen Pruni Persicae (*Tao Ren*), tip-nipped and skinned, and Radix Panacis Ginseng (*Ren Shen*), 1.5 *liang* each, and Rhizoma Cyperi Rotundi (*Xiang Fu Zi*), one half *jin*. Powder the above. First soak the Radix Rehmanniae with juice extracted from the ginger. Then soak the dregs of the ginger with the juice from the Radix Rehmanniae, running out of the juice being the measure (of the process) in both (cases). Put all 11 ingredients together, dry in the sun, powder finely, make into pills with vinegar paste, and take on an empty stomach with ginger soup.

For absence of menses, (use) Cortex Magnoliae Officinalis (*Hou Po*), 3 *liang*. Boil in 3 *sheng* of water down to 1 *sheng*, divide into 3 doses, and take on an empty stomach. For amenorrhea of all kinds that is due to cold contending in the interior, (use) *Si Wu Tang* plus Rhizoma Curcumae Zedoariae (*Peng Zhu*) and processed dry Rhizoma Zingiberis (*Zhi Gan Jiang*), 1 slice each. Boil with 3 slices of fresh Rhizoma Zingiberis (*Sheng Jiang*). In unmarried women, dry Rhizoma Zingiberis should be deleted.

For menstrual flow as copious as profuse vaginal bleeding, (use) 1 packet of *Si Wu Tang*, 3 *qian* of powdered Rhizoma Cyperi Rotundi (*Xiang Fu Mo*), 1 piece of blast-fried dry Rhizoma Zingiberis (*Pao Gan Jiang*), and a small amount of Radix Glycyrrhizae (*Gan Cao*). Boil with some 100 grains of millet, divide into 2 doses, and take on an empty stomach. For abdominal pain before menstruation, take half a dose of *Lai Fu Dan* (Return & Recover Elixir) with *Qi Qi Tang* (Seven Qi Decoction)[4] from the *Ju Fang (Collected Formulas)*. For a copious menstrual flow which is unable to terminate in due time, add to *San Bu Wan* (Three Supplements Pills) Radix Cyperi Rotundi (*Suo Cao Gen*), Plastrum Testudinis (*Gui Ban*), and Rhizoma Ciboti Barometz (*Jin Mao Gou Ji*. And for) copious menstrual flow, (use) stir-fried Radix Scutellariae Baicalensis (*Huang Qin*), stir-fried Radix Albus Paeoniae Lactiflorae (*Bai Shao Yao*), and processed Plastrum Testudinis (*Gui Ban*), 1 *liang* for each of the above, stir-fried Cortex Phellodendri (*Huang Bai*), 3 *qian*, Cortex Cedrelae (*Chun Pi*), 7.5 *qian*, and Rhizoma Cyperi Rotundi (*Xiang Fu*), 2.5 *qian*. Powder the above and make into pills with wine paste.

For counterflow menstrual blood (with) fishy smell of blood, spitting of blood, or vomiting of blood, take Succus Allii Tuberosi (*Jiu Zhi*) and effect will follow instantly.

A person who suffered from accumulated phlegm damaging the channels with amenorrhea and raving at night was prescribed Fructus Trichosanthis Kirlowii (*Gua Lou Zi*), 1 *qian*, Rhizoma Coptidis Chinensis (*Huang Lian*), one half *qian*, Fructus Evodiae Rutecarpae (*Wu Zhu Yu*), 10 pieces, Semen Pruni Persicae (*Tao Ren*), 5 pieces, Massa Medica Fermentata Cum Semenis Oryzam Sativam (*Hong Qu*), a small amount, Fructus Amomi (*Sha Ren*), 3 *qian*, and Fructus Crataegi (*Shan Zha*), 1 *qian*. The above were powdered and made into pills with Succus Zingiberis (*Jiang Zhi*) cake.

A person who suffered for a long time from yin vacuity with blocked channels and vessels[4], short and inhibited voiding of urine, and generalized aching pain was prescribed *Si Wu Tang* plus Rhizoma Atractylodis (*Cang Zhu*), Radix Achyranthis Bidentatae (*Niu Xi*), Pericarpium Citri Reticulatae (*Chen Pi*), and Radix Glycyrrhizae (*Sheng Gan Cao*). In addition, *Cang Suo Wan* (Atractylodes & Cyperus Pills)[5] plus Herba Xanthii Sibirici (*Cang Er*) and wine-processed Radix Paeoniae Lactiflorae (*Shao Yao*) were made into pills. These pills were swallowed with a decoction made from the former formula.

For menstrual flow earlier than due time as a result of heat, (use) *Si Wu Tang* plus Radix Scutellariae Baicalensis (*Huang Qin*), Rhizoma Coptidis Chinensis (*Huang Lian*), and Rhizoma Cyperi Rotundi (*Xiang Fu*). For menstruation preceded by pain, (use) *Xiao Wu Chen Tang* (Minor Lindera & Cyperus Decoction)[6] plus Fructus Citri Seu Ponciri (*Zhi Qiao*), Pericarpium Viridis Citri Reticulatae (*Qing Pi*), Radix Scutellariae Baicalensis (*Huang Qin*), and Rhizoma Ligustici Wallichii (*Chuan Xiong*). This is a prescription for those with qi repletion (only). The above are boiled and taken on an empty stomach.

---

[4] This consists of Radix Panacis Ginseng (*Ren Shen*), mix-fried Radix Glycyrrhizae (*Zhi Gan Cao*), Cortex Cinnamomi (*Rou Gui*), 1 *liang* for each of the above, and Rhizoma Pinelliae Ternatae (*Ban Xia*), 5 *liang*. Powder; 3 *qian* per dose. Boil with 3 slices of ginger and take before a meal.

[5] This consists of Rhizoma Cyperi Rotundi (*Xiang Fu*), stir-fried with child's urine, and Rhizoma Atractylodis (*Cang Zhu*), 2 *liang* each, Pericarpium Citri Reticulatae (*Chen Pi*) and Sclerotium Poriae Cocoris (*Fu Ling*), 1.5 *liang* each, Fructus Citri Seu Ponciri (*Zhi Qiao*), Rhizoma Pinelliae Ternatae (*Ban Xia*), Rhizoma Arisaematis (*Nan Xing*), and mix-fried Radix Glycyrrhizae (*Zhi Gan Cao*), 1 *liang* for each of the above. Make into pills with Succus Zingiberis (*Jiang Zhi*) cake.

[6] This consists of Radix Linderae Strychnifoliae (*Wu Yao*), pitted, 10 *liang*, mix-fried Radix Glycyrrhizae (*Zhi Gan Cao*), 1 *liang*, and Rhizoma Cyperi Rotundi (*Xiang Fu*), 20 *liang*. Powder; 1 *qian* per dose.

Chapter Two

Childbirth & Pregnancy

A woman invariably miscarried around the 3rd month of pregnancy. The pulse on the left hand was large but weak and felt choppy when pressure was applied. This led to the recognition that her blood was scant. Because she was young at age, it was only (necessary to) supplement the central qi in order to allow the blood to build itself up. It was early summer and (I) bid her to take a thick decoction made of *Bai Zhu Tang* (Atractylodes Decoction)[1] with 1 *qian* of powdered Radix Scutellariae Baicalensis (*Huang Qin*). Administration of tens of doses preserved (the fetus) and ensured safe delivery.

This caused (me) to think that, in most cases, falling (fetus, *i.e.,* miscarriage) is due to internal heat with vacuity. (With pregnancy,) heat becomes more serious day by day as does vacuity. It is necessary to weigh which (factor) is graver and which lighter.[2] Pregnancy

---

[1] There are at least seven formulas with this same name. The most likely one seems to be the one composed of Rhizoma Atractylodis Macrocephalae (*Bai Zhu*), Radix Panacis Ginseng (*Ren Shen*), Fructus Piperis Cubebae (*Bi Cheng Qie*), Fructus Terminaliae Chebulae (*He Zi*), Flos Caryophylli (*Ding Xiang*), Semen Alpiniae Katsumadai (*Cao Dou Kou*), Radix Astragali Membranacei (*Huang Qi*), Radix Praeparatus Aconiti Carmichaeli (*Fu Zi*), Sclerotium Poriae Cocoris (*Fu Ling*), Fructus Germinatus Hordei Vulgaris (*Mai Ya*), Lignum Aquilariae Agallochae (*Chen Xiang*), Pericarpium Citri Reticulatae (*Chen Pi*), Radix Saussureae Seu Vladimiriae (*Mu Xiang*), Fructus Immaturus Citri Seu Ponciri (*Zhi Shi*), and Radix Glycyrrhizae (*Gan Cao*). However, it is equally possible that this refers simply to a soup made from Rhizoma Atractylodis Macrocephalae alone.

[2] This implies that the treatment of heat should be given priority and that vacuity should be treated secondarily.

(during the first) 3 months is ascribed to ministerial fire in the upper.[3] That is why miscarriage easily takes place (then). If not, why are Radix Scutellariae Baicalensis (*Huang Qin*), prepared Folium Artemisiae Argyii (*Shu Ai*), and Gelatinum Corii Asini (*E Jiao*) the medicinals to calm the fetus?

One method of ascertaining pregnancy in women with menstrual signs for 3 months (consists of) taking a spoonful of a thick decoction made from raw, powdered Rhizoma Ligustici Wallichii (*Chuan Xiong Mo*) on an empty stomach. If (something) stirs gently in the abdomen, a fetus is proved.

Before delivery, it is necessary to clear heat and nurture blood. If, in the 8th or 9th month of pregnancy, a woman contracts dyspnea as a result of fire stirring and upward counterflow of the fetal (qi, one should,) without delay, powder and take Radix Scutellariae Baicalensis (*Tiao Qin*), Rhizoma Cyperi Rotundi (*Xiang Fu*), and the like. Put Radix Scutellariae Baicalensis in water and choose those that look heavier for use.

(A formula) to secure the fetus (consists of) Radix Rehmanniae (*Di Huang*), one half *qian*, Radix Et Apex Angelicae Sinensis (*Dang Gui Shen Wei*), Radix Panacis Ginseng (*Ren Shen*), Radix Albus Paeoniae Lactiflorae (*Bai Shao Yao*), and Pericarpium Citri Reticulatae (*Chen Pi*), 1 *qian* for each of the above, Rhizoma Atractylodis Macrocephalae (*Bai Zhu*), 1.5 *qian*, Radix Scutellariae Baicalensis (*Huang Qin*) and Rhizoma Ligustici Wallichii (*Chuan Xiong*), one half *qian* each, Rhizoma Coptidis Chinensis (*Huang Lian*) and stir-fried Cortex Phellodendri (*Huang Bai*), each a small amount, Radix Glycyrrhizae (*Gan Cao*), 3 *fen*, Ramus Et Folium Lonicerae Japonicae (*Sang Shang Yang Er Teng*) with 7 round leaves, *i.e.*, *Jin Yin Teng*, and Semen Oryzae Sativae (*Nuo Mi*), 14 grains. Slice, boil, and take. In case of blood vacuity with disquieted (fetus),

---

[3] Ministerial fire is the fire generated in the kidney or liver. However, it tends to move upward causing disturbances of various kinds. During the first months of pregnancy, the fetus is believed to lie in the upper burner, where fire, or rather ministerial fire, is raging.

use Gelatinum Corii Asini (*E Jiao*). In case of (abdominal) pain, use Fructus Amomi (*Suo Sha*).

Shu Tai Wan (Bind the Fetus Pills), which are taken in the 8-9th months (of pregnancy, consist of) Radix Scutellariae Baicalensis (*Huang Qin*), 1 *liang* in summer, 7 *liang* in spring and autumn, one half *liang* in winter, stir-fried with wine, Pericarpium Citri Reticulatae (*Chen Pi*), 1 *liang*, Rhizoma Atractylodis Macrocephalae (*Bai Zhu*), 2 *liang*, fire prohibited (*i.e.*, kept away from fire), and Sclerotium Poriae Cocoris (*Fu Ling*), 7.5 *qian*, fire prohibited. Powder the above and make into pills with gruel.

Shu Tai Yin (Bind the Fetus Drink, consist of) Pericarpium Arecae (*Da Fu Pi*), 3 *qian*, Radix Panacis Ginseng (*Ren Shen*), one half *qian*, Pericarpium Citri Reticulatae (*Chen Pi*), one half *qian*, Rhizoma Atractylodis Macrocephalae (*Bai Zhu*), 1 *liang*, Radix Albus Paeoniae Lactiflorae (*Bai Shao Yao*), 1 *qian*, Ramus Et Folium Perillae Frutescentis (*Zi Su Jing Ye*), 1 *qian*, mix-fried Radix Glycyrrhizae (*Zhi Gan Cao*), 3 *fen*, Radix Et Apex Angelicae Sinensis (*Dang Gui Shen Wei*), 1 *qian*, with Fructus Citri Seu Ponciri (*Zhi Qiao*) and Fructus Amomi (*Suo Sha*) allowed to be added, all the above as one dose. Boil with 5 leaves of Chinese green onion and 7 leaves of Buxus Microphullae (*Huang Yang Shu*). Take before a meal. Taking about 10 doses in the 8-9th months (of pregnancy) will avail tremendously. In summer, Rhizoma Coptidis Chinensis (*Huang Lian*) may be added but not in winter. In spring, Rhizoma Ligustici Wallichii (*Chuan Xiong*) may be added. In the presence of complicated patterns, discretion is required to deal with (this).

In the 9th month (of pregnancy), administer Radix Scutellariae Baicalensis (*Huang Qin*), 1 *liang* appropriate for cooling (purposes), deleted (or) reduced by half for weak and feeble persons, stir-fried Fructus Citri Seu Ponciri (*Zhi Qiao*), 7.5 *qian*, Rhizoma Atractylodis Macrocephalae (*Bai Zhu*), 1 *liang*, and Talcum (*Hua Shi*), 7.5 *qian*, used only in case of scant urine 10 days before delivery. Powder the above, make into pills the size of Chinese parasol seeds with gruel; 30 pills per dose taken on an empty stomach with hot boiled water. Taking more is prohibited for fear of damaging the original qi. If 2 *qian* of mix-fried Radix Glycyrrhizae (*Zhi Gan Cao*) are added in the decoction and taken before a meal, (this formula) is also called *Shu Tai Yin.*

Da Sheng San (Expedite Delivery Powder), taken from the 9th month (of pregnancy), 30-50 doses allowed, prevents abdominal pain and ensures easy delivery. (It consists of) Radix Scutellariae Baicalensis (*Huang Qin*), Radix Panacis Ginseng (*Ren Shen*), Rhizoma Atractylodis Macrocephalae (*Bai Zhu*), Talcum (*Hua Shi*), Fructus Citri Seu Ponciri (*Zhi Qiao*), Folium Buxus Microphyllae (*Huang Yang Tou*), Rhizoma Cyperi Rotundi (*Xiang Fu Mi*), Pericarpium Citri Reticulatae (*Chen Pi*), Radix Glycyrrhizae (*Gan Cao*), Pericarpium Arecae (*Da Fu Pi*), Fructus Perillae Frutescentis (*Zi Su*), and Radix Albus Paeoniae Lactiflorae (*Bai Shao Yao*). In spring, add Rhizoma Ligustici Wallichii (*Chuan Xiong*). In case of qi vacuity, double the amounts of Radix Panacis Ginseng and Rhizoma Atractylodis Macrocephalae. In case of qi repletion, double the amounts of Rhizoma Cyperi Rotundi and Pericarpium Citri Reticulatae. In case of blood vacuity, double the amounts of Radix Angelicae Sinensis (*Dang Gui*) and Radix Rehmanniae (*Di Huang*). In case of a replete form, double the amount of Fructus Perillae Frutescentis. In case of quick temper, double the amount of Rhizoma Coptidis Chinensis (*Huang Lian*). In case of abundant heat, double the amount of Radix Scutellariae Baicalensis. In case of damp phlegm, double the amount of Talcum and add Rhizoma Pinelliae Ternatae (*Ban Xia*). In case of food accumulation, add Fructus Crataegi (*Shan Zha*) in double amount. In case of quick hungering after meals, double the amount of Folium Buxus Microphyllae. If there is heat and also in summer, increase Radix Scutellariae Baicalensis (*Huang Qin*). If there is phlegm, add Rhizoma Pinelliae Ternatae (*Ban Xia*). In case of abdominal pain, add Radix Saussureae Seu Vladimiriae (*Mu Xiang*) and Cortex Cinnamomi (*Guan Gui*) which are supervised by Radix Scutellariae Baicalensis. In winter months, Radix Scutellariae Baicalensis should not be used.

An Tai Wan (Calm the Fetus Pills, consist of) Rhizoma Atractylodis Macrocephalae (*Bai Zhu*), Radix Scutellariae Baicalensis (*Huang Qin*), and stir-fried Massa Medica Fermentata (*Shen Qu*). Take in the shape of pills made with gruel. Radix Scutellariae Baicalensis calms the fetus, for it is a medicinal for the upper and middle burners, able to downbear and make fire go downwards. Fructus Amomi (*Suo Sha*, also) calms the fetus and treats pain because it can move qi. Before delivery, to calm the fetus, Rhizoma Atractylodis Macrocephalae and Radix Scutellariae Baicalensis are wonderful medicinals. Semen Leonuri Heterophylli (*Chong Wei Zi*) quickens blood and moves qi, doing wonders for supplementing yin. For that reason it has acquired the name of benefiting the mother herb. Since it supplements qi while moving it, it prevents stagnation before delivery and vacuity after delivery.

In the 4-5th months of pregnancy, in case of sudden gripping abdominal pain, char and powder 14 pieces of Fructus Zizyphi Jujubae (*Da Zao*) and take with child's urine. In case of stirring fetus (manifest) merely by lumbago, the fetus turning and giving impact on the heart, or incessant (vaginal) bleeding, boil Folium Artemisiae Argyii (*Ai Ye*) the size of a hen's egg in 4 *sheng* of wine down to 2 *sheng* and take as 2 doses. This does great wonders.

(In case of) stirring fetus with abdominal pain, the fetus's life being uncertain, administration of the following medicinals can calm the fetus if it is alive or precipitate it if it is already dead: Radix Angelicae Sinensis (*Dang Gui*), 4 *liang*, and Rhizoma Ligustici Wallichii (*Chuan Xiong*), 9 *liang*. Boil in 4 *sheng* of wine down to 3 *sheng* and take.

Disharmonious fetal qi making its way upward with cardiac and abdominal distention, fullness, and pain is called fetal suspension. (For it,) there is a formula, *Zi Su Yin* (Perilla Drink), which also treats failure to deliver the child for days running due to qi bind caused by fright and apprehension towards labor: Fructus Et Ramus Perillae Frutescentis (*Zi Su Lian Jing*), 1 *liang*, Radix Angelicae Sinensis (*Dang Gui*), 7 *qian*, Radix Panacis Ginseng (*Ren Shen*), Rhizoma Ligustici Wallichii (*Chuan Xiong*), Radix Albus Paeoniae Lactiflorae (*Bai Shao Yao*), and Pericarpium Citri Reticulatae (*Chen Pi*), one half *liang* for each of the above, Radix Glycyrrhizae (*Gan Cao*), 3 *qian*, Pericarpium Arecae (*Da Fu Pi*), one half *liang*, Rhizoma Zingiberis (*Jiang*), 4 slices, and Bulbus Allii Fistulosi (*Cong*, a piece) 7 *cun* long. Boil and take on an empty stomach.

(To treat fetal) excitement and unrest in pregnancy, obtain any amount of Fructus Amomi (*Suo Sha*), stir-fry well over a small fire, strip of its skin, powder, and take brewed with heated wine. Once the place of the stirring fetus in the womb feels extremely hot, the fetus will become calm. This offers miraculous effect.

(In case of) death in utero with mother's qi expired, take [4 characters missing] or Succus Leonuri Heterophylli (*Yi Mu Cao Zhi*. The dead child) will be precipitated immediately. In case of death in utero due to footling presentation, take powdered Radix Angelicae Sinensis (*Dang Gui*) brewed with wine. In case of death in utero with the mother's qi bordering on expiration, powder Terra Flava Usta (*Fu Long Gan*), brew with water, and take. Another formula (is made by) boiling 1 *liang* of Cinnabar (*Zhu Sha*) in water for a short time, powder, brew with wine, and take. (It offers) instant effect.

(In case of) threatening to give birth before the months and days of pregnancy are complete, extract 2 *sheng* of juice from Rhizoma Acori Graminei (*Shi Chang Pu*) by pounding and pour down the throat. In case of pregnant swelling fullness from the feet up to the abdomen with inhibited urination and moderate thirst, powder 5 *liang* of Sclerotium Polypori Umbellati (*Zhu Ling*) and take a square *cun* coin with boiled water, 3 times a day. In case of coughing in pregnancy, stir-fry Bulbus Fritillariae (*Bei Mu*), powder, make into pills with granulated sugar, and melt in the mouth in the night. (This is) remarkable.

For food damage in pregnancy, it is very troublesome to prescribe medication and the only safe choices are *Mu Xiang Wan* (Saussurea Pills) and *Bai Zhu San* (Atractylodes Powder). This (condition) requires prohibitions of the mouth (*i.e.*, dietary prohibitions).

Conception (under the condition of) menstrual gathering[4] justifies the fear of disquieted fetal qi, slight abdominal pain, ache in the lower back, or no liking for food. It is treated with *An Tai Yin* (Calm the

---

[4]   This implies blood clots in the menstrual flow.

Fetus Drink): Rhizoma Atractylodis Macrocephalae (*Bai Zhu*), 1 *qian*, Radix Panacis Ginseng (*Ren Shen*), one half *qian*, Radix Angelicae Sinensis (*Dang Gui*), 1 *qian*, Radix Albus Paeoniae Lactiflorae (*Basi Shao Yao*), 1 *qian*, prepared Radix Rehmanniae (*Shu Di Huang*), 1 *qian*, Rhizoma Ligustici Wallichii (*Chuan Xiong*), 5 *fen*, Pericarpium Citri Reticulatae (*Chen Pi*), 5 *fen*, Radix Glycyrrhizae (*Gan Cao*), 3 *fen*, Fructus Amomi (*Suo Sha*), 2 *fen*, Fructus Perillae Frutescentis (*Zi Su*), 3 *fen*, and Radix Scutellariae Baicalensis (*Tiao Qin*), 5 *fen*, the above as one dose. Boil in water with 1 slice of ginger and take before a meal. If several doses of this formula are taken regularly after the 5-7th months of pregnancy, it ensures the safety of the pregnant woman through to delivery. It is particularly good if taken in the 7-8th months with 7 pieces each of Pericarpium Arecae (*Da Fu Pi*) and Folium Buxus Microphyllae (*Huang Yang Tou*).

During the month before delivery, (use) Radix Angelicae Sinensis (*Quan Shen Dang Gui*), 1 *qian*, Rhizoma Ligustici Wallichii (*Chuan Xiong*), 1 *qian*, Radix Angelicae (*Bai Zhi*), 5 *fen*, Radix Scutellariae Baicalensis (*Tiao Qin*), 1 *qian*, Pericarpium Citri Reticulatae (*Chen Pi*), 1 *qian*, Rhizoma Cyperi Rotundi (*Xiang Fu*), 1 *qian*, and Radix Glycyrrhizae (*Gan Cao*), 3 *fen*. Boil the above and take brewed with 1 *qian* of *Yi Yuan San* (Boost the Original Powder). For persons with body vacuity, add 1 *qian* of Radix Panacis Ginseng (*Ren Shen*).

For fetal suspension with abdominal distention, stomachache, and fetal (*i.e.*, uterine) pain, (use) the fetus-protecting *Zi Su Yin* (discussed above. In case of) swelling in pregnancy due to abundant dampness, stir-fry 1 *he* (*i.e.*, 0.1 *sheng*) of Fructus Gardeniae Jasminoidis (*Shan Zhi*) and swallow with thin gruel.

A formula in the *San Yin Fang* (*Three Causes Formulas*), *Li Yu Tang* (Carp Decoction), treats enlarged abdomen with complicated water qi[5] in pregnancy. (It consists of) Rhizoma Atractylodis Macrocephalae (*Bai Zhu*), 5 *liang*, Radix Albus Paeoniae Lactiflorae (*Bai Shao Yao*) and Radix Angelicae Sinensis (*Dang Gui*), 3 *liang* each, and Sclerotium Poriae

---

[5]   Water qi means swelling in this case.

Cocoris (*Fu Ling*), 4 *liang*. Grate the above. Boil 1 carp after dressed as for an ordinary dish, collect the soup, removing the fish. Boil and take 4 *qian* (of the powdered medicinals) per dose in 1.5 cups of the fish soup with 7 slices of ginger and a small amount of Pericarpium Citri Reticulatae (*Chen Pi*).

When conception is first perceived, if one carries about a purple purse containing 1 *liang* of Realgar (*Xiong Huang*), a girl fetus will change to a boy. Another method (consists of) tying a bowstring round the waist for 2 months at the beginning (of pregnancy) and a girl fetus will change to a boy. This is a secret method with few knowing it.

Fetal leakage[6] is ascribed to qi vacuity, blood vacuity, and blood heat. To calm the fetus in pregnancy, boil 2 *liang* of Fructus Germinatus Hordei Vulgaris (*Da Mai Ya*) in 1.5 cups of water down to 1 cupful. Take warm for 3 times or brewed with honey. Another formula (consists of) *Si Wu Tang* (Four Materials Decoction) plus Radix Achyranthis Bidentatae (*Niu Xi*), Rhizoma Curcumae Zedoariae (*Peng Zhu*), blast-fried Cortex Cinnamomi (*Pao Guan Gui*), and Flos Carthami Tinctorii (*Hong Hua*), all in equal amounts. Boil in water, the ratio of water to the medicinals being 7 to 3, down to 1/2 and take on an empty stomach. (Yet) another formula (is made by) putting a fingertipful of carbonate of lead (*Shao Fen*) into a date (*Zao*), wrap the date with a wet piece of paper, and roast. Chew and swallow on an empty stomach with limeless wine, 3-4 dates per day. (This formula) can also precipitate a dead fetus.

A formula to precipitate a dead fetus (is made by) boiling and taking *Fo Shou San* (Buddha's Hand Powder)[7] plus 3 pieces of Secretio Moschi Moschiferi (*She Xiang*) or *Dang Men Zi* (by another name) and 1 *qian* of powdered Radix Et Rhizoma Rhei (*Da Huang Mo*). In severe cases,

---

[6] *I.e.*, vaginal bleeding in pregnancy

[7] This consists of Rhizoma Ligustici Wallichii (*Chuan Xiong*) and Radix Angelicae Sinensis (*Dang Gui*) inlarge doses.

take with tile-baked, powdered Tabanus (*Mang Chong*) and Hirudo (*Shui Zhi*).

For swelling in pregnancy, (use) *Li Yu Tang* plus *Ren Shen Bai Zhu Wu Ling San* (Ginseng & Atractylodes Five *Ling* Powder).[8] Hideous obstruction (*i.e.,* nausea or morning sickness) should be treated as phlegm, usually with *Er Chen Tang* (Two Aged Decoction) with powdered Rhizoma Atractylodis Macrocephalae (*Bai Zhu*) put in. Make into pills with water and take with what (substance) one likes and water. Another formula (consists of) Rhizoma Cyperi Rotundi (*Xiang Fu Zi*), 2 *qian*, Fructus Amomi (*Sha Ren*), Sclerotium Poriae Cocoris (*Fu Ling*), and Radix Glycyrrhizae (*Gan Cao*), 1 *qian* for each of the above. If (the patient) likes acrid (substances), add Flos Caryophylli (*Ding Xiang*). Powder and take dry.

Cravings for a (certain) substance in pregnancy indicates vacuity of one viscus. Suppose there is vacuity of the liver. (In that case,) the liver is only able to nourish the fetus with nothing more for other purposes or for the liver itself. Therefore, in case of liver vacuity, (the patient) likes sour substances.

For fetal heat in the month before delivery, use *San Bu Wan* (Three Supplements Pills) plus stir-fried Rhizoma Cyperi Rotundi (*Xiang Fu*) and Radix Albus Paeoniae Lactiflorae (*Bai Shao Yao*). Make into pills with cake. Besides, *San Bu Wan* made into pills with *Di Huang Gao* (Rehmannia Paste) can be administered to suppress heat. (And,) in the 8-9th months of pregnancy, it is necessary to normalize the qi with Fructus Citri Seu Ponciri (*Zhi Qiao*) and Ramulus Perillae Frutescentis (*Su Zi Jing*).

A woman, nearly 30 years of age, who had been pregnant for 2 months suffered from a disease of uncontrollable retching and vomiting, spinning head, and visual dizziness. Five to seven days after administration of Radix Panacis Ginseng (*Ren Shen*), Rhizoma Atracty-

---

[8] See Note 9, Ch. 5, Bk. 1. Plus Radix Panacis Ginseng (*Ren Shen*) and Rhizoma Atractylodes Macrocephalae (*Bai Zhu*).

lodis Macrocephalae (*Bai Zhu*), Rhizoma Ligustici Wallichii (*Chuan Xiong*), Pericarpium Citri Reticulatae (*Chen Pi*), and Sclerotium Poriae Cocoris (*Fu Ling*), (her condition) became all the more serious with the pulse being wiry, particularly so on the left hand, and, in addition, weak. This was the disease of hideous obstruction. Excited by angry qi, the liver qi was counterflowing and the fetal qi was also embraced. (In this case,) supplementation with Radix Panacis Ginseng and Rhizoma Atractylodis Macrocephalae was diametrically inappropriate. (Therefore, I) administered only 24 pills of *Yi Qing Wan* (Suppress the Green-Blue Pills) taken with *Fu Ling Tang* (Poria Decoction).[9] Five packets achieved some degree of improvement. The pulse was slightly rapid, the mouth was dry with a bitter taste in it, and a sour taste appeared in the mouth after taking even a little gruel. This was because stagnant qi around the diaphragm was not yet completely moved. (Hence) she was bid to boil Rhizoma Ligustici Wallichii (*Chuan Xiong*), Pericarpium Citri Reticulatae (*Chen Pi*), Fructus Gardeniae Jasminoidis (*Shan Zhi*), fresh Rhizoma Zingiberis (*Sheng Jiang*), and Sclerotium Poriae Cocoris (*Fu Ling*) and take (this decoction) with 50 pills of *Yi Qing Wan*.

After a little more than 10 doses (of the above) had been taken, (nearly) all her remaining symptoms were overcome. Her food intake was as large as half her ordinary, but a hungry feeling was liable to quickly follow meals. This was because liver heat was not yet (completely) leveled. Then (she was bid to) take 20 pills of *Yi Qing Wan* with boiled water. Twenty days later, she was relieved. On examination, although the pulse on both hands was calm and harmonious, the pulse on the left hand was very weak. This showed inevitable miscarriage. By now the liver qi was already leveled, and, therefore, Radix Panacis Ginseng (*Ren Shen*) and Rhizoma Atractylodis Macrocephalae (*Bai Zhu*) could be used. Then (I) began to prescribe these and other medicinals to supplement as a part of a formula in

---

9   There are more than 10 formulas with this same name. The most likely one is composed of Sclerotium Poriae Cocoris (*Fu Ling*), 4 *liang*, Cortex Cinnamomi (*Gui Xin*) and Rhizoma Atractylodis Macrocephalae (*Bai Zhu*), 3 *liang* each, and mix-fried Radix Glycyrrhizae (*Zhi Gan Cao*), 2 *liang*; 3 *qian* per dose. Powder and boil.

order to anticipate the vacuity following miscarriage. (The formula) was administered for 1 day and the fetus aborted by itself. (The woman) was safe and sound.

A woman with a thin form and quick temper, free from internal heat, was thirsty, desiring water in the 3rd month of pregnancy when it was hot summer. (She was) accordingly administered *Si Wu Tang* plus Radix Scutellariae Baicalensis (*Huang Qin*), Pericarpium Citri Reticulatae (*Chen Pi*), Radix Glycyrrhizae (*Sheng Gan Cao*), and Caulis Akebiae Mutong (*Mu Tong*. After) several doses were taken, (she) recovered. Later she gave birth to a child. At the age of 2, (the child) suddenly contracted malaria. This was due to fetal toxins not yet completely eliminated because the medicinals administered during pregnancy had been inadequate. If sores or scabies grew (on the child, the malaria) would heal without the need for treatment. This (later) turned out to be true.

Radix Scutellariae Baicalensis (*Huang Qin*) is a divine medicinal for calming the fetus, but, ignorant of this, vulgar physicians, afraid of its cold (nature), dare not use it, saying that (only) warm medicinals are capable of nurturing the fetus. It should be understood that it is necessary to clear heat before delivery and that, when heat is cleared, blood will circulate along the channels, having no chance to move frenetically. Thus (Radix Scutellariae Baicalensis) nurtures the fetus.

Before delivery, (one) should use *Si Wu Tang*. If, (however,) the patient is thin and weak with blood vacuity, do not use it because Radix Paeoniae Lactiflorae (*Shao Yao*) fells the liver. For strong persons during their youth, it may be used nonetheless.

Difficult presentation may be caused by vacuity of qi and blood. There is a rather detailed discussion (of this) in the *Ge Zhi Yu Lun (Extra Treatises Based on Investigation & Inquiry)* and the *Da Quan Liang Fang (Great Compendium of Fine Formulas)* provides formulas to choose from. The cause of difficult delivery may be negligence in the 8th and 9th months of pregnancy or stagnant qi unable to convey or turn (the child). The birthing woman should be made strong (immediately) after the delivery is completed. The birthing woman may be helped to sit still against an(other) woman sitting on the bed for 2-3 watches and she should not be allowed to lie down to sleep until the lochia has run out. Otherwise, malign blood may enter the heart and cause instant death. In addition, there is a moxa method to treat difficult delivery in women. Moxa the tip of the small toe of the right foot of the woman with a cone the size of a grain of wheat made from prepared Folium Artemisiae Argyii (*Shu Ai*). Five cones moxaed, (the child will) come out.

A formula to hasten delivery (consists of) Radix Angelicae (*Bai Zhi*), Pulvis Fumi Carbonisati (*Bai Cao Shuang*), and Talcum (*Hua Shi*). Powder and take with *Xiong Gui Tang* (Ligusticum & *Dang Gui* Decoction). This also treats retention of the placenta if taken brewed with Succus Zingiberis (*Jiang Zhi*) and wine. Other efficacious choices can be found in the *Fu Ren Da Quan Liang Fang* (*Great Compendium of Fine Formulas for Women*).

A formula to ensure easy delivery (is made by) collecting Herba Leonuri Heterophylli (*Yi Mu Cao*) in the 6th (lunar) month and drying it in the sun with its roots preserved. Powder and make into pills the size of pellets with honey. Towards labor, dissolve in boiled water and take. It is no less remarkable if taken after boiled down to a paste. A formula to hasten delivery (is made by) powdering equal amounts of Radix Angelicae (*Bai Zhi*) and Pulvis Fumi Carbonisati (*Bai Cao Shuang*). Take with boiled water towards delivery. This is particularly remarkable if taken together with *Yi Yuan San* (Boost the Original Powder). Besides, it also treats transverse and footling presentation. It should be mixed with child's urine and a small amount of vinegar and (then) soaked in boiling water. One dose only and two lives will be immediately saved. Another formula (is made by) powdering Semen Plantaginis (*Che Qian Zi*) and taking 2 *qian* brewed with wine.

For death in utero due to footling presentation, (use) powdered Radix Angelicae Sinensis (*Dang Gui*). Take brewed with wine. A formula to hasten delivery (is made by) boiling *Fo Shou San*, brew with *Yi Yuan San*, and take as necessary. *Cun Jin San* ([One] Inch [Bar of] Gold Powder) treats difficult delivery. (Obtain) the head of a used writing brush (made from) rabbit hair, burn to ash and grind finely. Mix with

1 cup of Succus Rhizomatis Nelumbinis Nuciferae (*Ou Zhi*) and take. (The child) will be delivered instantly. If the birthing woman is vacuous and weak, one may fear that the lotus-root juice might stir up wind. In that case, (one) can heat it in a silver vessel over a fire and take hot. Another formula (is made by) mixing and stirring well oil, honey, and urine. (This is good for) difficult delivery. It is particularly remarkable if taken with powdered Herba Leonuri Heterophylli (*Yi Mu Cao*).

A formula for difficult delivery (consists of) Fructus Amomi (*Suo Sha*), vinegar-boiled Rhizoma Cyperi Rotundi (*Xiang Fu*), Fructus Citri Seu Ponciri (*Zhi Qiao*), Radix Glycyrrhizae (*Gan Cao*), and Talcum (*Hua Shi*). Take with boiled water. A thin and even pulse (foretells) easy delivery, and a large, floating, and moderate (*i.e.*, relaxed/retarded) pulse shows dissipated qi and (hence foretells) difficult delivery. (In that case,) childbirth is likened to tugging a boat over a dam. In addition, *Niu Xi Gao* (Achyranthes Paste) and *Di Huang Gao* (Rehmanniae Paste) treat difficult delivery.

(To treat) dysentery towards childbirth, ash-burn Fructus Gardeniae Jasminoidis (*Zhi Zi*), any amount, powder finely, and take 1 square *cun* coin with hot water on an empty stomach. A severe case needs no more than 5 doses. When childbirth is going to take place in a cold month, distention and fullness below the navel that deters the hands from touching is due to cold entering the child's gate. Take (Zhang) Zhong-jing's *Yang Rou Tang* (Mutton Decoction).[10] A formula to hasten delivery (consists of) swallowing Semen Capparis Pterocarpae (*Ma Bing Lang*) towards delivery and the child will soon be delivered with one piece of the seed in each palm.

---

[10] This is composed of mutton (*Yang Rou*) without fat, 3 *jin*, Radix Angelicae Sinensis (*Dang Gui*), Cortex Cinnamomi (*Gui Xin*), Rhizoma Ligustici Wallichii (*Chuan Xiong*), Radix Glycyrrhizae (*Gan Cao*), and Radix Ledebouriellae Sesloidis (*Fang Feng*), 2 *liang* for each of the above, Radix Paeoniae Lactiflorae (*Shao Yao*), 3 *liang*, and fresh Rhizoma Zingiberis (*Sheng Jiang*), 4 *liang*. Powder the above. First cook the mutton well, then put in the other ingredients, and continue to boil. Divide into 3 doses after removing the dregs.

Difficult delivery is commonly seen only in those with depression and oppression and the leisured, the rich, and the noble who are well attended. It is seldom seen in the poor and humble. The ancient formula, *Shou Tai Yin* (Thin the Fetus Drink)[11] probably does not afford a never-failing approach. A clan cousin of mine, who was beset by (the past experience of) difficult delivery, had chosen to abort each time she had a child. I took great pity on her. Seeing that she was fat and labored (with difficulty) doing her wifely chores, (I) knew that she was vacuous of qi and had been sitting for too long. (Therefore,) non-circulation of qi made the vacuity still worse. Because of qi vacuity in the mother, the child in the uterus was unable to move itself. It was necessary to supplement the qi of the mother. Then the child may become strong and easily delivered. (I) bid her to let me know when she was in her 5-6th months of pregnancy. Then (I) prescribed her tens of doses of *Zi Su Yin* (Perilla Drink) from the *Da Quan Liang Fang (Great Compendium of Fine Formulas)* with certain qi-supplementing medicinals added. Because of this, she gave birth to a baby boy extremely rapidly. Subsequently (I) have prescribed this formula with additions and subtractions in accordance with the mother's character and the seasons, and none of the takers have failed to respond well. (In other words,) the birthing mothers felt no pain during labor and were immune to disease. On this account, (I) have named this formula *Da Sheng San* (Expedite Delivery Powder).

---

[11] This consists of Fructus Citri Seu Ponciri (*Zhi Qiao*), Radix Scutellariae Baicalensis (*Huang Qin*) and Rhizoma Atractylodis Macrocephalae (*Bai Zhu*).

Chapter Three

Postpartum Conditions

So sublime and consummate is the feminine origin that tens of thousands of things arise and generate out of it. This is common knowledge. In newly birthed women, good blood is not necessarily depleted, foul blood is not necessarily accumulated, and the viscera and bowels are not necessarily cold. What use are medicinals? If only drink and food and everyday life are constantly adjusted and taken good care of, there is no possibility for disease to arise. Even if a disease arises, it is necessary to trace the cause and to determine which channel is involved. A qi disease should be treated by treating the qi, and a blood disease should be treated by treating the blood. How indiscreet are (the authors of) the *Ju Fang (Collected formulas)* that (they) should have designed the formula *Hei Shen San* (Black Spirit Powder)[1] with exaggerated indiscrimination! Each time I have met a birthing woman with no disease, I have told her to give up *Hei Shen San*, big eggs, salt, and various kinds of meat and to merely have gruel to nurse and balance herself. Occasionally, they are allowed to have a little yellow croaker which should be cooked sweet and bland. Not till a month after is the woman allowed to have a little meat. Even eggs should be broken and boiled well. This is greatly capable of nurturing the stomach and dispelling phlegm.

One postpartum regulating and balancing formula (consists of) Radix Angelicae Sinensis (*Dang Gui*), 1 *liang*, Rhizoma Ligustici Wallichii (*Chuan Xiong*), 1 *liang*, Radix Angelicae (*Bai Zhi*), Cortex Cinnamomi (*Guan Gui*), Rhizoma Curcumae Zedoariae (*E Zhu*), and Cortex Radicis Moutan (*Mu Dan Pi*), 5 *fen* for each of the above, Sclerotium Poriae Cocoris (*Fu Ling*), 1 *qian*, and Radix Glycyrrhizae (*Gan Cao*), 3 *fen*. Boil the above and take. In case of abdominal pain, add Rhizoma Corydalis Yanhusuo (*Xuan Hu Suo*). In case of fever, add Radix Scutellariae Baicalensis (*Huang Qin*) and Radix Bupleuri (*Chai Hu*). In case of inability to ingest food, add Fructus Amomi (*Suo Sha*) and Pericarpium Citri Reticulatae (*Chen Pi*).

Qing Hun San (Clear the *Hun* Powder) treats postpartum blood faintness: Lignum Sappanis (*Su Mu*), one half *liang*, Radix Panacis Ginseng (*Ren Shen*), 1 *liang*, and child's urine. Boil the above 3

---

[1] This consists of one half *sheng* of black soybeans (*Hei Dou*), winesoaked prepared Radix Rehmanniae (*Shu Di*), wine-processed Radix Angelicae Sinensis (*Dang Gui*), Cortex Cinnamomi (*Rou Gui*), blast-fried Rhizoma Zingiberis (*Pao Jiang*), mix-fried Radix Glycyrrhizae (*Zhi Gan Cao*), Radix Paeoniae Lactiflorae (*Shao Yao*), and Pollen Typhae (*Pu Huang*), 4 *liang* for each of the above. Powder; 2 *qian* per dose. Boil with wine and child's urine.

ingredients together with water and wine and take. Postpartum blood faintness is a gradual result of vacuity fire carrying blood (upward. One may also) burn Colla Cornu Cervi (*Lu Jiao*) to ash, grind very finely after fire toxins are liberated[2], brew in good wine, and pour down (the patient's throat). Consciousness will be regained in no time. This moves blood extremely quickly. Another method (consists of) cutting Herba Allii Tuberosi (*Jiu Cai*) very finely. Put into a bottle with a nozzle, pour hot vinegar (into it), seal (the opening of) the bottle promptly, and then insert the nozzle into the nose of the birthing woman. This cures visual dizziness.

Before delivery, the mother tends to suffer from (blood) stagnation and after delivery from (blood) vacuity. (Therefore,) postpartum, it is necessary to greatly supplement blood, and the various patterns that may ever arise should be treated as a branch. Postpartum, no disease whatever should be treated by effusing the exterior. To supplement vacuity postpartum, (use) Radix Panacis Ginseng (*Ren Shen*) and Rhizoma Atractylodis Macrocephalae (*Bai Zhu*), 1 *qian* each, Radix Scutellariae Baicalensis (*Huang Qin*), one half *qian* [Radix Astragali Membranacei {*Huang Qi*} in a {variant} edition {later editor}], Pericarpium Citri Reticulatae (*Chen Pi*), 5 *fen*, Rhizoma Ligustici Wallichii (*Chuan Xiong*), 5 *fen*, mix-fried Radix Glycyrrhizae (*Zhi Gan Cao*), 3 *fen*, and Radix Et Apex Angelicae Sinensis (*Dang Gui Shen Wei*), 5 *fen*. If there is heat, add 3 *fen* of dry Rhizoma Zingiberis (*Gan Jiang*) and 1 *qian* of Sclerotium Poriae Cocoris (*Fu Ling*).

To disperse postpartum blood clots, (use) Talcum (*Hua Shi*), 3 *qian*, Myrrha (*Mo Yao*), 3 *qian*, Resina Daemonoropsis Draconis (*Qi Lin Jie*), 2 *qian*, (and, if that is) not available, Cortex Radicis Moutan (*Mu Dan Pi*) instead, 1 *qian*. Powder the above and make into pills with vinegar paste. (To treat) postpartum retention of lochia, powder Feces Trogopterori Seu Pteromi (*Wu Ling Zhi*), make into pills with Massa Medica Fermentata (*Shen Qu*) paste, and take with Rhizoma Atractylodis Macrocephalae (*Bai Zhu*) and Pericarpium Citri Reticulatae (*Chen Pi*)

---

[2] Heated, *i.e.*, stir-fried, medicinals should be cooled in many cases before use. This cooling was believed to liberate fire toxins acquired in the process of heating.

soup. Resina Daemonoropsis Draconis and Feces Trogopterori Seu Pteromi are extremely good for dispersing postpartum blood clots.

(To treat) postpartum persistent flow of lochia with lower abdominal pain, mix Feces Trogopterori Seu Pteromi (*Wu Ling Zhi*) and powdered Rhizoma Cyperi Rotundi (*Xiang Fu Mo*) with vinegar (and make) into pills. In severe cases, add Semen Pruni Persicae (*Tao Ren*) with tips preserved. Postpartum abdominal pain with fever invariably reveals malign blood. It is imperative to expel it.

For postpartum fever, (use) *Si Wu Tang* (Four Materials Decoction) with additions and subtractions. For fever, counterflow retching, retching and vomiting, extremely abundant phlegm, and perspiration arising with vomiting 7-8 days after delivery as a result of great fright and scare, (use) *Ba Wu Tang* (Eight Materials Decoction) plus Radix Astragali Membranacei (*Huang Qi*) and, if accompanied by lower abdominal pain, Cortex Cinnamomi (*Gui*).

Postpartum wind stroke[3] should never in any case be treated as wind. For postpartum wind stroke, (use) Herba Seu Flos Schizonepetae Tenuifoliae (*Jing Jie Sui*) and stir-fried Radix Angelicae Sinensis (*Dang Gui*) in equal amounts. Powder; 2-3 *qian* per dose. Take with spraying-on-bean wine. [This also treats blood faintness. {later editor}] (But for) postpartum blood confounding and blood faintness, administer *Qing Hun San* (Clear the *Hun* Powder): Folium Lycopi Lucidi (*Ze Lan Ye*) and Radix Panacis Ginseng (*Ren Shen*), 2.5 *qian* each, Herba Seu Flos Schizonepetae Tenuifoliae (*Jing Jie*), 1 *liang*, Rhizoma Ligustici Wallichii (*Chuan Xiong*), one half *liang*, and Radix Glycyrrhizae (*Gan Cao*), 2 *qian*. Powder the above and take brewed with equal amounts of water and wine.

For postpartum abdominal pain or loose bowels, administer *Qing Liu Wan* (Green-Blue Six Pills) with a decoction of spleen-supplementing

---

[3]   This covers a wide spectrum of conditions, from colds to tetany. Its signs include, for example, fever, aversion to cold, dry retching, spontaneous sweating, headache, dyspnea, clenched jaw, loss of consciousness, and opisthotonos.

and blood-supplementing medicinals. For postpartum diarrhea, use Rhizoma Atractylodis Macrocephalae (*Bai Zhu*), Rhizoma Ligustici Wallichii (*Chuan Xiong*), Sclerotium Poriae Cocoris (*Fu Ling*), dry Rhizoma Zingiberis (*Gan Jiang*), Radix Scutellariae Baicalensis (*Huang Qin*), Talcum (*Hua Shi*), Pericarpium Citri Reticulatae (*Chen Pi*), and Radix Albus Paeoniae Lactiflorae (*Bai Shao Yao*). Stir-fry, slice, boil, and take.

Postpartum great fever necessarily requires dry Rhizoma Zingiberis (*Gan Jiang*). In a moderate case, use bland Sclerotium Poriae Cocoris (*Fu Ling*) to percolate the heat. No bitter, cold, exterior-effusing medicinals whatever are allowed to be used. It may be asked why dry Rhizoma Zingiberis is used in the presence of great heat? The answer is that this kind of heat is not repletion heat. (Dry ginger) is able to lead blood medicinals to generate blood. However, it should not be used alone but always in combination with yin-supplementing medicinals. This embodies the subtlety and intricacy by which nature is created and transformed. Who under heaven can produce things as they are but the supreme spirit?

Postpartum fever and aversion to cold is always ascribed to qi and blood vacuity. An insufficient pulse[4] on the left hand (justifies) more blood-supplementing medicinals than qi-supplementing ones, while an insufficient pulse on the right hand (justifies) more qi-supplementing medicinals than blood-supplementing ones. Postpartum aversion to cold and fever with abdominal pain requires expelling malign blood. Herba Leonuri Heterophylli (*Yi Mu Cao*) and Semen Leonuri Heterophylli (*Chong Wei Zi*) treat the various before delivery and postpartum diseases.

If *Si Wu Tang* is administered postpartum, Radix Albus Paeoniae Lactiflorae (*Bai Shao Yao*) should be deleted, since, with its sourness and cold, it fells the engendering and expediting qi. However, it may be used in a strong person at a young age.

---

[4]   A short, slow, choppy, weak, or thin pulse, for example, is an insufficient pulse.

For postpartum absence of breast milk, (use) Medulla Tetrapanacis Papyriferi (*Tong Cao*), Herba Dianthi (*Qu Mai*), Radix Platycodi Grandiflori (*Jie Geng*), Pericarpium Viridis Citri Reticulatae (*Qing Pi*), Radix Bupleuri (*Chai Hu*), Radix Angelicae (*Bai Zhi*), Radix Rubrus Paeoniae Lactiflorae (*Chi Shao Yao*), Radix Trichosanthis Kirlowii (*Tian Hua Fen*), Fructus Forsythiae Suspensae (*Lian Qiao*), and Radix Glycyrrhizae (*Gan Cao*). Boil in water and take sip by sip with the stomach still full after a meal (and) while stroking the breasts with one hand. If the child is lost, postpartum aversion to cold and fever (even) with absence of breast milk requires dispersing milk. Stir-fry and grind 2 *liang* of Fructus Germinatus Hordei Vulgaris (*Mai Ya*). Brew with boiled water and take as 4 doses.

Postpartum water swelling necessarily requires greatly supplementing qi and blood as the ruling (method) with a small amount of Rhizoma Atractylodis (*Cang Zhu*) and Sclerotium Poriae Cocoris (*Fu Ling*) as assistants in order that water should be disinhibited by itself. Postpartum, vanquished blood may take advantage of vacuity to pour into the channels and connecting vessels, eroding the soil[5] to develop water with puffy swelling in the four limbs, face, and eyes. (In that case), no matter what, do not use water qi conducting medicinals. First of all, administer 3-5 doses of *Wu Pi San* (Five Skins Powder) plus Cortex Radicis Moutan (*Mu Dan Pi*) and then 20-30 doses of *Tiao Jing San* (Balance the Menses Powder) from the *Ju Fang (Collected Formulas)*. This is effective. The blood will move by itself and the swelling will be dispersed. *Wu Pi San* (consists of) Radix Acanthopanacis (*Wu Jia Pi*), Cortex Radicis Lycii (*Di Gu Pi*), Cortex Rhizomatis Zingiberis (*Sheng Jiang Pi*), Cortex Radicis Mori Albi (*Sang Bai Pi*), and Cortex Sclerotii Poriae Cocoris (*Fu Ling Pi*)[6]. Add Cortex Radicis Moutan (*Mu Dan Pi*), boil, and take. *Tiao Jing San* (consists of) Radix Angelicae Sinensis (*Dang Gui*), Cortex Cinnamomi (*Rou Gui*), and Succinum (*Hu Bo*), 1 *qian* for each of the above, Secretio Moschi Moschiferi (*She Xiang*) and

---

[5]   The spleen is ascribed to earth and, for that reason, is sometimes called soil. Further, the flesh is also ascribed to earth or soil because it is ruled by the spleen.

[6]   The dosage should be 1 *qian*.

Herba Cum Radice Asari Sieboldi (*Xi Xin*), 5 *fen* each, Myrrha (*Mo Yao*), 1 *qian*, and Radix Rubrus Paeoniae Lactiflorae (*Chi Shao*), 1 *qian*. Powder the above, 5 *fen* (per dose), taken brewed with a small amount of Succus Zingiberis (*Jiang Zhi*) and warm wine.

For postpartum incessant (vaginal) bleeding, boil 3 *liang* of Pollen Typhae (*Pu Huang*) in 3 *sheng* of water down to 1 *sheng* and take. Postpartum blood faintness, oppression of the heart, and qi expiration[7], (use) Flos Carthami Tinctorii (*Hong Hua*), 1 *liang*. Grind the above into powder, divide into 2 doses, (ready) 2 cups of wine, boil 1 cup (with the medicinal), and take together with the other. In case of clenched jaw, pry (the teeth open) and pour (the decoction) down (the patient's throat). For various postpartum wind (patterns, use) half a cup of juice from Herba Xanthii Sibirici (*Cang Er Cao Zhi*). Take warm. This also treats toothache. For postpartum rash (the size of) chestnut kernels all over the body with fire-like fever, mash Semen Pruni Persicae (*Tao Ren*) by grinding with the lard of a pig killed in the last month and apply. For postpartum blood faintness bordering on expiration, (use) Rhizoma Pinelliae Ternatae (*Ban Xia*, and make) water pills the size of soybeans. Insertion (of these pills) into the nose brings resurrection immediately.

To precipitate a dead child or the placenta retained after delivery, (use) Secretio Moschi Moschiferi (*She Xiang*), one half *qian*, and powdered Cortex Cinnamomi (*Guan Gui Mo*), 3 *qian*. Take with warmed wine, and in no time, (the child or placenta) will be sent out as if pushed by a hand. A person had a miscarriage, but discharged no tangible things. (I, therefore, prescribed) *Si Wu Tang* plus Nitre (*Xiao*).

A woman, aged 18, who had difficult delivery and gave birth (only) after 7 days. (Then) she suffered from diarrhea, thirst, panting, a red face with purple macules, lower abdominal distention, and urinary stoppage. She was prescribed Radix Achyranthis Bidentatae (*Niu Xi*), Semen Pruni Persicae (*Tao Ren*), Radix Angelicae Sinensis (*Dang Gui*),

---

[7] Expiration or qi expiration means weak breath or loss of consciousness. It is also sometimes means death.

Flos Carthami Tinctorii (*Hong Hua*), Caulis Akebiae Mutong (*Mu Tong*), Talcum (*Hua Shi*), Radix Glycyrrhizae (*Gan Cao*), Rhizoma Atractylodis Macrocephalae (*Bai Zhu*), Pericarpium Citri Reticulatae (*Chen Pi*), and Sclerotium Poriae Cocoris (*Fu Ling*). These were boiled and taken with *Yi Mu Cao Gao* (Leonurus Paste)[8] No improvement was shown. Then (she was) prescribed Radix Achyranthis Bidentatae (*Du Niu Xi*) which was to be drunk after being boiled down to a paste. Approximately during the first watch in the night, (she) had a violent evacuation of a bucketful of stool. Her urination was freed and recovery ensued. (However,) because thirst arose, *Si Jun Zi Tang* (Four Gentlemen Decoction) was administered plus Radix Angelicae Sinensis (*Dang Gui*) and Radix Achyranthis Bidentatae (*Niu Xi*) taken brewed with *Yi Mu (Cao) Gao* (Leonurus Paste).

A woman who, as a result of postpartum fright and anxiety, contracted a disease of heavy-headedness, a sensation of a weight sagging in the cardiac region of the chest, susceptibility to fright, and trance and restlessness as if over the waves was prescribed Fructus Immaturus Citri Seu Ponciri (*Zhi Shi*), Fructus Germinatus Hordei Vulgaris (*Mai Ya*), Massa Medica Fermentata (*Shen Qu*), Bulbus Fritillariae (*Bei Mu*), Herba Cyperi Rotundi (*Hou Suo*), 1.5 *qian* for each of the above, Rhizoma Curcumae (*Jiang Huang*), 1.5 *qian*, Rhizoma Pinelliae Ternatae (*Ban Xia*), 2 *qian*, Semen Pruni Persicae (*Tao Ren*), Cortex Radicis Moutan (*Mu Dan Pi*), Semen Trichosanthis Kirlowii (*Gua Lou Zi*), 1 *qian* for each of the above, and Flos Carthami Tinctorii (*Hong Hua*), 5 *fen*. The above were powdered and made into pills with ginger cake. After administration, the substance in the chest disappeared but the susceptibility to fright and trance were not eliminated.

Then the prescription (consisted of) Cinnabar (*Chen Sha*), Tuber Curcumae (*Yu Jin*), and Rhizoma Coptidis Chinensis (*Huang Lian*), 3 *qian* for each of the above, Radix Angelicae Sinensis (*Dang Gui*), Radix Polygalae Tenuifoliae (*Yuan Zhi*), and Sclerotium Pararadicis Poriae Cocoris (*Fu Shen*), 2 *qian* for each of the above, Margarita (*Zhen Zhu*),

---

[8] This has only one ingredient, Herba Leonuri Heterophylli (*Yi Mu Cao*). Pound thoroughly and then simmer down to a paste; one half to 1 *qian* per dose.

Radix Panacis Ginseng (*Ren Shen*), Radix Glycyrrhizae (*Sheng Gan Cao*), and Rhizoma Acori Graminei (*Chang Pu*), 1.5 *qian* for each of the above, Calculus Bovis (*Niu Huang*), Fel Ursi (*Xiong Dan*), and Lignum Aquilariae Agallochae (*Chen Xiang*), 1 *qian* for each of the above, Flos Carthami Tinctorii (*Hong Hua*), 5 *qian*, gold foil (*Jin Bo*), 1 foil, and bile(-processed) Rhizoma Arisaematis (*Dan Xing*), 3 *qian*. The above were powdered and made into pills with the blood of a pig's heart. After administration, susceptibility to fright and trance improved.

Then the prescription (consisted of) Fructus Immaturus Citri Seu Ponciri (*Zhi Shi*), Rhizoma Pinelliae Ternatae (*Ban Xia*), Rhizoma Curcumae (*Jiang Huang*), Fructus Crataegi (*Shan Zha*), Massa Medica Fermentata (*Shen Qu*), Fructus Germinatus Hordei Vulgaris (*Mai Ya*), Pericarpium Citri Reticulatae (*Chen Pi*), and Fructus Gardeniae Jasminoidis (*Shan Zhi*), 5 *qian* for each of the above, and Rhizoma Atractylodis Macrocephalae (*Bai Zhu*), 1 *liang*. The above were powdered and made into pills with ginger cake. Taking this (formula) assisted the stomach in dispersing food and phlegm.

Then the prescription (consisted of) Calculus Bovis (*Niu Huang*), 2 *qian*, Rhizoma Acori Graminei (*Chang Pu*), 2.5 *qian*, Cinnabar (*Zhu Sha*) and Tuber Curcumae (*Yu Jin*), 3 *qian* each, Radix Polygalae Tenuifoliae (*Yuan Zhi*) and Succinum (*Hu Bo*), 2.5 *qian* each, Margarita (*Zhen Zhu*), Flos Carthami Tinctorii (*Hong Hua*), and Lignum Aquilariae Agallochae (*Chen Xiang*), 1 *qian* for each of the above, Rhizoma Coptidis Chinensis (*Huang Lian*), Radix Panacis Ginseng (*Ren Shen*), and bile(-processed) Rhizoma Arisaematis (*Dan Xing*), 5 *qian* for each of the above, and Radix Angelicae Sinensis (*Dang Gui*, no amount given). The above were powdered and made into pills with the blood of a pig's heart. Taking this (formula) settled the heart and calmed the spirit.

Then the prescription was Lacca Sinica Exiccata (*Gan Qi*), 3 *qian*, stir-fried till smoke was seen no longer, Rhizoma Sparganii (*San Leng*) and Rhizoma Curcumae Zedoariae (*E Zhu*), 7.5 *qian* each, Rhizoma Atractylodis (*Cang Zhu*), Pericarpium Viridis Citri Reticulatae (*Qing Pi*), Pericarpium Citri Reticulatae (*Chen Pi*), and iron dust (*Zhen Sha*), 1 *liang* for each of the above, Cortex Magnoliae Officinalis (*Hou Po*) and Radix Angelicae Sinensis (*Dang Gui*), one half *liang* each, and Rhizoma Cyperi

Rotundi (*Sheng Xiang Fu*), 2 *liang*. The above were powdered and made into pills with cake. If this formula had not been administered, a decoction of the following medicinals might have been administered after granary-emptying: Rhizoma Atractylodis Macrocephalae (*Bai Zhu*), 4 *qian*, Pericarpium Citri Reticulatae (*Chen Pi*), Radix Scutellariae Baicalensis (*Huang Qin*), Radix Albus Paeoniae Lactiflorae (*Bai Shao Yao*), and Rhizoma Cyperi Rotundi (*Xiang Fu Zi*), 2 *qian* for each of the above, Sclerotium Poriae Cocoris (*Fu Ling*), 1.5 *qian*, Radix Angelicae Sinensis (*Dang Gui*), Tuber Ophiopogonis Japonicae (*Mai Men Dong*), and Pericarpium Viridis Citri Reticulatae (*Qing Pi*), 1 *qian* for each of the above, Fructus Citri Seu Ponciri (*Zhi Qiao*), 6 *fen*, Lignum Aquilariae Agallochae (*Chen Xiang*) and Radix Glycyrrhizae (*Sheng Gan Cao*), 5 *fen* each. The above are to be divided into 6 doses. These (medicinals) eliminate chest fullness, clear heat, and percolate (water) with their bland flavor.

To treat child pillowing pain in women[9], boil Fructus Crataegi (*Tang Qiu Zi*) down to a thick decoction, brew with granulated sugar, and take. This offers instant effect. Whether before or after delivery, (this kind of pain) is usually due to blood vacuity.

A woman, nearly 30 years of age, who had given birth recently in the first (lunar) month of the year suffered from hypertonicity of the left leg and right hand, dyspnea, inability to sleep with black qi[10] appearing around the mouth, on the nose, and in the face, and a wiry pulse at the superficial level but choppy at the deep level (and) particularly so on the right hand. Suspecting that her spleen had been subjected to dampness, (I) asked whether she had been cruelly thirsty and had craved water during pregnancy. She replied that in the 3rd month of pregnancy she was fond of tea water. On account of this, (I) prescribed Radix Scutellariae Baicalensis (*Huang Qin*), Herba Seu Flos Schizonepetae Tenuifoliae (*Jing Jie*), Radix Saussureae Seu Vladimiriae (*Mu Xiang*),

---

[9] This refers to lower abdominal pain supposedly due to the fetus in the womb pillowing its head on that place.

[10] Qi here means complexion or color.

Talcum (*Hua Shi*), Rhizoma Atractylodis Macrocephalae (*Bai Zhu*), Semen Arecae Catechu (*Bing Lang*), Pericarpium Citri Reticulatae (*Chen Pi*), Rhizoma Atractylodis (*Cang Zhu*), Radix Glycyrrhizae (*Gan Cao*), and Radix Paeoniae Lactiflorae (*Shao Yao*). From the 5th dose onward, Semen Pruni Persicae (*Tao Ren*) was added. Another 4 doses were administered, and a sloshing sound was heard in the abdomen. Then the stools were evacuated full of crystal-like lumps, the largest being the size of the yolk of a hen's egg and the smallest being the size of tadpoles, tens in number. After that, hypertonicity was settled and dyspnea stopped. Then Herba Seu Flos Schizonepetae Tenuifoliae, Semen Arecae Catechu, and Talcum were deleted from the formula and Radix Angelicae Sinensis (*Dang Gui Shen*) and Sclerotium Poriae Cocoris (*Fu Ling*) were added to balance and rectify the blood vessels. Ten doses administered, recovery was achieved.

It has been observed that the urinary bladder damaged by a careless midwife may give rise to dribbling urination. A Madam Xu, who was young, contracted this condition. (I) thought that, since broken bones or flesh which are external injuries can be mended, it is also possible to heal the bladder even though it is inside the abdomen. On examination, her pulse was extremely vacuous. At this, I said to myself, that it is clear that those with difficult delivery are usually persons with blood vacuity and that, after experiencing difficult delivery, qi and blood vacuity become all the more serious. Therefore (I) prescribed the superlatively supplementing medicinals; Rhizoma Atractylodis Macrocephalae (*Bai Zhu*) and Radix Panacis Ginseng (*Ren Shen*) as the sovereigns and Semen Pruni Persicae (*Tao Ren*), Pericarpium Citri Reticulatae (*Chen Pi*), Radix Astragali Membranacei (*Huang Qi*), and Sclerotium Poriae Cocoris (*Fu Ling*) as the assistants. These were boiled in a soup of pig's or sheep's urinary bladders. (The patient) was bid to take this when extremely hungry. The dosage was 1 *liang* (of the medicinals). A month later, recovery was achieved. In all probability, qi and blood quickly succeeded in engendering, thus making it possible to put right the bladder. If there had been (even) a little delay, success would have been hardly possible.

Chapter Four

Diseases Ascribed to Qi & Blood

A woman suffered from dead blood, food accumulation, and phlegm rheum forming into lumps, sometimes stirring in the two lateral costal regions, sometimes causing abdominal rumbling and a clamoring stomach, with dizziness and generalized fever, (all this) occurring intermittently. [The formulas can be found in the chapter of lumps, {*i.e.*, Ch. 80, Bk. 5. later editor}]

To treat pain in the sea of blood[1] in women, (use) Radix Angelicae Sinensis (*Dang Gui*), 1 *qian*, Radix Glycyrrhizae (*Gan Cao*) and Radix Saussureae Seu Vladimiriae (*Mu Xiang*), 5 *qian* each, Rhizoma Cyperi Rotundi (*Xiang Fu*), 2 *qian*, and Radix Linderae Strychnifoliae (*Wu Yao*), 1.5 *qian*, all as one dose. Boil in water and take before a meal. For blood and qi pain in females, rub Rhizoma Curcumae Zedoariae (*E Zhu*) in wine and take .

A woman had a blood lump (in the abdomen) like a plate. It was impossible (for her) to take drastic medicinals because of pregnancy. (Therefore, I prescribed) Rhizoma Cyperi Rotundi (*Xiang Fu*), 4 *liang*, vinegar-boiled Semen Pruni Persicae (*Tao Ren*), 1 *liang*, skinned and tip-nipped, vinegar-boiled Pumice (*Hai Shi*), 2 *liang*, and Rhizoma Atractylodis Macrocephalae (*Bai Zhu*), 1 *liang*, (all the above) made into pills with Massa Medica Fermentata (*Shen Qu*) paste.

For unbearable blood and qi stabbing heart pain in females, (use) powdered Radix Saussureae Seu Vladimiriae (*Mu Xiang Mo*). Take brewed with wine. For blood and qi entering the brain giving rise to spinning and oppression of the head and inability to recognize people, (use) tender Folium Xanthii Sibirici (*Cang Er*). Dry in the shade,

---

[1] *I.e.*, the liver

powder, and take brewed with wine. If a woman suffers from abdominal pain caused by concretions and conglomerations or in case of qi attacking and block, use Rhizoma Cyperi Rotundi (*Xiang Fu*), 1 *liang*, boiled with vinegar, Radix Angelicae Sinensis (*Dang Gui*), 1 *liang*, blast-fried, skinned Rhizoma Sparganii (*Bai San Leng*), 1 *liang*, blast-fried Rhizoma Sparganii (*Hei San Leng*), 1 *liang*, Rhizoma Curcumae Zedoariae (*Hei E Zhu*), 1 *liang*, Myrrha (*Mo Yao*), Gummum Olibani (*Ru Xiang*), and Rhizoma Ligustici Wallichii (*Chuan Xiong*), 5 *qian* for each of the above, Folium Laminariae Japonicae (*Kun Bu*) and Herba Sargassi (*Hai Zao*), 1 *liang* each, both stir-fried, Semen Arecae Catechu (*Bing Lang*), 5 *qian*, Pericarpium Viridis Citri Reticulatae (*Qing Pi*), 1 *liang*, stripped of its pulp, Lacca Sinica Exiccata (*Gan Qi*), 5 *qian*, stir-fried till smoke is seen no more, and Radix Saussureae Seu Vladimiriae (*Mu Xiang*), Lignum Aquilariae Agallochae (*Chen Xiang*), and Fructus Amomi (*Suo Sha*), 5 *qian* for each of the above. Powder the above and make into pills the size of Chinese parasol tree seeds with paste made from vinegar; 60-70 pills per dose taken on an empty stomach either with boiled water or with boiled saltwater. Raw, cold, oily, and fatty substances are prohibited.

To treat blood and qi pain of the lower back and abdomen, (use) Radix Angelicae Sinensis (*Dang Gui*) and Rhizoma Corydalis Yanhusuo (*Xuan Hu*) in equal amounts. Powder coarsely; 3 *qian* per dose. Boil with 3 slices of ginger. A formula to treat all kinds of diseases caused by blood stasis (consists of) Rhizoma Cyperi Rotundi (*Xiang Fu*), 4 *liang*, boiled with vinegar, Semen Pruni Persicae (*Tao Ren*), calcined Concha Arcae Inflatae (*Wa Long Zi*), 2 *liang*, boiled in vinegar for 1 day and 1 night, and Cortex Radicis Moutan (*Mu Dan Pi*), wine-steamed Radix Et Rhizoma Rhei (*Da Huang*), Radix Angelicae Sinensis (*Dang Gui*), Rhizoma Ligustici Wallichii (*Chuan Xiong*), and Flos Carthami Tinctorii (*Hong Hua*), 5 *qian* for each of the above. Powder the above and make into pills with cake. For absence of menses with abdominal gripping pain, (use) Radix Aconiti (*Tai Wu*), 2 *liang*, Radix Angelicae Sinensis (*Dang Gui*), and Rhizoma Curcumae Zedoariae (*E Zhu*), 1 *liang* each. Powder and take 2 *qian* with wine on an empty stomach.

A woman's menses had been absent for 2 months with abdominal pain and fever. (For such a case,) the menstrual disorder will heal on its own when blood is moved and cooled. (In such cases, use) *Si Wu Tang* (Four Materials Decoction) plus Radix Scutellariae Baicalensis (*Huang Qin*), Flos Carthami Tinctorii (*Hong Hua*), Semen Pruni Persicae (*Tao Ren*), Rhizoma Cyperi Rotundi (*Xiang Fu*), Rhizoma Corydalis Yanhusuo (*Xuan Hu Suo*), and others.

A woman, more than 40 years of age, with a white facial complexion, a thin form, and quick temper, had had an overwhelming disappointment. Three months later, (she developed) a mass over the ribs in the flank below the breast which grew steadily to screen the heart accompanied by moderate pain, oppression of the diaphragm, food intake reduced by 3/4, a bitter taste in the mouth in the mornings, and the pulse on both hands faint, short, and choppy. I was aware of her absence of menses and dreaded treating her. I pondered till midnight. Since the woman was still strong enough to go out and see the doctor, dress, and speak as usual, I concluded that she still had stomach qi. Therefore, I prescribed Radix Panacis Ginseng (*Ren Shen*), Rhizoma Atractylodis Macrocephalae (*Bai Zhu*), Radix Angelicae Sinensis (*Dang Gui*), and Rhizoma Ligustici Wallichii (*Chuan Xiong*) with certain qi(-supplementing) medicinals as assistants to make a large dose. She was made to take (the decoction) 4 times that night. Externally, *Da Hu Bo Gao* (Great Succinum Paste)[2] was applied over the mass to prevent it from growing further. In more than a month, above 100 doses of supplementing formulas were administered, and her food intake had increased to half of her norm. (I) then continued with the same prescriptions. Another month passed and her pulse gradually became replenished. Again the same formula was administered together with approximately 100 pills of *Run Xia Wan* (Moisten & Precipitate Pills).[3]

---

[2] This consists of 1 *liang* each of powdered Radix Et Rhizoma Rhei (*Da Huang*) and slaked lime (*Po Xiao*). Pound garlic and this powder well into a paste and then apply as a dressing.

[3] There are four formulas with this same name. The most likely one is composed of 1 *jin* of Pericarpium Citri Rubri (*Ju Hong*), 4 *liang* of Radix Glycyrrhizae (*Gan Cao*), and one half *liang* of salt. Boil well, dry in the sun, and powder for use.

The menses lasted but 2 days, and the pulse improved by 4/5 in terms of the choppy (quality). It was already getting hot and the menstrual flow was always a purple color. (She) was administered the same preceding formula with Rhizoma Sparganii (*San Leng*) added and still taken with *Run Xia Wan* and, in addition, with 15 pills of *Yi Qing Wan* (Suppress the Green-Blue Pills) as assistant. After another month, the mass was found without notice to have reduced to half. Her menstrual flow returned to but half a day short of normal duration, and her food intake was restored to normal with good taste. Only eating meat gave her an unpleasant feeling. I bid her stop the medication and put off treatment till the next spring when wood would become effulgent.

In the sixth (lunar) month of the succeeding year, it was unexpectedly reported to me that, all of a sudden, the mass had arose again in a night and was 1½ fingers larger than the old. Her pulse was a little wiry and a little weaker on the left hand than on the right, but its rate was normal. According to her telling, the mass caused slight oppression when the stomach was full but stopped after food moved away (from the stomach). I thought that there must be some heart-stirring matter stimulating the mass. Inquiry confirmed (my supposition). Then (I) prescribed the previous formula with stir-fried Radix Scutellariae Baicalensis (*Huang Qin*) and stir-fried Rhizoma Coptidis Chinensis (*Huang Lian*) added in addition to small amounts of Caulis Akebiae Mutong (*Mu Tong*) and fresh Rhizoma Zingiberis (*Sheng Jiang*) as assistants and Rhizoma Sparganii (*San Leng*) deleted. These were boiled and taken with *Run Xia Wan*. Externally, *Hu Bo Gao* was applied. Half a month later, the menses appeared and the qi mass was dispersed. This was (a case of) lung metal being burned by fire, wood conquering earth to some extent, and earth being no longer able to transport. (Thus) the clear and the turbid interfered with one another. The remainder of the old mass had not been effaced because blood and qi had not yet been fully restored. Whenever even a dot of turbid qi lodged, the old mass would re-appear. Since blood and qi had been supplemented, the lungs were now free from evils. (Thus) wood qi yielded, earth qi was rectified, turbid qi was moved away, and the mass was dispersed.

A maiden servant, aged 40, had a reflective character and was liable to worry. Her menses was absent for 3 months and, in the middle of the lower abdomen, there was a mass gradually growing to the size of a cake. All the pulses were choppy and heavy but not altogether out of harmony. The mass caused acute pain when pressed, and, upon palpation, it seemed to be half a *cun* above (*i.e.*, around. I) had prescribed 4-5 times *Xiao Shi Wan* (Niter Pills)[4] from the *Qian Jin (Thousand [Pieces of] Gold)* when she unexpectedly informed me that her nipples had turned black and contained breast milk and that she must be pregnant. I told her that a choppy pulse was a definite argument against pregnancy. (I) prescribed 2 more doses and the pulse became a little too hollow. I realized that (my prescription) was too drastic. (Therefore,) I bid her to stop the formula and prescribed *Si Wu Tang* with Rhizoma Atractylodis Macrocephalae (*Bai Zhu*) in double amount and with Pericarpium Citri Reticulatae (*Chen Pi*) and mix-fried Radix Glycyrrhizae (*Zhi Gan Cao*) added as assistants. After 30 doses were taken, the pulse became replenished and (I) again administered *Xiao Shi Wan* 4-5 times.

(One day) she unexpectedly told me that the mass had shrunk a great deal. I bid her to stop the medication. Half a month later, the menses came with severe pain and nearly half a *sheng* of black blood precipitated, in which there were scores of pepper-corn-like clots. The mass reduced by half and she came for more medication. I explained to her that, as the mass was already broken, no attacking (formula) was needed any longer. (I assured her that) if only she abode by the prohibitions, the mass would disappear altogether with the menses the next month. Later, (my words) turned out to be true.

---

[4] This consists of 1 *liang* of Nitre (*Xiao Shi*), 1.5 *liang* of Radix Et Rhizoma Rhei (*Da Huang*), 3-7 pieces of Semen Crotonis (*Ba Dou*), and 3 *fen* each of Radix Praeparatus Aconiti Carmichaeli (*Fu Zi*) and blast-fried Rhizoma Zingiberis (*Pao Jiang*). Powder and make into pills with honey.

Chapter Five

Flooding & Leaking (*i.e.*, Uterine Bleeding)

Qi vacuity, blood vacuity, and blood heat (are the causes of) profuse uterine bleeding. (Li) Dong-yuan designed treatment methods (for this condition). However, he never spoke of heat but (solely) argued for cold (as the cause). Students should give new consideration (to his teaching). The classic states, Yin being vacuous and yang contending is spoken of as (blood) flooding. Looking from this (angle), the problem becomes quite clear.

In an emergency case, (one) should treat the branch (with) Radix Angelicae (*Bai Zhi*) soup brewed with Pulvis Fumi Carbonisati (*Bai Cao Shuang*). For a (more) severe case, carbonized Petriolus Trachycarpi (*Zong Lu Pi Hui*, brewed with Radix Angelicae soup) proves extremely remarkable. Later on, use *Si Wu Tang* (Four Materials Decoction) plus Radix Glycyrrhizae (*Gan Cao*) and fresh Rhizoma Zingiberis (*Sheng Jiang*) to balance and rectify. For a case due to taxation, use the simultaneously upbearing and supplementing medicinals, Radix Panacis Ginseng (*Ren Shen*) and Radix Astragali Membranacei (*Huang Qi*). For a case due to cold, (use) dry Rhizoma Zingiberis (*Gan Jiang*), while for a case due to heat, (use) Radix Scutellariae Baicalensis (*Huang Qin*). In case of excessively profuse bleeding, first administer 1 dose of powdered Feces Trogopterori Seu Pteromi (*Wu Ling Zhi Mo*). However, it is necessary to distinguish between cold and heat (for treatment to be effective). Feces Trogopterori Seu Pteromi is able not only to move (the blood) but (also) to check (bleeding).

A woman who suffered from flooding (*i.e.*, profuse uterine bleeding) was prescribed Radix Angelicae (*Bai Zhi*) and Rhizoma Cyperi Rotundi (*Xiang Fu*) in equal amounts. These were powdered and taken in the shape of pills.

Another formula (is made by) obtaining the raw skull of a dog. Burn (this) to ash with nature preserved and take brewed with wine or together with other medicinals. (Yet) another formula (is made by) cooking Feces Trogopterori Seu Pteromi (*Wu Ling Zhi*) till half done, powder, and take brewed with wine. In case of either qi vacuity or blood vacuity, use *Si Wu Tang* with Radix Panacis Ginseng (*Ren Shen*) and Radix Astragali Membranacei (*Huang Qi*) added.

Leaking (*i.e.*, dribbling uterine bleeding) is due to heat with vacuity. (For this, use) *Si Wu Tang* plus Rhizoma Coptidis Chinensis (*Huang Lian*). To treat (both) profuse and dribbling uterine bleeding, add Rhizoma Cyperi Rotundi (*Xiang Fu*), Radix Angelicae (*Bai Zhi*), Radix Scutellariae Baicalensis (*Huang Qin*), Gelatinum Corii Asini (*E Jiao*) and dry Rhizoma Zingiberis (*Gan Jiang*) to *Si Wu Tang*. There are also cases of profuse bleeding due to blood heat. (For these, use) large doses of *Jie Du Tang* (Resolve Toxins Decoction).[1] (And) to treat profuse bleeding, (one can) take *Si Wu Tang* brewed with carbonized Herba Xanthii Sibirici (*Cang Er Hui*).

There are cases of profuse and dribbling uterine bleeding caused by great fright and fear. (In this case,), it is usually qi that drives and precipitates (the blood. For this, use) Rhizoma Cyperi Rotundi (*Xiang Fu*), stir-fried till black, 1 *qian*, stir-fried Radix Albus Paeoniae Lactiflorae (*Bai Shao Yao*), 1 *qian*, Rhizoma Ligustici Wallichii (*Chuan Xiong*), 5 *fen*, prepared Radix Rehmanniae (*Shu Di Huang*), 1 *qian*, Radix Astragali Membranacei (*Huang Qi*), 5 *fen*, Rhizoma Atractylodis Macrocephalae (*Bai Zhu*), 1 *qian*, Radix Sanguisorbae (*Di Yu*), 5 *fen*, stir-fried Pollen Typhae (*Pu Huang*), 5 *fen*, Radix Panacis Ginseng (*Ren Shen*), 5 *fen*, Rhizoma Cimicifugae (*Sheng Ma*), 3 *fen*, and Radix Angelicae Sinensis (*Dang Gui*), 1 *qian*. Boil and take. In severe cases, take with 1 *qian* of carbonized Petriolus Trachycarpi (*Zong Mao Hui*) brewed in.

---

[1] This consists of Radix Et Rhizoma Rhei (*Da Huang*), Fructus Citri Seu Ponciri (*Qiao*), Fructus Forsythiae Suspensae (*Lian Qiao*), and Radix Glycyrrhizae (*Gan Cao*), 1 *qian* for each of the above, Rhizoma Coptidis Chinensis (*Huang Lian*), Radix Scutellariae Baicalensis (*Huang Qin*), stir-fried Fructus Gardeniae Jasminoidis (*Zhi Zi*), and Radix Ledebouriellae Sesloidis (*Fang Fen*), 3 *qian* for each of the above, Cortex Phellodendri (*Huang Bai*), and Radix Rubrus Paeoniae Lactiflorae (*Chi Shao Yao*), each 2 *qian*.

In case of incessant, profuse uterine bleeding, take one half *sheng* of Succus Radicis Cirsii Japonici (*Sheng Ji Gen Zhi*) and (the bleeding) will surely be stanched. Another formula (consists of) Rhizoma Cyperi Rotundi (*Xiang Fu*), char-fried till black and powdered, 2 *liang*, and Fructus Forsythiae Suspensae (*Lian Qiao*), 5 pieces, burnt to ash and powdered. Take 3 *qian* per dose together with some 10 pills of the *Ju Fang's (Collected Formulas) Zhen Ling Dan (Zhen* Miraculous Elixir)[2] brewed with a thin gruel (made from) old, mildewed millet. Another formula (is made by) powdering Radix Scutellariae Baicalensis (*Huang Qin*. Then) heat the iron weight of a steelyard and quench in wine. Take the powder with the wine. (And) for blood in the urine for no (identifiable) reason, powder Os Draconis (*Long Gu*) and take a square *cun* coinful brewed with wine.

---

[2]   *Zhen* is the name of one of eight *gua* or trigrams of the *Yi Jing (Classic of Change)*. It consists of a solid line, broken line, and a solid line reading up from the bottom. It symbolizes the east in orientation, thunder amongst natural phenomena, the emperor in society, spring in the seasons, and wood in the five phases and is one of the yang trigrams. Because of this, *Zhen* here means something flourishing and wonderful.

The processing method of these pills is as follows: Calcine Limonitum (*Yu Yu Liang*) with vinegar repeatedly till it disintegrates. Then stir-fry. Process Hematitum (*Dai Zhe Shi*) the same way as above and put these 2 ingredients together with Fluoritum (*Zi Shi Ying*) and Hallyositum Rubrum (*Chi Shi Zhi*) into a pot which is then covered and sealed closely with salt mud. Burn 10 *jin*, i.e., 5 kg of charcoal and heat the pot till all the charcoal is used up. Bury the pot in the ground for 2 days. Then mix the processed ingredients with 2 *liang* of ground Gummum Olibani (*Ru Xiang*), 2 *liang* of ground Myrrha (*Mo Yao*), 2 *liang* of ground Feces Trogopterori Seu Pteromi (*Wu Ling Zhi*), and 1 *liang* of water-ground Cinnabar (*Zhu Sha*). Finally make into pills the size of Gorgon fruit seeds with cooked glutinous rice.

Chapter Six

Strangury & Inhibited Urination

For all kinds of incessant strangury, inhibited voiding of dark-colored urine with pain, and fetus pressing on the bladder, wash and extract 1 *he* of juice from tender Herba Oxalis Corniculatae (*Suan Jiang Cao*), mix with 1 *he* of wine, and take on an empty stomach. This is very remarkable. For the disease of inhibited urination, (use) Radix Achyranthis Bidentatae (*Niu Xi*), 5 *liang*. Boil in 3 *sheng* of wine down to one half *sheng*, remove the dregs, and then take as 3 doses. This also treats blood bind with hardness and pain (in the genitals. But) for blood strangury, obtain a handful of Caulis Bambusae In Taeniis (*Zhu Ru*), boil, and take while warm on an empty stomach. It offers an effect instantly.

Chapter Seven

Fetus Pressing on the Bladder

Fetus pressing on the bladder may be caused by refraining from urinating for (too long a) time. (For this, use) powdered Talcum (*Hua Shi*). Take 2 *qian* brewed with Bulbus Allii Fistulosi (*Cong Tou*) soup.

A woman, aged 40, suffered from fetus pressing on the bladder in the 9th month of pregnancy with inability to void for as long as 3 days and sudden swelling of the lower legs. (The suffering was so great) she could not stand living any longer. Her pulse was slender and choppy on the right hand but a little less inharmonious on the left. This was impugned to overeating and the fetal ligation being damaged by qi and thus unable to lift itself up. Consequently, (the fetus) sagged down to press on the bladder which was turned to one side, and the qi, blocked by (the bladder), became tense. Therefore, the portal did not allow exit (of urine). This is largely the case with the disorder of fetus pressing on the bladder. Accordingly, I designed a formula to supplement the blood and nurture the qi. It does not only put right the fetal ligation, enabling (it) to lift itself up, but prevents its sagging. Only thus is a cure justifiably guaranteed.

(The formula consisted of) Radix Panacis Ginseng (*Ren Shen*), Radix Et Apex Angelicae Sinensis (*Dang Gui Shou Wei*), Radix Albus Paeoniae Lactiflorae (*Bai Shao Yao*), Rhizoma Atractylodis Macrocephalae (*Bai Zhu*), Pericarpium Citri Reticulatae (*Chen Pi*) with its white inner layer preserved, mix-fried Radix Glycyrrhizae (*Zhi Gan Cao*), Rhizoma Pinelliae Ternatae (*Ban Xia*), and fresh Rhizoma Zingiberis (*Sheng Jiang*). These were boiled to a thick decoction and administered for 4 doses. At daybreak next day, the dregs of these 4 doses were boiled together as 1 dose. (The patient) was forced to take it all at once and then her throat was probed to provoke vomiting of the decoction. After urination was totally unblocked with voiding of black water, Pericarpium Arecae (*Da Fu Pi*), Fructus Citri Seu Ponciri (*Zhi Qiao*), fresh Folium Allii Fistulosi (*Qing Cong Ye*), and Fructus Amomi (*Suo Sha Ren*) were added to the above formula. Twenty doses were administered to prevent before delivery and postpartum vacuity. It turned out later that (she was) safe through delivery and stayed healthy afterward.

A woman who was pregnant suffered from the disorder of the fetus pressing on the bladder. The pulse on both hands was a little choppy and, when pressure was applied, was wiry. It was a little less inharmonious on the left. This (condition) was contracted from worry and frustration. A choppy pulse indicates scant blood with abundant qi, and a wiry pulse indicates rheum. With scant blood, the fetus is weak, unable to lift itself up, while in the presence of abundant qi and rheum, the middle burner is not clear and constricts. Conscious of where to escape from, the fetus must go down and, therefore, is inclined to sag. (She was) prescribed *Si Wu Tang* (Four Materials Decoction) plus Radix Panacis Ginseng (*Ren Shen*), Rhizoma Atractylodis Macrocephalae (*Bai Zhu*), Rhizoma Pinelliae Ternatae (*Ban Xia*),

Pericarpium Citri Reticulatae (*Chen Pi*), Radix Glycyrrhizae (*Sheng Gan Cao*), and fresh Rhizoma Zingiberis (*Sheng Jiang*). These were boiled and taken on an empty stomach. Subsequently, her throat was probed with fingers to provoke vomiting of the decoction. A little while later, when her qi calmed down, another dose was administered. The same (administration was performed) once again the next morning. (After) 8 doses had been taken, recovery ensued. (I) was not certain whether this method held good or not and later tried it on several more persons, also achieving effect (in these). Its concluding results, (however,) remain to be further proved.

Chapter Eight

Red & White Vaginal Discharge

(This) is governed by damp heat. The red is ascribed to blood, and the white is ascribed to qi and to phlegm. Vaginal discharge and dribbling uterine bleeding both may be (due to) accumulated phlegm in the stomach flowing down to seep into the urinary bladder. (In this case,) it is appropriate to apply upbearing. (Unfortunately,) few realize this.

In fat persons, phlegm is the common (cause. For this, use) Pumice (*Hai Shi*), Rhizoma Pinelliae Ternatae (*Ban Xia*), Rhizoma Arisaematis (*Nan Xing*), Rhizoma Atractylodis (*Cang Zhu*), stir-fried Cortex Phellodendri (*Huang Bai*), Rhizoma Ligustici Wallichii (*Chuan Xiong*), Cortex Cedrelae (*Chun Gen Pi*), and Pulvis Indigonis (*Qing Dai*). In thin persons, the disorder of vaginal discharge is rarely seen and, if they do contract it, it is ascribed to heat. (For this, use) Cortex Phellodendri (*Huang Bai*), Talcum (*Hua Shi*), Cortex Cedrelae (*Chun Pi*), Rhizoma Ligustici Wallichii (*Chuan Xiong*), Pumice (*Hai Shi*), and Pulvis Indigonis (*Qing Dai*). Take in the shape of pills. Another formula (is made by) powdering Semen Zanthoxyli Bungeani (*Jiao Mu*) and taking with thin gruel.

In severe cases, ejection must be applied to treat the upper in order to upraise the qi, while *Er Chen Tang* (Two Aged Decoction) plus Rhizoma Atractylodis (*Cang Zhu*) and Rhizoma Atractylodis Macrocephalae (*Bai Zhu*) must be administered to treat the lower. In addition, Concha Arcae Inflatae (*Wa Long Zi*) must be introduced.

From another point of view, red and white vaginal discharge are both ascribed to blood, but they should be classified either as discharge from the large or from the small intestine. One formula (consists of) char-frying and powdering Fructus Viticis Negundae (*Huang Jing Zi*). This is to be taken with thin gruel. It treats white vaginal discharge and heart pain as well.

Among Master Luo's methods, either *Shi Zao Tang* (Ten Dates Decoction)[1], *Shen You Wan* (God Bless Pills), or *Yu Zhu San* (Jade Candle Powder)[2] are applicable. It is not allowed to administer drastically attacking (medicinals). However, repletion cases do allow for this. For blood vacuity, (use) *Si Wu Tang* (Four Materials Decoction) with additions and subtractions. In case of qi vacuity, administer from time to time Radix Panacis Ginseng (*Ren Shen*), Pericarpium Citri Reticulatae (*Chen Pi*), and Rhizoma Atractylodis Macrocephalae (*Bai Zhu*). In case of severe dampness, use *Gu Chang Wan* (Secure the Intestines Pills): Cortex Ailanthi Altissimae (*Chun Gen Bai Pi*), 2 *liang*, and stir-fried Talcum (*Hua Shi*), 1 *liang*. Powder, grind, and make into pills with gruel. (In case of) stirring ministerial fire, add a small amount of stir-fried Cortex Phellodendri (*Huang Bai*) to the medicinals.

---

[1] This consists of Flos Daphnis Genkwae (*Yuan Hua*), Radix Euphorbiae Kansui (*Gan Sui*), and Herba Euphorbiae Pekinensis (*Da Ji*), all in equal amounts; 1 *qian* per dose. Boil with 10 dates.

[2] This consists of Radix Angelicae Sinensis (*Dang Gui*), Rhizoma Ligustici Wallichii (*Chuan Xiong*), prepared Radix Rehmanniae (*Shu Di*), Radix Albus Paeoniae Lactiflorae (*Bai Shao*), Radix Et Rhizoma Rhei (*Da Huang*), Mirabilitum (*Mang Xiao*), and Radix Glycyrrhizae (*Gan Cao*), all in equal amounts. Powder and take; 8 *qian* per dose.

In case of efflux[3], add Os Draconis (*Long Gu*) and Hallyositum Rubrum (*Chi Shi Zhi*). In case of stagnation[3], add Flos Althaeae Rosae (*Kui Hua*. If the patient is) impetuous in temper, add Rhizoma Coptidis Chinensis (*Huang Lian*). In cold months, introduce a small amount of Rhizoma Zingiberis (*Jiang*) and Radix Praeparatus Aconiti Carmichaeli (*Fu Zi*). One should follow the opportunity to adapt to change. (In any case,) one should refrain from thick flavored (food) by all means.

Another formula consists of Rhizoma Alpiniae Officinari (*Liang Jiang*), Radix Paeoniae Lactiflorae (*Shao Yao*), and Rhizoma Coptidis Chinensis (*Huang Lian*), 2.4 *qian* for each of the above, (all) burnt to ash. Mix with 1 *liang* of Cortex Cedrelae (*Chun Pi*), powder all the above, make into pills with gruel, and take with thin gruel.

For vaginal discharge due to phlegm qi, (use) Rhizoma Atractylodis (*Cang Zhu*), Rhizoma Cyperi Rotundi (*Xiang Fu*), Talcum (*Hua Shi*), Concha Mactrae Quadrangularis (*He Fen*), Rhizoma Pinelliae Ternatae (*Ban Xia*), and Sclerotium Poriae Cocoris (*Fu Ling*).

A woman suffered from white vaginal discharge with the complication of painful wind. (She was prescribed) Rhizoma Pinelliae Ternatae (*Ban Xia*), Sclerotium Poriae Cocoris (*Fu Ling*), Rhizoma Ligustici Wallichii (*Chuan Xiong*), Pericarpium Citri Reticulatae (*Chen Pi*), Radix Glycyrrhizae (*Gan Cao*), Rhizoma Atractylodis (*Cang Zhu*), rice water soaked Rhizoma Arisaematis (*Nan Xing*), wine-washed and sun-dried Cortex Phellodendri (*Huang Bai*), and wine-washed Radix Achyranthis Bidentatae (*Niu Xi*).

A woman suffered in the upper from head wind with runny nose. (For this she was prescribed) Rhizoma Arisaematis (*Nan Xing*), Rhizoma Atractylodis (*Cang Zhu*), wine-processed Radix Scutellariae Baicalensis (*Huang Qin*), Flos Magnoliae Liliflorae (*Xin Yi*), and Rhizoma Ligustici Wallichii (*Chuan Xiong*. In addition, she suffered) in the lower from white vaginal discharge. (For this, she was prescribed) Rhizoma

---

[3] Because red and white vaginal discharge is ascribed to the intestines, efflux here refers to loose bowels while stagnation to dry, bound stools or constipation.

Arisaematis (*Nan Xing*), Rhizoma Atractylodis (*Cang Zhu*), Cortex Phellodendri (*Huang Bai*), char-fried Rhizoma Atractylodis Macrocephalae (*Bai Zhu*), Talcum (*Hua Shi*), Rhizoma Pinelliae Ternatae (*Ban Xia*), and Concha Ostreae (*Mu Li*).

A formula for pink and white vaginal discharge (consists of) Plastrum Testudinis (*Gui Ban*) and Fructus Gardeniae Jasminoidis (*Zhi Zi*), 2 *liang* each, stir-fried Cortex Phellodendri (*Huang Bai*), 1 *liang*, Radix Albus Paeoniae Lactiflorae (*Bai Shao Yao*), 7.5 *qian*, Rhizoma Cyperi Rotundi (*Xiang Fu*), 5 *qian*, dry Rhizoma Zingiberis (*Gan Jiang*), 2.5 *qian*, Fructus Corni Officinalis (*Shan Zhu Yu*), Radix Sophorae Flavescentis (*Ku Shen*), and Cortex Cedrelae (*Chun Pi*), 5 *qian* for each of the above, and Bulbus Fritillariae (*Bei Mu*), 3.5 *qian*. Powder the above and make into pills with wine paste. (While) a formula for red and white vaginal discharge (consists of) wine-roasted Plastrum Testudinis (*Gui Ban*), 2 *liang*, stir-fried Cortex Phellodendri (*Huang Bai*), 1 *liang*, stir-fried Rhizoma Zingiberis (*Jiang*), 1 *qian*, and Fructus Gardeniae Jasminoidis (*Zhi Zi*), 2.5 *qian*. Powder the above and make into pills with wine paste. Take twice daily, 70 pills per dose.

A formula for white vaginal discharge during pregnancy (consists of) Rhizoma Atractylodis (*Cang Zhu*), 3 *qian*, Radix Angelicae (*Bai Zhi*), 2 *qian*, stir-fried Rhizoma Coptidis Chinensis (*Huang Lian*), 1.5 *qian*, stir-fried Radix Scutellariae Baicalensis (*Huang Qin*), 3 *qian*, stir-fried Cortex Phellodendri (*Huang Bai*), 1 *qian*, Radix Albus Paeoniae Lactiflorae (*Bai Shao Yao*), 2.5 *qian*, stir-fried Cortex Cedrelae (*Chun Gen Pi*), 1.5 *qian*, and Fructus Corni Officinalis (*Shan Zhu Yu*), 1.5 *qian*. (However,) to treat white vaginal discharge due to bound phlegm, use *Xiao Wei Dan* (Minor Stomach Elixir), several pills taken when half empty/half full. When depression and accumulation is opened, it is appropriate to administer a supplementing formula (consisting of) Rhizoma Atractylodis Macrocephalae (*Bai Zhu*), 1 *liang*, Radix Scutellariae Baicalensis (*Huang Qin*), 5 *qian*, Flos Rubrus Et Albus Althaeae Rosae (*Hong Bai Kui Hua*), one half *qian* each, and Radix Albus Paeoniae Lactiflorae (*Bai Shao Yao*), 7.5 *qian*. Powder the above, steam in the shape of cake, and make into pills; 20 pills (per dose) taken with a decoction of *Si Wu Tang* on an empty stomach. White vaginal discharge requires Talcum

(*Hua Shi*), Rhizoma Arisaematis (*Nan Xing*), Cortex Phellodendri (*Huang Bai*), and Radix Scutellariae Baicalensis (*Tiao Qin*).

Gu Chang Wan (Secure the Intestines Pills) treat damp qi diarrhea, blood in the stools, and white vaginal discharge. They are used to dry dampness below when treating illness requiring removal of old accumulations from the stomach and intestines, but it should not be used alone. They are administered with a particular decoction in accordance with the disease. Powder (the ingredients) together with Cortex Cedrelae (*Chun Gen Pi*) and make into pills with paste. Another formula, cool and drying, (consists of) Cortex Cedrelae (*Chun Bai Pi*), 4 *liang*, and Talcum (*Hua Shi*), 2 *liang*, powdered and made into pills with paste.

To treat white vaginal discharge due to damage by the seven affects with a rapid pulse, (use) stir-fried Rhizoma Coptidis Chinensis (*Huang Lian*), 5 *qian*, wine-steamed Cacumen Biotae Orientalis (*Bian Bai*), 5 *qian*, stir-fried Cortex Phellodendri (*Huang Bai*), 5 *qian*, Rhizoma Cyperi Rotundi (*Xiang Fu*), 1 *liang*, stir-fried with vinegar, Rhizoma Atractylodis Macrocephalae (*Bai Zhu*), 1 *liang*, Radix Angelicae (*Bai Zhi*), 2 *qian*, ash-burnt with nature preserved, stir-fried Cortex Cedrelae (*Chun Pi*), 2 *liang*, and Radix Albus Paeoniae Lactiflorae (*Bai Shao Yao*), 1 *liang*. Make the above into pills with gruel and take.

To treat red and white vaginal discharge caused by overwhelming dampness, (use) Rhizoma Atractylodis (*Cang Zhu*), 1 *liang*, stir-fried with salt, Radix Albus Paeoniae Lactiflorae (*Bai Shao Yao*), 1 *liang*, Fructus Citri Seu Ponciri (*Zhi Qiao*), 3 *qian*, stir-fried Cortex Cedrelae (*Chun Bai Pi*), 3 *liang*, roasted, dry Rhizoma Zingiberis (*Gan Jiang*), 2 *qian*, Radix Sanguisorbae (*Di Yu*), 5 *qian*, Radix Glycyrrhizae (*Gan Cao*), 3 *qian*, and stir-fried Talcum (*Hua Shi*), 1 *qian*. Powder the above, make into pills with gruel, and take with thin gruel.

To treat women with red and white vaginal discharge, first administer *Si Wu Tang* with additions and subtractions. Then ash-burn a lacquered (wood) article with nature preserved, powder, and take 5 *qian* with limeless wine on an empty stomach. One dose can check (the discharge). Another formula treats years old persistent disease of vaginal discharge: Radix Albus Paeoniae Lactiflorae (*Bai Shao Yao*), 3 *liang*, and dry Rhizoma Zingiberis (*Gan Jiang*), 5 *qian*. Stir-fry the above till yellow and powder; 2 *qian* (per dose) taken on an empty stomach with thin gruel. (To treat) vaginal disease of dribbling discharge of five colors with marked emaciation, burn Carapax Amydae (*Bie Jia*) till yellow, powder, and take 2 *qian* on an empty stomach with thin gruel.

A fat woman suffered from vaginal discharge. (She was prescribed) Pumice (*Hai Shi*), 4 *liang*, Rhizoma Arisaematis (*Nan Xing*), Radix Scutellariae Baicalensis (*Huang Qin*), Rhizoma Atractylodis (*Cang Zhu*), and Rhizoma Cyperi Rotundi (*Xiang Fu*), 3 *liang* for each of the above, Rhizoma Atractylodis Macrocephalae (*Bai Zhu*), Cortex Cedrelae (*Chun Gen Pi*), and Massa Medica Fermentata (*Shen Qu*), 1.5 *liang* for each of the above, Radix Angelicae Sinensis (*Dang Gui*), 2 *liang*, Radix Angelicae (*Bai Zhi*), 1.2 *liang*, Rhizoma Ligustici Wallichii (*Chuan Xiong*), 1.25 *liang*, Sclerotium Poriae Cocoris (*Fu Ling*), 1.5 *liang*, Radix Albus Paeoniae Lactiflorae (*Bai Shao Yao*) and Cortex Phellodendri (*Huang Bai*), 1 *liang* each, and Talcum (*Hua Shi*), 1.5 *liang*. Powder the above and make into pills with Massa Medica Fermentata (*Shen Qu*) paste.

The disease of vaginal discharge is governed by damp heat. Flos Albus Althaeae Rosae (*Bai Kui Hua*) treats white vaginal discharge, while Flos Rubrus Althaeae Rosae (*Hong Kui Hua*) treats red vaginal discharge. Copious and enduring vaginal discharge disease requires upbearing medicinals used in combination with damp heat (removing) ones. If (the patient) is emotionally agitated, add Rhizoma Coptidis Chinensis (*Huang Lian*).

Chapter Nine

Conception

Inability to conceive in fat (persons) is caused by the fat within the body blocking the uterus and leading to amenorrhea. (To treat this,) use phlegm-conductors. Inability to conceive in thin (persons) is a result of the uterus being devoid of blood and (consequent) inability of the essence qi to concentrate. (To treat this,) use blood-nurturing and yin-nurturing formulas such as *Si Wu Tang* (Four Materials Decoction).

My niece, replete both in form and qi, did not bear a child until rather long after marriage. After administration of *Shen Xian Ju Bao Dan* (Immortal Collect Treasure Elixir)[1], *yong ju* broke out on (her) back. Her condition was quite dangerous. Her pulse was found to be large, rapid, and choppy. (I) promptly prescribed more than a 100 doses of *Si Wu Tang* with additions and subtractions to supplement yin blood. Luckily she had a sturdy physique and was easy to salvage. If she had had a flimsy physique, it would have been too late to regret.

---

[1] This consists of Myrrha (*Mo Yao*), Succinum (*Hu Po*), roasted Radix Saussureae Seu Vladimiriae (*Mu Xiang*), and Radix Angelicae Sinensis (*Dang Gui*), 1 *liang* for each of the above, Cinnabar (*Zhu Sha*) and Secretio Moschi Moschiferi (*She Xiang*), 1 *qian* each, and Gummum Olibani (*Ru Xiang*), 1 *fen*. Powder the above and make into pills the size of Chinese parasol tree seeds with honey; 20 pills per dose.

Chapter Ten

Sterilization

Boil 1 *sheng* of fermented wheat flour in 5 *sheng* of limeless wine down to 3.5 *sheng*. Filter out the dregs with a silk cloth and then take as 3 doses. On the eve of the menstrual flow, take 1 dose in the evening, another at the 5th watch, and a third at daybreak the next morning. Then the menses comes, and sterilization will be realized for (one's) entire life.

Chapter Eleven

Miscellaneous Diseases in Females

Generally speaking, the various miscellaneous diseases are treated in the same way as for males.

For genital swelling in females, grate and stir-fry one half *jin* of Fructus Immaturus Citri Seu Ponciri (*Zhi Shi*) till hot, wrap with an old cloth, and iron (the affected part with it). Change when it becomes cool. For malign sores in the genitals, apply good Sulphur (*Liu Huang*) powder as a dressing. It is extremely remarkable. In case of wet papules, acetate of lead (*Qian Fen*) may be added. Another formula (is made by) powdering and applying Alumen (*Ku Fan*). This is also applicable for genital sores in males.

For pain in the secret part in females, iron with stir-fried salt wrapped in a black cloth. For cold genitals, powder Flos Syzygii Aromatici (*Mu Ding Xiang*), fill in a gauze bag the size of a small finger, insert into the genitals, and healing will follow. A medicinal to warm the inside (consists of) powdered Fructus Cnidii Monnieri (*She Chuang Zi Mo*). Mix evenly with a small amount of wheat flour (into a pill) the size of a date, wrap with a silk cloth, and insert (into the vagina).

For feces exiting through the urethra, (use) *Wu Ling San* (Five *Ling* Powder) to separate and disinhibit water and grains. For dream communication with ghosts, take powdered Cornu Cervi (*Lu Jiao Mo*) brewed with wine. For hair not black in females, smear (the hair with) Oleum Musae Basjoo (*Ba Jiao You*). For wind[1] itching and dormant papules with incessant itching in females, powder Herba Xanthii Sibirici (*Cang Er*) and Semen Platycaryae Strobilaceae (*Hua Guo Zi*) and take 2-3 *qian* with spraying-on-beans wine.

According to a discussion in the *Da Quan Liang Fang (Great Compendium of Fine Formulas)*, dream communication with ghosts in females is ascribed to vacuity of the viscera and bowels and the spirit failing to keep to (its abode). Therefore, ghost qi is given a chance to cause disease. The manifestations include not wanting to see people, (talking to oneself) as if in a dialogue, and sometimes talking and laughing but sometimes weeping and lamenting. A slow and hidden or bird-pecking pulse image is an indicator of disease caused by ghost evils. In addition, the pulse keeping on with no intermissions and not knowing the measure of its number with no change in complexion are also its indicators. Ghosts are intangible, but when one acts on them, one can communicate (with them). This is because, if (one's) thinking is perversive, the ghost will be acted upon and summoned up. It clings to evil qi and enters the human body to link with the spirit. Therefore, it sometimes appears in dreams. Usually, the treatment method is to employ evil-dispelling medicinals like Cinnabar (*Zhu Sha*), Secretio Moschi Moschiferi (*She Xiang*), Realgar (*Xiong Huang*), Ramulus Euonymi Alati (*Gui Jian*), and tiger skull (*Hu Tou Gu*). These can offer a cure.

---

[1]　Wind is often used not only to describe the cause of disease but also to suggest rapid or sudden breaking out of rash.

Book Eight

Pediatrics

Master Qian's formulary is the forefather of formulas for children. His formula designs are exceedingly good. If physicians are able to abide by and make (appropriate) expansion and reduction of them, they will never fail to be efficacious when used. In treating miscellaneous disorders in children, the medicinals used are usually the same as for adults, only the dosage should be smaller. Therefore, there is no point dwelling on (this further). In suckling infants, there is usually abundant damp heat. In infants, food accumulation and phlegm heat, a disease due to milk damage, is, by and large, a disease of the liver and spleen. Because infants are easily angered, liver disease is the commonest of all (in them). The liver is never anything but superabundant, while the kidneys are never anything but insufficient. There are two causes of disease (in children). One is overeating, and the other is warmth. Infants are subject to cold in winter months and to heat in summer months.

Chapter One

Neonatal (Diseases)

In utero, there are foul substances in the mouth of the child. After delivery, before the (first) cry is issued, (the mouth) should be cleaned by swabbing with the fingers wrapped with silk cloth. Then (they should be) treated with the (following) Radix Glycyrrhizae (*Gan Cao*) method. Freshly born, the child should not be fed with breast milk (for the time being). Obtain a piece of Radix Glycyrrhizae (*Gan Cao*), 1 finger long, roast it till crisp, and boil in 2 *he* (of water). Then dab (the decoction) into the child's mouth and the child will soon eject the foul fluids in the chest. Concha Corbiculae Fulmineae (*Xian Qiao*) can check (this vomiting if necessary). Later on, when (the child) is hungry and thirsty, administer 2 more doses. (However,) administer no more than 1 *he* (even) if the foul fluids are not totally vomited. After ejection of the foul fluids, the child will grow intelligent and be free from disease.

Three days after birth, (it is time) to open the child's stomach and intestines with a thick fluid made of ground rice. If the newborn is made to melt a small amount of beans in the mouth, about 2 beans given at short intervals, it can be fed with breast milk 6-7 days (after birth). After birth, boil a pig's gallbladder in 5 *sheng* of water down to 1 *sheng*, (allow to) settle, and bathe the child with the clear solution, and it will be immune to sores and scabies. If, after birth, the child does not suckle milk and (has) urinary stoppage, boil 3 *he* of breast milk down to a thick decoction in a silver or stone vessel with 1 *cun* of Bulbus Allii Fistulosi (*Cong*) sliced into 4 pieces. Pour (this) down (its throat) and cure will follow in no time.

If, on the 7th day after birth, the child suddenly contracts umbilical wind[1] with pursed lips[2], not one out of a hundred cases survives. At the juncture, there are invariably millet-like papules over the tongue. Scrape these with a silk cloth wet with warm, boiled water, and the child will be saved. This works wonders. After birth, under the tongue there may (also) be a membrane like seeds of a pomegranate attaching to the root of the tongue, making the child unable to speak. This can be taken off, (during which process) there may arise slight bleeding. In case of incessant bleeding, absorb this with Crinis Carbonisatus (*Fa Hui*) or apply a mixture of wine with powdered Alum (*Bai Fan*) and soot from under the cauldron.

For clenched jaw on the 10th day after birth, finely grind a small amount of Calculus Bovis (*Niu Huang*), brew with 1 character of Succus Bambusae (*Dan Zhu Li*), mix with pig's milk and wine, and drop into the child's mouth. If, within a 100 days after birth, wind damage[3] arises in the child with nasal congestion which does not yield to medication, this is the result of exposure to blowing wind after bathing. Brew powdered Rhizoma Arisaematis (*Tian Nan Xing*) in ginger juice and apply on the fontanel. Retain this till the nasal congestion has disappeared.

---

[1] This refers to tetanus in newborns. It is so called because it is believed to be caused by invasion of wind through the navel. Its manifestations mainly include clenched jaw, arched back, rigid nape of the neck, sensitivity to light, sound, and touch, and, in extreme cases, choking which eventually leads to death.

[2] This is a typical and critical sign of umbilical wind. It means clenched jaw but suggests more, including, for example, refusal to suckle milk, spasms of the lips, and inability to speak.

[3] *I.e.*, flu or colds

Chapter Two

Acute & Chronic Fright Wind

Zhen Jing Wan (Settle Fright Pills) settle (susceptibility to) fright, tranquilize the spirit, abate heat, transform phlegm, and check cough. (They consists of) Margarita (*Zhen Zhu*), 1 *qian*, Succinum (*Hu Po*), 3 *qian*, gold foil (*Jin Bo*), 10 foils, bile(-processed) Rhizoma Arisaematis (*Dan [Nan] Xing*), 5 *qian*, Calculus Bovis (*Niu Huang*), 2 *qian*, Secretio Moschi Moschiferi (*She Xiang*), 5 *fen*, dry Succus Bambusae Textilis (*Tian Zhu Huang*) and Realgar (*Xiong Huang*), 3 *qian* each, and Cinnabar (*Chen Sha*), 3.5 *qian*. Powder the above and make into pills the size of Chinese parasol tree seeds with ginger paste; 6 pills per dose taken with a soup of Herba Menthae (*Bo He*) with ginger and honey.

Da Tian Nan Xing Wan (Major Arisaematis Pills) treat acute and chronic fright wind with drooling, tidal fever, spasms, clenched teeth, drawing between the mouth and eyes, etc: (These consist of) bile(-processed) Rhizoma Arisaematis (*Dan Xing*), 5 *qian*, Rhizoma Gastrodiae Elatae (*Tian Ma*), Radix Panacis Ginseng (*Ren Shen*), Radix Ledebouriellae Sesloidis (*Fang Feng*), 2.5 *qian* for each of the above, Calculus Bovis (*Niu Huang*) and Gummum Olibani (*Ru Xiang*), 1 *qian* each, Cinnabar (*Zhu Sha*), 2 *qian*, dried Buthus Martensi (*Quan Xie*), 14 pieces, Secretio Moschi Moschiferi (*She Xiang*), 1 *qian*, and Borneolum (*Nao Zi*), 5 *fen*. Make into pills the size of Semen Euryalis Ferocis (*Qian Shi*) with heated honey. Take with a soup of Herba Seu Flos Schizonepetae Tenuifoliae (*Jing Jie*) and Herba Menthae (*Bo He*).

Acute and chronic fright wind with fever, clenched jaw, deep-lying heat in the palms of the hands and the soles of the feet, phlegm heat, coughing with phlegm, and phlegm dyspnea (require) the combined use of a heavy formula for ejection, a small dose of *Gua Di San* (Melon Pedicle Powder), with powdered Radix Sophorae Flavescentis (*Ku Shen*) and Semen Phaseoli Calcarati (*Chi Xiao Dou*) taken with sour pickle, and afterwards, *Tong Shen San* (Communicate with the Divinity

Powder) taken in the shape of honey pills. To calm wind, Anoplophora Chinensis (*Sang Nu*) on the mulberry tree can occasionally be administered after being dried in the shade and ground. This kind of Anoplophora is yellow and white compared with that (occurs) on the poplar tree.

To treat fright (wind) in infants with heat, (use) Radix Panacis Ginseng (*Ren Shen*), Sclerotium Poriae Cocoris (*Fu Ling*), Radix Albus Paeoniae Lactiflorae (*Bai Shao Yao*), wine-fried Rhizoma Atractylodis Macrocephalae (*Bai Zhu*), and fresh Rhizoma Zingiberis (*Sheng Jiang*). Boil and take. In summer months, add Rhizoma Coptidis Chinensis (*Huang Lian*), Radix Glycyrrhizae (*Sheng Gan Cao*), and Folium Bambusae (*Zhu Ye*).

There are formulas current that can treat both kinds of fright (wind), but (one) should not by any means make use of them unwarrantedly. Fright (wind) is classified as two patterns. One is acute fright (wind) governed by hot phlegm requiring drainage. The other is chronic fright which is governed by spleen vacuity and, more often than not, ends in death. (In that case,) the required treatment is to supplement the spleen. In acute (cases), the only appropriate treatment is to downbear fire, precipitate phlegm, and nurture the blood. In chronic (cases), the only remedy is *Zhu Sha An Shen Wan* (Cinnabar Calm the Spirit Pills) whose modifications can be sought among blood(-supplementing) medicinals. (Li) Dong-yuan explains that, for chronic fright (wind), one should first replenish spleen earth before dissipating wind evils.

Hei Long Wan (Black Dragon Pills) treat the two patterns of acute and chronic fright wind. (They consist of) bile(-processed) Rhizoma Arisaematis (*Dan Xing*), 1 *liang*, Chlorite Schist (*Meng Shi*), 1 *liang*, Cinnabar (*Chen Sha*), 3 *qian*, Resina Alois (*Lu Hui*), and dry Succus Bambusae Textilis (*Tian Zhu Huang*), 5 *qian* for each of the above, ash-burnt Scolopendra Subspinipes (*Wu Gong*), 1.5 *qian*, Bombyx Batryticatus (*Jiang Can*), 5 *qian*, and Pulvis Indigonis (*Qing Dai*), 5 *qian*. Mix the above with Radix Glycyrrhizae (*Gan Cao*) paste into pills the size of cock's heads. Take after dissolving in a soup of ginger, honey, and Herba Menthae (*Bo He*) for acute fright wind or in a soup of Radix

Platycodi Grandiflori (*Jie Geng*) and Rhizoma Atractylodis Macrocephalae (*Bai Zhu*) for chronic fright wind.

A child under 1 month old bordering on fright (wind) is bound to die once struck by wind. Smear the five hearts[1] with Cinnabar (*Zhu Sha*) mixed with fresh water into a thick solution. This is miraculously efficacious.

For fright wind, obtain 1 intact scorpion, strip it of its feet, and roast with 4 leaves of Herba Menthae (*Bo He*) as a wrapping over a fire till the leaves are parched. Grind together with the leaves and administer as 4 doses with boiled water. For wind drooling[2] in adults, this is taken all as 1 dose. For subjection to fright in the womb developing into fright (wind) under 1 month old, finely grind Cinnabar (*Zhu Sha*), mix with a small amount of Calculus Bovis (*Niu Huang*) and pig's milk into a thin fluid, and then put into the mouth (of the child). This is even more remarkable if Secretio Moschi Moschiferi (*She Xiang*) is also added. Incipient fright (wind) requires *Fang Feng Dao Chi San* (Ledebouriella Conduct the Red Powder). This consists of dry Radix Rehmanniae (*Sheng Gan Di Huang*), Rhizoma Ligustici Wallichii (*Chuan Xiong*), Caulis Akebiae Mutong (*Mu Tong*), Radix Ledebouriellae Sesloidis (*Fang Feng*), and Radix Glycyrrhizae (*Gan Cao*), all in equal amounts. Take 3 *qian* boiled with Folium Bambusae (*Zhu Ye*). Afterwards, administer *Ning Shen Gao* (Tranquilize the Spirit Paste, which consists of) cored Tuber Ophiopogonis Japonicae (*Mai Men Dong*), 1 *liang*, pure Secretio Moschi Moschiferi (*She Xiang*), 1 *qian*, Sclerotium Poriae Cocoris (*Fu Ling*), and Cinnabar (*Zhu Sha*), 1 *liang* each. Powder the above and make into small cakes with heated honey. Take after dissolving in Herba Menthae (*Bo He*) soup before sleep; 1 cake per night.

---

[1] The five hearts referred to here are the centers of the soles, palms, and the midpoint between the eyebrows. One should note that according to another interpretation, the five hearts include the cardiac region instead of the midpoint between the eyes.

[2] This refers to tetany with arched back rigidity, clenched jaw, and drooling due to wind stroke.

Ancient physicians have warned that fright spasms in infants are usually a heat pattern and that they will become a crushing pattern if, once they are met, fright wind medicinals are (recklessly) employed, such as Radix Aconiti Coreani (*Bai Fu Zi*), dried Buthus Martensi (*Quan Xie*), Bombyx Batryticatus (*Jiang Can*), and Radix Aconiti (*Chuan Wu*). Later a formula for fright wind was developed. It merely includes *Dao Chi San* (Conduct the Red Powder)[3] plus Radix Rehmanniae (*Di Huang*) and Radix Ledebouriellae Sesloidis (*Fang Feng*). The administration of 3 doses can conduct away evil heat from the heart channel and spasm will be checked. After that, administer *Ning Shen Gao*. This is miraculously efficacious.

Duo Ming San (Snatch Back Life Powder) can treat acute and chronic fright wind with a tide of phlegm and drool congested and stagnated in the throat, (thus) presenting an imminent threat to life. Its administration never fails to offer a cure, and its miraculous efficacy cannot be over-valued. (It is made as follows.) Put 1 *liang* of Chlorite Schist (*Qing Meng Shi*) into a crucible together with 1 *liang* of Mirabilitum (*Yan Xiao*, and) heat till red-hot over a charcoal fire until the Mirabilitum is no longer observable. (Then) take out and grind when the medicinals turn cool and to a golden color. For acute fright wind with phlegm and fever, take brewed with undiluted Succus Herbae Menthae (*Bo He Zhi*). For chronic fright wind with spleen vacuity, grind *Qing Zhou Bai Wan Zi* (Qing Zhou [County] White Pellets)[4], boil into a thin paste, mix with honey, and take (with *Duo Ming San*).

To treat acute and chronic fright wind on the point of death, a moxa method can also be taught. Moxa at the thumb between the nail and the flesh 3 cones of Folium Artemisiae Argyii (*Ai*), each the size of the

---

[3] This consists of Radix Rehmanniae (*Sheng Di*), Radix Glycyrrhizae (*Gan Cao*), and Caulis Akebiae Mutong (*Mu Tong*), all in equal amounts; 3 *qian* per dose boiled with Folium Bambusae (*Zhu Ye*).

[4] This consists of boiled, water-washed Rhizoma Pinelliae Ternatae (*Sheng Ban Xia*), 7 *liang*, Radix Aconiti (*Sheng Wu Tou*), one half *liang*, Rhizoma Arisaematis (*Sheng Nan Xing*), 3 *liang*, and Radix Aconiti Coreani (*Sheng Bai Fu Zi*). After a complicated process, these are made into pills with glutinous rice.

end of a chopstick, on the left hand for males and the right for females. At the same time, administer Cinnabar (*Chen Sha*), Herba Menthae (*Bo He*), Calomelas (*Qing Fen*), one half *qian* for each of the above, dried Buthus Martensi (*Quan Xie*), 1 piece stripped of its feet, and Semen Crotonis (*Ba Dou*), 1 piece, completely de-oiled. Powder together; one half character per dose. Boil crumbles of glutinous rice cake and take brewed with (the powder). In case of clenched teeth, pry them (open) and pour down (the patient's throat). When drool and phlegm issue through the mouth with diarrhea, cure is effected. If the vomiting and diarrhea is followed by chronic fright wind with clouded sleep and tugging and slackening of the hands and feet, grind into powder 5 *qian* of *Jin Ye Dan* (Gold Fluid Elixir)[5] and 3 *qian* of *Qing Zhou Bai Wan Zi*, administering 3 *fen* with raw ginger and thin gruel.

For fright wind, both the mother and the child may take *Si Jun Zi Tang* (Four Gentlemen Decoction) combined with *Er Chen Tang* (Two Aged Decoction) plus Herba Menthae (*Bo He*), Rhizoma Gastrodiae Elatae (*Tian Ma*), Herba Cum Radice Asari Sieboldi (*Xi Xin*), and dried Buthus Martensi (*Quan Xie*. While) *Ri Yu Dan* (Sun & Moon Elixir) treats acute and chronic fright wind in infants. (It is composed of) Cinnabar (*Zhu Sha*), 1 *liang*, Calomelas (*Qing Fen*), 1 *liang*, and Scolopendra Subspinipes (*Wu Gong*), 1 piece. Powder the above and make into pills the size of broomcorn millet with the insects inside the stalks of Herba Artemisiae Apiaceae (*Qing Hao*), 1 pill for 1 year of age taken with breast milk.

For acute and chronic fright wind in infants with congested and exuberant hot phlegm and fever, (use) Folium Menthae (*Bei Bo He Ye*) and Calcareous Spar (*Han Shui Shi*), 1 *liang* each, Pulvis Indigonis (*Qing Dai*), Bombyx Batryticatus (*Bai Jiang Can*), and Cinnabar (*Chen Sha*), 1 *qian* for each of the above, stir-fried dried Buthus Martensi (*Quan Xie*), 2 pieces, stir-fried Fructus Gleditschiae Sinensis (*Zhu Ya Zao Jiao*) 5 *fen*,

---

[5] The processing is as follows: Grind 10 *liang* of Sulphur (*Liu Huang*) in water, put in a ceramic container which is sealed with a mixture of water and Hallyositum Rubrum (*Chi Shi Zhi*), heat for 7 days over a small fire, grind when it is cool, and make into pills with cake.

Fructus Sophorae Japonicae (*Huai Jiao*), 5 *fen*, and Radix Ledebouriellae Sesloidis (*Fang Feng*), one half *qian*. Powder the above and pour down (the child's throat) with Medulla Junci Effusi (*Deng Xin*) soup mixed with breast milk.

For arched back rigidity and forward staring eyes caused by fright, pour down (the child's throat) Rhizoma Arisaematis (*Nan Xing*), Rhizoma Pinelliae Ternatae (*Ban Xia*), Succus Bambusae (*Zhu Li*), and Succus Zingiberis (*Jiang Zhi*) and moxa *Yin Tang* (M-HN-3).[6] In case of death from acute or chronic fright wind, chew 1 piece of Flos Syzygii Aromatici (*Mu Ding Xiang*) in the mouth, collect a small amount of crystallized urine (*Ren Zhong Bai*), mix these with the blood of the middle finger of the mother, and rub onto the teeth (of the child) and resurrection will follow in no time. Another method (consists of) applying the blood of a white, black-boned cock on the lips and resurrection will follow instantly.

Chapter Three

Gan Disease[1]

To treat *gan* disease with an enlarged belly, (use) Rhizoma Picrorrhizae (*Hu Huang Lian*), 1 *qian*, to eliminate fruit accumulation; vinegar-soaked Resina Ferulae Asafoetidae (*A Wei*), 1.5 *qian*, to eliminate meat accumulation; Massa Medica Fermentata (*Shen Qu*), 2 *qian*, to eliminate food accumulation; stir-fried Rhizoma Coptidis Chinensis (*Huang Lian*), 2 *qian*, to remove heat accumulation; and Secretio Moschi Moschiferi

---

[6]   Hall of Impression

[1]   This is one of the four major problems in children: fright wind, *gan*, measles, and polio. Its main manifestations include yellow facial complexion, emaciation, brittle hair, enlarged belly with prominent green-blue veins, and languor.

(*She Xiang*), 4 grains. Powder the above and make into pills the size of Semen Cannabis Sativae (*Ma Zi*) with pig bile; 20 pills per dose taken with Rhizoma Atractylodis Macrocephalae (*Bai Zhu*) soup.

Xiang Chan Wan (Fragrant Toad Pills) treat *gan* and are able to disperse worm accumulation, food accumulation, meat accumulation, and abdominal distention. (They consist of) blast-fried Rhizoma Sparganii (*San Leng*), blast-fried Rhizoma Curcumae Zedoariae (*Peng Zhu*), Pericarpium Viridis Citri Reticulatae (*Qing Pi*), Pericarpium Citri Reticulatae (*Chen Pi*), stir-fried Massa Medica Fermentata (*Shen Qu*), stir-fried Fructus Germinatus Hordei Vulgaris (*Mai Ya*), Radix Gentianae Scabrae (*Long Dan Cao*), and Semen Arecae Catechu (*Bing Lang*), 5 *qian* for each of the above, Rhizoma Picrorhizae (*Hu Huang Lian*), Fructus Meliae Toosendanis (*Chuan Lian Zi*), Fructus Quisqualis Indicae (*Shi Jun Zi*), and Rhizoma Coptidis Chinensis (*Huang Lian*), 4 *qian* for each of the above, Rhizoma Atractylodis Macrocephalae (*Bai Zhu*), 1 *liang*, Radix Saussureae Seu Vladimiriae (*Mu Xiang*), 2 *qian*, and dried toad (*Gan Chan*), 5 pieces. Powder the above (except for) the toads which are to be cooked well and then pounded before being mixed with the other (medicinals). Make with vinegar paste into pills the size of millet; 20 pills per dose taken with thin gruel.

Fei Er Wan (Fatten Children Pills) treat various kinds of *gan* accumulation disease[2] in children. (They consist of) Resina Alois (*Lu Hui*), ground separately, 3 *qian*, Rhizoma Picrorhizae (*Hu Huang Lian*), 3 *qian*, stir-fried Massa Medica Fermentata (*Shen Qu*), 4 *qian*, stir-fried Rhizoma Coptidis Chinensis (*Huang Lian*), Rhizoma Atractylodis Macrocephalae (*Bai Zhu*), and stir-fried Fructus Crataegi (*Shan Zha*), 5 *qian* for each of the above, and stir-fried Fructus Praeparatus Ulmi Macrocarpae (*Wu Yi*), 2.5 *qian*. Powder the above and make into pills the size of millet with pig bile; 15 pills per dose.

---

[2] In particular, this treats spleen *gan* which is characterized by a withered yellow facial complexion, emaciated flesh, somnolence, fatigue, frequent fever, impaired appetite, enlarged belly with glomus and fullness, frequent abdominal pain, food cravings, a perverse appetite for earth and coal, occasional vomiting and diarrhea of roundworms, and fishy stinking stools.

Lu Hui Wan (Aloe Pills) treat the five kinds of *gan*[3] with marked emaciation, worm gnawing, stomachache, and abdominal distention. (They consist of) Resina Alois (*Lu Hui*), Rhizoma Picrorhizae (*Hu Huang Lian*), and Radix Saussureae Seu Vladimiriae (*Mu Xiang*), 2.5 *qian* for each of the above, Semen Arecae Catechu (*Bing Lang*), 2 pieces, Pulvis Indigonis (*Qing Dai*), 2 *qian*, Fructus Praeparatus Ulmi Macrocarpae (*Wu Yi*), 1 *qian*, Secretio Moschi Moschiferi (*She Xiang*), 1 character, Fructus Quisqualis Indicae (*Shi Jun Zi*), 20 pieces, dry toad (*Gan Chan*), 1 piece, roasted with wine, and Pericarpium Viridis Citri Reticulatae (*Qing Pi*), stripped of its pulp and cut, 2.5 *qian*, parch-fried with 20 pieces of Semen Crotonis (*Ba Dou*) which are removed afterwards. Make the above into pills the size of broomcorn millet with pig bile; 15 pills per dose taken with thin gruel.

To treat *gan* yellowing (of the face) with food accumulation, (use) Rhizoma Atractylodis Macrocephalae (*Bai Zhu*), Rhizoma Coptidis Chinensis (*Huang Lian*), and carbonized Fructus Crataegi (*Ku Shan Zha*), all in equal amounts. Powder and make into pills with Massa Medica Fermentata (*Shen Qu*) paste; 15 (per dose) taken with boiled water. For *gan* mouth[4], administer 5 doses of *Wu Gan Bao Tong Wan* (Five *Gan*

---

[3] *I.e.*, liver, heart, lung, spleen, and kidney *gan*. Liver *gan* is manifested by emaciation, green-blue facial complexion, rocking of the head, rubbing of the eyes, night blindness, dry eyes, enlarged belly with prominent green-blue veins, purplish green-blue nails, and thin, green-blue stools or blood or pus in the stools. Heart *gan* is manifested by generalized heat, red facial complexion, spontaneous sweating, thirst, sores in the mouth, vexation of the heart with chest oppression, grinding of the teeth, no appetite, emaciation, and vomiting or diarrhea. Lung *gan* is characterized by qi counterflow coughing, dry skin with brittle hair, constant running of clear nasal mucus, aversion to cold with fever, sores in the nose and mouth, inflated abdomen, diarrhea of rice water like stool, reduced intake of milk and food, fishy smell in the mouth, and emaciation. The distinctive signs of kidney *gan* include skinny emaciation, bleeding gums, a foul smell in the mouth, reduced appetite, efflux diarrhea, and, in the extreme, ulceration of the anus and prolapse of the rectum. For more information about spleen *gan*, see Note 2 above.

[4] *I.e.*, sores in the mouth due to *gan*

Protect Children Pills)[5] with Fructus Praeparatus Ulmi Macrocarpae (*Wu Yi*), 2 *qian*, Fructus Quisqualis Indicae (*Shi Jun Zi*) and Cortex Radicis Meliae Azedarachis (*Ku Lian Gen*), 3 *qian* each. Powder together and make into pills the size of Semen Cannabis Sativae (*Ma Zi*) with gruel; 30 pills per dose taken with thin gruel. Another formula (is made) on the 5th day of the 5th (lunar) month of the year by obtaining Venum Bufonis Bufonis (*Xia Mo*). Mix (this) with powdered Cinnabar (*Zhu Sha*) and Secretio Moschi Moschiferi (*She Xiang*, and make) into pills the size of Semen Cannabis Sativae (*Ma Zi*); 1 pill (per dose) taken with breast milk on an empty stomach.

For *gan* diarrhea, administer powdered Hallyositum Rubrum (*Chi Shi Zhi*), one half *qian*, taken brewed with thin gruel. For brain *gan*[6] with itching of the eyebrows, tufted hair, and a yellow colored, emaciated face, drop the bile of the crucian carp (*Ji Yu*) into the nose (of the child). An effect follows in 3-5 days. For running horse *gan*[7], burn Periostracum Bombycis Mori (*Can Tui Zhi*) with nature preserved, mix with a small amount of Secretio Moschi Moschiferi (*She Xiang*), powder, make into pills with honey, and apply (as dressing). It is still

---

[5] This consists of Rhizoma Coptidis Chinensis (*Huang Lian*), char-fried Caput Anguilae Japonicae (*Bai Shan Tou*), replaceable by stir-fried Fructus Praeparatus Ulmi Macrocarpae (*Wu Yi*), Radix Gentianae Scabrae (*Long Dan Cao*), Realgar (*Xiong Huang*), Pericarpium Viridis Citri Reticulatae (*Qing Pi*), Galla Rhi Chinensis (*Wu Bei Zi*), stir-fried Feces Vespertilionis Superrantis (*Ye Ming Sha*), Cortex Radicis Meliae Azedarachis (*Ku Lian Gen*), stir-fried cocoon of Monema Flavescens (*Tian Jiang Zi*), Rhizoma Picrorhizae (*Hu Huang Lian*), Secretio Moschi Moschiferi (*She Xiang*), Pulvis Indigonis (*Qing Dai*), Fel Ursi (*Xiong Dan*), and Resina Alois (*Lu Hui*), 1 *liang* for each of the above, and Caput Bufonis Bufonis (*Chan Tou*), roasted till yellow, 1 piece. Powder the above and make into pills the size of Semen Cannibis Sativae (*Ma Zi*) with glutinous rice .

[6] This refers to *gan* with the complications of sores on the head, fever, loss of hair, baldness, dry nose and mouth, and dull eyes.

[7] This is an acute purulent lesion consisting of rapidly developing ulceration of the gums and membranes of the lips and mouth which may lead to blackening of the face with necrosis and even perforation of the cheeks.

better if a small amount of Alumen (*Ku Fan*) is added. For tooth gan[8], (use) Os Draconis (*Long Gu*), 3 *qian*, Calomelas (*Qing Fen*), 5 *fen*, Aerugo (*Tong Lu*), 5 *fen*, Secretio Moschi Moschiferi (*She Xiang*), 1 character, and Alumen (*Ku Fan*), 2 *qian*. Grind the above finely and apply. For tooth gan with ulceration of the mouth and gums, (use) Calomelas (*Qing Fen*), 1 *qian*, Alumen (*Ku Fan*), 2 *qian*, and powdered Cortex Phellodendri (*Huang Bai Mo*), 3 *qian*. First, wash clean the affected area with a swab of cloth wet with water and then apply the medicinals dry.

A child from a rich family, aged 14, had a yellow face and was good at eating (*i.e.*, had a large appetite) with rapid hungering (after eating). He ate nothing but meat. (He) had had diarrhea for 1 month and the pulse on both hands was large. Nonetheless, he was not very fatigued. If this were ascribed to damp heat, there would be fatigue and low food intake, but, on the contrary, his form was thin with large food intake and, in addition, absence of thirst. This must be dysentery caused by pathogenic worms. Examination of the stool revealed that this was indeed caused by roundworms. I instructed that a worm-eliminating formula be administered instead of accumulation-eliminating formulas (and) assured (his parents of his) recovery.

(However,) between spring and summer the next year, (he) had diarrhea with no abdominal pain but a dry mouth. This was a result of treating worms without treating *gan* the year before. Accordingly, (I) administered a formula for eliminating *gan* heat, (*i.e.,*) *Bai Zhu Tang*, boiled into a thick decoction. Three days later, the diarrhea was improved by half. Seeing that he was exceedingly thin, I instructed (him) to use Rhizoma Atractylodis Macrocephalae (*Bai Zhu*) as the sovereign and Radix Paeoniae Lactiflorae (*Shao Yao*) as the minister, together with Rhizoma Ligustici Wallichii (*Chuan Xiong*), Pericarpium Citri Reticulatae (*Chen Pi*), Rhizoma Coptidis Chinensis (*Huang Lian*), and Rhizoma Picrorhizae (*Hu Huang Lian*). These were to be mixed with a small amount of Resina Alois (*Lu Hui*) into pills and taken with boiled *Bai Zhu Tang*. Meat and sweets were prohibited, and recovery was expected to come by itself 3 years later.

---

[8] This refers to ulceration of the gums in *gan*.

Chapter Four

Pox & Papules

(These) are divided into qi vacuity and blood vacuity (types) and should be supplemented. In case of qi vacuity, use Radix Panacis Ginseng (*Ren Shen*), Rhizoma Atractylodis Macrocephalae (*Bai Zhu*), Sclerotium Poriae Cocoris (*Fu Ling*), and Radix Glycyrrhizae (*Gan Cao*) plus toxin-resolving medicinals. For blood vacuity, (use) *Si Wu Tang* (Four Materials Decoction) plus toxin-resolving medicinals. Wine-fried Rhizoma Coptidis Chinensis (*Huang Lian*) is a toxin-resolving medicinal. Once red spots appear, *Sheng Ma Ge Gen Tang* (Cimicifuga & Pueraria Decoction)[1] is prohibited because it is capable of making the exterior vacuous by effusing.

Vomiting, diarrhea, and low food intake are (signs of) internal repletion, and supplementation in case of internal repletion gives rise to *yong*. (While) sunken, hidden pox which are a dull whitish gray color show exterior vacuity. (For this,) use (Zhang) Zi-he's method of burning Pulvis Praeparatus Glycyrrhizae (*Ren Zhong Huang*).[2] In case of extremely black and sunken (pox, adopt the method of) burning human feces. Red, brilliant, prominent (pox) show exterior repletion. Administration of exterior(-supplementing) medicinals in case of exterior repletion leads to ulceration with refusal to form scabs. (While) the dual arising of vomiting and diarrhea with sunken, hidden (pox) shows dual vacuity of the exterior and interior.

---

[1] This consists of Rhizoma Cimicifugae (*Sheng Ma*), Radix Puerariae Lobatae (*Ge Gen*), Radix Paeoniae Lactiflorae (*Shao Yao*), and mix-fried Radix Glycyrrhizae (*Zhi Gan Cao*), all in equal amounts. Powder, boil, and take; 4 *qian* per dose.

[2] Simply burn Pulvis Praeparatus Glycyrrhizae (*Ren Zhong Huang*) with nature preserved and take with wine.

At the outset of pox sores or before their eruption, it is appropriate to administer to anyone who contracts them the following formula. It can reduce the number of pox if they would (otherwise) be numerous or improve (the condition) if it would (otherwise) be severe. The formula consists of a 3 *cun* long (piece) of Fructus Luffae Cylindricae (*Si Gua*, taken) near (*i.e.*, in front of) the base. Burn this to ash together with Luffa seeds and skin with nature preserved, powder, and take mixed with granulated sugar. It is equally good to add powdered Cinnabar (*Zhu Sha*).

A formula that resolves the pox sore toxins (consists of) Fructus Luffae Cylindricae (*Si Gua*), Rhizoma Cimicifugae (*Sheng Ma*), wine-processed Radix Paeoniae Lactiflorae (*Shao Yao*), Radix Glycyrrhizae (*Sheng Gan Cao*), Fructus Crataegi (*Tang Qiu*), Semen Glycineae Max (*Hei Dou*), Cornu Rhinoceroris (*Xi Jiao*), and Semen Phaseoli Calcarati (*Chi Xiao Dou*). Another formula that resolves pox sores which can be used both before and after their eruption (is made by) powdering Cinnabar (*Zhu Sha*) and taking this brewed with honey water. (This) may reduce the number of pox if they (otherwise) would be numerous or reduce (them) to nil if they (otherwise) would have been a small number.

If a child suffering from pox sore has diarrhea and thirst, giving (them) honey water, water melon, persimmon, and other raw, cold substances is absolutely not permitted. (In that case,) it is appropriate to administer *Mu Xiang San* (Saussurea Powder)[3] which can be found in Chen Wen-zhong's[4] formulary for children. Before the sore papules have

---

[3] This consists of Radix Saussureae Seu Vladimiriae (*Mu Xiang*), Pericarpium Arecae (*Da Fu Pi*), Cortex Cinnamomi (*Rou Gui*), Rhizoma Pinelliae Ternatae (*Ban Xia*), Pericarpium Viridis Citri Reticulatae (*Qing Pi*), Radix Bupleuri (*Chai Hu*), Radix Panacis Ginseng (*Ren Shen*), Sclerotium Rubrum Poriae Cocoris (*Chi Fu Ling*), Radix Glycyrrhizae (*Gan Cao*), Fructus Terminaliae Chebulae (*He Zi*), and Flos Caryophylli (*Ding Xiang*), all in equal amounts.

[4] Chen Wen-zhong was an outstanding doctor during the Southern Song Dynasty. He was director of the then Imperial Medical Academy. Two works by him survive, *Xiao Er Bing Yuan Fang Lun* (*Treatise on the Origin of Pediatric Diseases and [Their] Formulas*) and *You You Xin Shu* (*A New Book on Disorders in Children*), the second of which was

taken shape as a (distinctive) pattern, apply Radix Mirabilis Jalapae (*Yan Zhi*) on the rims of the eye-sockets. This can prevent pox sores. For festering pox sores with pus staining the clothes, burn to ash feces dropped in the last month of the year by an ox to reduce (the sick child's) sleep. This prevents pox sore *yong* from developing. When the pox scabs on the head and face scale off to discharge pus and blood, moisten these with pure butter (*Su You*) to prevent *xian*. For pox and papule sores with agitation of the heart and disturbed sleep, wash with a swab (soaked in) Succus Rhizomatus Cimicifugae (*Sheng Ma Zhi*).

For pox sores with qi vacuity and hence inability to erupt, (use) Radix Astragali Membranacei (*Huang Qi*), Radix Panacis Ginseng (*Ren Shen*), wine-processed Radix Paeoniae Lactiflorae (*Shao Yao*), Radix Angelicae Sinensis (*Dang Gui*), Rhizoma Ligustici Wallichii (*Chuan Xiong*), a bean-sized amount of wine- processed Flos Carthami Tinctorii (*Hong Hua*), Radix Saussureae Seu Vladimiriae (*Mu Xiang*), and Radix Lithospermi Seu Arnebiae (*Zi Cao*). But for qi repletion and phlegm depression keeping (the pox) from erupting, (use) Rhizoma Atractylodis (*Cang Zhu*), Radix Angelicae (*Bai Zhi*), Radix Ledebouriellae Sesloidis (*Fang Feng*), Rhizoma Cimicifugae (*Sheng Ma*), Radix Scutellariae Baicalensis (*Huang Qin*), Radix Rubrus Paeoniae Lactiflorae (*Chi Shao Yao*), Fructus Forsythiae Suspensae (*Lian Qiao*), and Radix Angelicae Sinensis hairs (*Dang Gui Xu*). For blood heat causing eruption of skinless sores with great momentum in the lower burner (accompanied by) thirst, (use) Radix Trichosanthis Kirlowii (*Tian Hua Fen*), Radix Scutellariae Baicalensis (*Huang Qin*), Radix Paeoniae Lactiflorae (*Shao Yao*), Radix Puerariae Lobatae (*Ge Gen*), Radix Glycyrrhizae (*Gan Cao*), Gypsum (*Shi Gao*), and Talcum (*Hua Shi*). For weakness of both the qi and blood with black, sunken pox, (use) wine-processed Radix Paeoniae Lactiflorae (*Shao Yao*), Radix Panacis Ginseng (*Ren Shen*), Radix Astragali Membranacei (*Huang Qi*), Radix Angelicae (*Bai Zhi*), Radix Saussureae Seu Vladimiriae (*Mu Xiang*), Cortex Cinnamomi (*Gui Pi*), Rhizoma Ligustici Wallichii (*Chuan Xiong*), and Radix Angelicae Sinensis (*Dang Gui*).

---

a product of collaboration with his colleague, Zheng Hui-qing.

For blood subjected to dampness with (the pox) on the head falling flat and whitish gray, (use) Flos Carthami Tinctorii (*Hong Hua*), Lignum Sappanis (*Su Mu*), Rhizoma Atractylodis Macrocephalae (*Bai Zhu*), Rhizoma Atractylodis (*Cang Zhu*), Radix Paeoniae Lactiflorae (*Shao Yao*), Radix Angelicae Sinensis (*Dang Gui*), and Rhizoma Ligustici Wallichii (*Chuan Xiong*) with a small amount of wine added. For post-eruption damage by external malign qi causing fallen poxes[5], (use) Radix Panacis Ginseng (*Ren Shen*), Radix Paeoniae Lactiflorae (*Shao Yao*), Fructus Forsythiae Suspensae (*Lian Qiao*), Apex Radicis Astragali Membranacei (*Huang Qi Shao*), Apex Radicis Glycyrrhizae (*Gan Cao Shao*), Radix Angelicae (*Bai Zhi*), wine-processed Radix Angelicae Sinensis (*Dang Gui*), Rhizoma Ligustici Wallichii (*Chuan Xiong*), and a small amount of Radix Saussureae Seu Vladimiriae (*Mu Xiang*).

In relationship to pox sores, patients should be differentiated into clear and turbid (types), and their brave and fearful (nature) should be determined in terms of form and qi. For either black or sunken (pox) due to qi vacuity keeping (the pox) from erupting thoroughly, use wine-fried Radix Astragali Membranacei (*Huang Qi*), Radix Panacis Ginseng (*Ren Shen*), and wine-processed Radix Lithospermi Seu Arnebiae (*Zi Cao*).

Based on the correct color (of the pox), if the above (treatment) methods are employed and the color of pox turns lighter, this is incorrect. (In that case), use Rhizoma Ligustici Wallichii (*Chuan Xiong*), Radix Angelicae Sinensis (*Dang Gui*), Radix Paeoniae Lactiflorae (*Shao Yao*), Flos Carthami Tinctorii (*Hong Hua*), wine, and the like. If these methods are employed but the color of the pox is turning purple, this is ascribed to heat. (In that case,) use Rhizoma Cimicifugae (*Sheng Ma*), Radix Puerariae Lobatae (*Ge Gen*), Radix Scutellariae Baicalensis (*Huang Qin*), Rhizoma Coptidis Chinensis (*Huang Lian*), Cortex Cinnamomi

---

[5] Fallen or sunken pox are due to wind intruding in the course of eruption of pox. They present with a pattern of generalized aching, mild inversion, constipation, urinary stoppage, and retarded advance of pox which may turn blackish purple or fall flat. The pox may also refuse to form scabs or ulcerate with diarrhea of pus and blood, fever, cloudedness, and cold hands and feet.

(*Gui*), Fructus Forsythiae Suspensae (*Lian Qiao*), and the like. In severe cases, use powdered Cornu Rhinoceroris (*Xi Jiao*) to greatly resolve pox toxins.

(Those with) ashen, white (*i.e.,* gray) colored (pox or) those who are quiet or fearful should be viewed as cold. Pox being in step (*i.e.,* progressing normally), those who are brave, agitated, or have eruption should be viewed as heat. (Pox) which are all white in color and like bean shell on the verge of shrivelling are a result of drinking excessive water during their initial stage. Pox which are out of step are popularly called fallen pox. This (all) does not matter much. Simply administer exterior-replenishing medicinals and attend to the patient's urination and defecation. In case of constipation, just free evacuation. In case of urinary stoppage, just free urination. There may be cases where, at the outset, vexation, agitation, delirious ravings, frenetic thirst, and massive drinking arise. (If the patient) is actually allowed to drink, later (the pox) will not develop in step. (If this occurs), immediately administer cool medicinals to resolve the branch. Formulas like *Yi Yuan San* (Boost the Original Powder) can also be used.

Itching, sunken (pox) should be classified into vacuity and repletion (types) by examining their form, color, and the pulse. Repletion is shown by a strong pulse and vigorous qi[6], while vacuity is shown by a weak pulse and fearful qi. In case of vacuity itching, add blood-cooling medicinals to exterior- replenishing formulas. In case of repletion itching possibly with constipation, administer cool and cold medicinals, like a small amount of Radix Et Rhizoma Rhei (*Da Huang*), to precipitate the bound stool. For a moderate case with fearful qi, mix diluted honey and powdered Talcum (*Hua Shi*) and moisten the sores with (this mixture) with a feather.

Sparse (pox) are not toxic, but dense (pox) are toxic. Administer cool medicinals to resolve (the toxins). More than 10 doses will do no harm, and this prevents the trouble of eye injury later. Dry (pox) require abating fire. Wet (pox) require draining dampness. To abate fire, use

---

[6]   Qi here means both breathing and one's bearing or affect.

a light formula of Herba Seu Flos Schizonepetae Tenuifoliae (*Jing Jie*), Rhizoma Cimicifugae (*Sheng Ma*), Radix Glycyrrhizae (*Gan Cao*), Radix Puerariae Lobatae (*Ge Gen*), etc. Draining dampness (in this case means) draining dampness from the muscles and superficial interstices with wind medicinals such as Radix Angelicae (*Bai Zhi*) and Radix Ledebouriellae Sesloidis (*Fang Feng*). Pox sores impairing the eyes necessarily require Fructus Gardeniae Jasminoidis (*Shan Zhi*), Semen Cassiae Torae (*Jue Ming*), Radix Rubrus Paeoniae Lactiflorae (*Chi Shao Yao*), Radix Angelicae Sinensis hairs (*Dang Gui Xu*), Radix Scutellariae Baicalensis (*Huang Qin*), Rhizoma Coptidis Chinensis (*Huang Lian*), Radix Ledebouriellae Sesloidis (*Fang Feng*), Fructus Forsythiae Suspensae (*Lian Qiao*), Rhizoma Cimicifugae (*Sheng Ma*), and Radix Platycodi Grandiflori (*Jie Geng*). Powder and take in small doses.

Dull eyes will become bright by themselves in 100 days when qi and blood are restored to normal. Pox *yong*, usually the product of exterior repletion and blood heat, should be treated (differently) depending on whether (they are) located above or below. This does not allow for even a day's delay (in treatment). Suppuration necessarily requires (pus)-expelling, cool medicinals as the rulers, (such as) Radix Rubrus Paeoniae Lactiflorae (*Chi Shao Yao*), Nodus Radicis Glycyrrhizae (*Gan Cao Jie*), Fructus Forsythiae Suspensae (*Lian Qiao*), and Radix Platycodi Grandiflori (*Jie Geng*). To conduct (these ingredients) upward, use Rhizoma Cimicifugae (*Sheng Ma*) and Radix Puerariae Lobatae (*Ge Gen*). To conduct (them) downward, use Semen Arecae Catechu (*Bing Lang*) and Radix Achyranthis Bidentatae (*Niu Xi*. The above ingredients) should be assisted by Bulbus Fritillariae (*Bei Mu*), Herba Lonicerae Japonicae (*Ren Dong Cao*), Radix Angelicae (*Bai Zhi*), Fructus Trichosanthis Kirlowii (*Gua Lou*), and the like. In case of dry stools, use Radix Et Rhizoma Rhei (*Da Huang*. And) in case of fever, use Radix Scutellariae Baicalensis (*Huang Qin*) and Cortex Phellodendri (*Huang Bai*). Black pox sores are ascribed to blood heat and the ruling (method) is to cool the blood. White (pox sores) are ascribed to qi vacuity and the ruling (method) is to supplement the qi. (Pox which are) black and sunken in the center but white around (the) edges and retarded in advancing should be treated with a combined (method). At the initial stage, spontaneous sweating does not matter much, for it arises as a (natural) result of damp heat fuming and steaming.

Pox is classified into qi, blood, vacuity, and repletion (patterns). It should be observed daily. In most cases, some amount of insufficient qi and blood is found. Vacuity requires Radix Astragali Membranacei (*Huang Qi*). This should be aided by blood-engendering and quickening medicinals and assisted by small amounts of wind medicinals. Repletion requires Radix Albus Paeoniae Lactiflorae (*Bai Shao Yao*) and Radix Scutellariae Baicalensis (*Huang Qin*) as the sovereigns. These should be assisted by Radix Angelicae (*Bai Zhi*) and Fructus Forsythiae Suspensae (*Lian Qiao*). If ascribed to cold, Master Chen (Wen-zhong)'s formula[7] may also be used. Either before or after eruption, it is appropriate to administer *Shen Su Yin* (Ginseng & Perilla Drink).

Generally speaking, the adjusting and resolving method (consists of) quickening the blood and adjusting the qi, calming the exterior and harmonizing the center. This can be realized by using warm and cool medicinals in combination which are lightening[8], clearing, and toxin-eliminating. Warm medicinals include, for example, Radix Angelicae Sinensis (*Dang Gui*), Radix Astragali Membranacei (*Huang Qi*), and Radix Saussureae Seu Vladimiriae (*Mu Xiang*). Cool medicinals include, for example, Radix Peucedani (*Qian Hu*), Radix Puerariae Lobatae (*Ge Gen*), and Rhizoma Cimicifugae (*Sheng Ma*). Those used as assistants include, for example, Rhizoma Ligustici Wallichii (*Chuan Xiong*), Radix Paeoniae Lactiflorae (*Shao Yao*), Fructus Citri Seu Ponciri (*Zhi Qiao*), Radix Platycodi Grandiflori (*Jie Geng*), Caulis Akebiae Mutong (*Mu Tong*), Radix Lithospermi Seu Arnebiae (*Zi Cao*), and Radix Glycyrrhizae (*Gan Cao*). During the initial stage, spontaneous

---

[7] I.e., *Mu Xiang San* (Saussurea Powder). See Note 5 above.

[8] Lightening and clearing mean effusing or dissipating by so-called light medicinals. For example, fever and headache are treated with Herba Ephedrae (*Ma Huang*) which resolves the exterior by means of diaphoresis and Radix Puerariae Lobatae (*Ge Gen*) which resolves fire in the muscles. Exterior cold and interior heat with sore throat, etc. are treated with Herba Menthae (*Bo He*), Semen Arcti Lappae (*Niu Bang Zi*) and Radix Platycodi Grandiflori (*Jie Geng*). Urinary and fecal block and abdominal urgency with rectal pressure are treated with Fructus Trichosanthis Kirlowii (*Gua Lou*), Radix Platycodi Grandiflori (*Jie Geng*), and Radix Asteris Tatarici (*Zi Wan*). All these treatments are called lightening.

sweating does not matter much, for it is a result of the fuming and steaming of damp heat.

A dressing for pox *yong* (consists of) Bulbus Fritillariae (*Bei Mu*), Rhizoma Arisaematis (*Nan Xing*), Bombyx Batryticatus (*Jiang Can*), Radix Trichosanthis Kirlowii (*Tian Hua Fen*), Radix Angelicae (*Bai Zhi*), Radix Aconiti (*Cao Wu*), Radix Et Rhizoma Rhei (*Da Huang*), and Fructus Gleditschiae Sinensis (*Zhu Ya Zao Jiao*), all in equal amounts, and Calcareous Spar (*Han Shui Shi*) in double amount. Powder the above and apply after mixing with vinegar.

A male, more than 20 years of age, suffered from pox sores. After the pox had withered, there suddenly arose clenched jaw, rigidity of the limbs without ability to stretch or contract, and periumbilical pain from time to time. This pain was followed by cold sweating like rain, and the sweating ended with relief of the pain. This was intermittent and the pulse was wiry, taut, and urgent like a drawn bowstring. Inquiry revealed that this fellow had been exceedingly taxed and overworked, and (I) concluded that taxation fatigue must have damaged the blood. What's more, because he lived in the mountains, the abundant wind cold there had taken advantage of vacuity to inflict an affection before he suffered from eruption of the pox. This made the blood vacuity all the more serious. It was necessary to use warm medicinals to nurture blood and acrid, cool medicinals to dissipate wind. Accordingly, (I) prescribed Radix Angelicae Sinensis (*Dang Gui Shen*) and Radix Albus Paeoniae Lactiflorae (*Bai Shao Yao*) as the sovereigns, Rhizoma Ligustici Wallichii (*Chuan Xiong*), Pericarpium Viridis Citri Reticulatae (*Qing Pi*), and Ramus Uncariae Cum Uncis (*Gou Teng*) as the ministers, Rhizoma Atractylodis Macrocephalae (*Bai Zhu*) and Pericarpium Citri Reticulatae (*Chen Pi*) as the assistants, and Radix Glycyrrhizae (*Gan Cao*), Cortex Cinnamomi (*Gui Pi*), southern Radix Saussureae Seu Vladimiriae (*Nan Mu Xiang*), and Radix Scutellariae Baicalensis (*Huang Qin*) as the envoys. (These) were boiled with a small amount of Flos Carthami Tinctorii (*Hong Hua*) and taken and a cure was effected.

My nephew had eruption of pox at 6-7 years of age with generalized fever, moderate thirst, and loose stools. The (attending) physician prescribed *Mu Xiang San* with 10 pieces of Flos Caryophylli (*Ding*

Xiang) added. I noticed that the eruption was retarded. It was true that this should be ascribed to qi weakness caused by loose stools, but because all the discharge was stinking stasis, the discharge might be caused by steaming heat rather than cold. When (I) immediately stopped the (medication, my nephew) had already taken 1 dose. (Then he) was administered *Huang Lian Jie Du Tang* (Coptis Revolve Toxins Decoction)[9] with Rhizoma Atractylodis Macrocephalae (*Bai Zhu*) added. Nearly 10 doses succeeded in resolving (the toxins). The diarrhea was checked and the pox erupted. (However,) he frequently had moderate heat in the muscles with *yong* growing on the hands and feet. Then cooling supplementation was administered. In a month, recovery resulted.

A person, aged 17, had pox with fever, severe cloudedness, and fatigue. (Their) pulse was large and a little rapid. (They) were prescribed a large dose of Radix Panacis Ginseng (*Ren Shen*), Rhizoma Atractylodis Macrocephalae (*Bai Zhu*), Radix Scutellariae Baicalensis (*Huang Qi*), Radix Angelicae Sinensis, and Pericarpium Citri Reticulatae (*Chen Pi*. These) were boiled into a thick decoction and drunk. (After) 20 doses had been taken, the pox erupted. Another 20 doses were administered and purulent pimples broke out with not a dot of skin over the whole body intact. Some suggested using Master Chen (Wen-zhong)'s formula, but I answered that this was merely vacuity without cold and (instructed the patient) to continue using the above formula. Recovery was effected after 60 doses.

---

[9] This consists of Rhizoma Coptidis Chinensis (*Huang Lian*), 3 *liang*, Cortex Phelloden-dri (*Huang Bai*) and Radix Scutellariae Baicalensis (*Huang Qin*), 2 *liang* each, and Fructus Gardeniae Jasminoidis (*Shan Zhi Zi*), 14 pieces. Divide into 2 doses, boil, and take.

Chapter Five

Vomiting & Diarrhea

Vomiting and diarrhea in infants are treated with Master Qian's *Yi Huang San* (Boost the Yellow Powder)[1] and *Bai Zhu San* (Atractylodes Powder) as the ruling (formulas) with certain additions and subtractions in accordance with conditions. For vomiting and diarrhea in children in summer months, *Yi Yuan San* (Boost the Original Powder) is best of all. Incessant vomiting and diarrhea in infants is likely to develop into chronic fright wind. (For it), Master Qian's five supplementing medicinals[2] for the five diarrheas are applicable. To treat vomiting and diarrhea and jaundice, (use) Rhizoma Sparganii (*San Leng*), Rhizoma Curcumae Zedoariae (*E Zhu*), Pericarpium Citri Reticulatae (*Chen Pi*), Pericarpium Viridis Citri Reticulatae (*Qing Pi*), Massa Medica Fermentata (*Shen Qu*), Fructus Germinatus Hordei Vulgaris (*Mai Ya*), Rhizoma Coptidis Chinensis (*Huang Lian*), Radix Glycyrrhizae (*Gan Cao*), Rhizoma Atractylodis Macrocephalae (*Bai Zhu*), and Sclerotium Poriae Cocoris (*Fu Ling*). Powder the above and take with thin gruel. In case of breast milk damage resulting in vomiting and diarrhea, add Fructus Crataegi (*Shan Zha*). In case of seasonal qi resulting in vomiting and diarrhea, add Talcum (*Hua Shi*). (And) in case of fever, add Herba Menthae (*Bo He*).

Vomiting and diarrhea with abdominal pain and vomiting of milk and diarrhea are both (due to) cold. (This requires) adjusting the spleen

---

[1] This consists of Pericarpium Citri Reticulatae (*Chen Pi*), Flos Caryophylli (*Ding Xiang*), Fructus Terminaliae Chebulae (*He Zi*), Pericarpium Viridis Citri Reticulatae (*Qing Pi*), and mix-fried Radix Glycyrrhizae (*Zhi Gan Cao*).

[2] This may refer to *Wu Wei Yi Gong San* (Five Flavor Wonder-Working Powder) which is composed of Radix Panacis Ginseng (*Ren Shen*), Rhizoma Atractylodis Macrocephalae (*Bai Zhu*), Sclerotium Poriae Cocoris (*Fu Ling*), Radix Glycyrrhizae (*Gan Cao*), and Pericarpium Citri Reticulatae (*Chen Pi*).

and stomach with *Ping Wei San* (Level the Stomach Powder). If this is mixed with heated honey and combined with the same amount of *Su He Xiang Wan* (Liquid Styrax Pills)[3], it forms the so-called *Wan An Gao* (Cure All Paste. It) is taken with thin gruel. *Wan An Wan* (Cure All Pills) invigorate the stomach, promote food intake, and check vomiting and diarrhea. (They consist of) Rhizoma Atractylodis Macrocephalae (*Bai Zhu*), Sclerotium Poriae Cocoris (*Fu Ling*), and Radix Panacis Ginseng (*Ren Shen*), 3 *qian* for each of the above, Pericarpium Citri Reticulatae (*Chen Pi*), Rhizoma Atractylodis (*Cang Zhu*), Cortex Magnoliae Officinalis (*Hou Po*), Sclerotium Polypori Umbellati (*Zhu Ling*), and Rhizoma Alismatis (*Ze Xie*), 5 *qian* for each of the above, dry Rhizoma Zingiberis (*Gan Jiang*), 3 *qian*, Cortex Cinnamomi (*Guan Gui*), 2 *qian*, and Radix Glycyrrhizae (*Gan Cao*), 2.5 *qian*. Powder the above and make into pills the size of Chinese parasol tree seeds with heated honey; 5 pills per dose dissolved in thin gruel and taken before a meal.

Chapter Six

Dysentery

For dysentery in infants, (use) Rhizoma Coptidis Chinensis (*Huang Lian*), Radix Scutellariae Baicalensis (*Huang Qin*), Pericarpium Citri Reticulatae (*Chen Pi*), and Radix Glycyrrhizae (*Gan Cao*). Boil and take. In case of red dysentery, add Semen Pruni Persicae (*Tao Ren*) and Flos Carthami Tinctorii (*Hong Hua*). In case of white dysentery, add

---

[3] This consists of Rhizoma Atractylodis Macrocephalae (*Bai Zhu*), Radix Saussureae Seu Vladimiriae (*Mu Xiang*), Cornu Rhinoceroris (*Xi Jiao*), stir-fried Rhizoma Cyperi Rotundi (*Xiang Fu*), Cinnabar (*Zhu Sha*), roasted Fructus Terminaliae Chebulae (*He Zi*), Lignum Santali Albi (*Tan Xiang*), Benzoinum (*An Xi Xiang*), Lignum Aquilariae Agallochae (*Chen Xiang*), Secretio Moschi Moschiferi (*She Xiang*), Flos Caryophylli (*Ding Xiang*), Fructus Piperis Longi (*Bi Ba*), Borneolum (*Bing Pian*), Gummum Olibani (*Xun Lu Xiang*), and Oleum Styracis Liquidis (*Su He Xiang You*).

powdered Talcum (*Hua Shi*). To treat infants with food accumulation and dysentery purely of blood, (use) stir-fried Massa Medica Fermentata (*Shen Qu*), Rhizoma Atractylodis (*Cang Zhu*), Talcum (*Hua Shi*), Radix Albus Paeoniae Lactiflorae (*Bai Shao Yao*), Radix Scutellariae Baicalensis (*Huang Qin*), Rhizoma Atractylodis Macrocephalae (*Bai Zhu*), Pericarpium Citri Reticulatae (*Chen Pi*), Radix Glycyrrhizae (*Gan Cao*), and Sclerotium Poriae Cocoris (*Fu Ling*). Boil and take with *Bao He Wan* (Protect & Harmonize Pills). To treat infants with uncheckable, enduring dysentery with inability to disperse water and grain, powder Fructus Citri Seu Ponciri (*Zhi Qiao*) and administer 2 *qian* with thin gruel. (To treat) red dysentery in infants, pound Halitum (*Qing Yan*) into a liquid and administer half a cupful per dose.

Chapter Seven

Various Kinds of Worms

(To treat) roundworms attacking the heart, boil Semen Coicis Lachryma-jobi (*Yi Yi Ren*) into a very thick decoction and take. Another formula (consists of) roasting Fructus Quisqualis Indicae (*Shi Jun Zi*) in a fire and take any amount with a decoction made of its shells. Related to (abdominal) pain due to roundworms, a rhyme quoted in Master Tang's formulary[1] says:

Worms are bred out of a habit of careless eating.
Worms growing inside, muscle and flesh become emaciated.
A great deal of sweets rapaciously taken,
Great pain relentlessly arises.

---

[1] Before the time of Zhu Dan-xi, there were several outstanding doctors with the same surname Tang. However, all of their works are lost. Therefore, the translator fails to identify this Master Tang. Among those doctors surnamed Tang, Tang Min-wang and his grandson, Tang Heng, specialized in pediatrics and Zhu might be referring to one of them.

Worry and crying and fear of medicine
Only make the flesh gradually wasted.
Philtrum, nose tip, and lower lip blacken,
These infallibly serve as a sign and token.
But, with foam dried and pain settled, back worms must fall,
Worms removed and no more disease is seen at all.

The formula to be used is *An Shen San* (Calm the Spirit Powder. This consists of) Lacca Sinica Exiccata (*Gan Qi*), 2 *qian*, stir-fried till smoke is no longer seen, Realgar (*Xiong Huang*), 5 *qian*, and Secretio Moschi Moschiferi (*She Xiang*), 1 *qian*. Powder the above, one half *qian* for 3 years of age, taken on an empty stomach with Cortex Radicis Meliae Azedarachis (*Ku Lian Gen*) soup.

All the methods to remove worms stipulate that medication be administered at the beginning of the month. (At that time,) worms have their heads upwards, (and) medication is surely efficacious. To treat tapeworms, obtain a handful of eastward-growing Cortex Radicis Punicae Granati (*Shi Liu Gen*), wash, and grate. (Then) boil in 3 *sheng* of water down to not more than half a bowlful and take warm early in the morning at the 5th watch. After all the worms are eliminated, take gruel to supplement (the stomach).

Hua Chong Wan (Transform [*i.e.*, Dissolve] Worms Pills, consist of) stir-fried Fructus Carpesii Abrotanoidis (*He Shi*), Semen Arecae Catechu (*Bing Lang*), carbonate of lead (*Hu Fen*), and Cortex Radicis Meliae Azedarachis (*Ku Lian Gen*), 5 *qian* (for each of the above), and Alum (*Bai Fan*), half crude, half calcined, 3 *qian*. Powder the above and make with paste into pills the size of red beans; 30 pills per dose taken with Succus Zingiberis Moigae (*Jiu Jiang*) and raw oil. Another (formula) to treat roundworms gnawing the heart with vomiting of water (is made by) powdering Fructus Carpesii Abrotanoidis (*He Shi*) and making into pills with honey; 30 pills taken with either boiled honey water or boiled vinegar water. (Yet another) formula to treat roundworms (consists of) using Cortex Radicis Meliae Azedarachis (*Lian Shu Gen*) as the sovereign and *Er Chen Tang* (Two Aged Decoction) as the assistant. Boil and take.

Children's vomiting of roundworms in winter months is usually due to stomach cold and stomach vacuity (forcing them) out. (For this, use) Master Qian's *Bai Zhu San* (Atractylodes Powder) with 2 pieces of Flos Caryophylli (*Ding Xiang*) added. Pills to treat worms (consist of) Rhizoma Picrorrhizae (*Hu Huang Lian*), 1 *qian*, Semen Arecae Catechu (*Bing Lang*), 1 *qian*, Pericarpium Citri Reticulatae (*Chen Pi*), 1 *qian*, Massa Medica Fermentata (*Shen Qu*), Tuber Curcumae (*Yu Jin*), Rhizoma Pinelliae Ternatae (*Ban Xia*), and Rhizoma Atractylodis Macrocephalae (*Bai Zhu*), 2 *qian* for each of the above, and Fructificatio Polypori Mylittae (*Lei Wan*), 1 *qian*. Powder the above and make into pills with paste.

Chapter Eight

Abdominal Distention & Pain

(For this, use) Semen Raphani Sativi (*Luo Bo Zi*), Ramulus Perillae Frutescentis (*Zi Su Geng*), dry Radix Puerariae Lobatae (*Gan Ge*) [dry Rhizoma Zingiberis {*Gan Jiang*} instead in a {variant} edition {later editor}], and Pericarpium Citri Reticulatae (*Chen Pi*), all in equal amounts, and Radix Glycyrrhizae (*Gan Cao*), in half amount. In case of low food intake, add Rhizoma Atractylodis Macrocephalae (*Bai Zhu*). Boil and take. Food accumulation and abdominal hardness in children invariably requires Fructus Perillae Frutescentis (*Zi Su*) and Semen Raphani Sativi (*Luo Bo Zi*). For abdominal pain in children due to liking to eat (too much) *zong zi*, use Rhizoma Coptidis Chinensis (*Huang Lian*) and distiller's grains (*Bai Jiu Yao*). Relief will follow. These may be taken in the shape of pills after being powdered. *Hei Long Wan* (Black Dragon Pills, also) treat abdominal pain in children. (They consist of) Terra Flava Usta (*Fu Long Gan*), 1 *liang*, Radix Panacis Ginseng (*Ren Shen*), Sclerotium Poriae Cocoris (*Fu Ling*), Rhizoma Atractylodis Macrocephalae (*Bai Zhu*), and Pulvis Fumi Carbonisati (*Bai Cao Shuang*), 5 *qian* for each of the above, Radix Glycyrrhizae (*Gan Cao*), 2 *qian*, and dry Rhizoma Zingiberis (*Gan Jiang*), 3 *qian*. Powder the above and make into pills the size of Chinese parasol tree seeds with gruel; 5 pills per dose taken with Pericarpium Citri Reticulatae (*Chen Pi*) soup.

Chapter Nine

Various Kinds of Accumulations

(The following) diffusing medicinals[1] treat the various kinds of accumulation and stagnation in children: Rhizoma Curcumae Zedoariae (*E Zhu*), Pericarpium Viridis Citri Reticulatae (*Qing Pi*), and Pericarpium Citri Reticulatae (*Chen Pi*), 5 *qian*, Flos Daphnis Genkwae (*Yuan Hua*), 3 *qian*, Semen Crotonis Tiglii (*Jiang Zi*), 15 pieces, de-oiled and ground separately, and Semen Arecae Catechu (*Bing Lang*), 5 *qian*. Powder (all the above except Semen Crotonis) which is put in later and make with vinegar into pills the size of millet; 7 pills for 1 year of age taken with ginger soup. *Xiao Ji Wan* (Disperse Accumulation Pills) eliminate accumulation lumps in children. (They consist of) Os Cyrtiospiriferis Sinensis (*Shi Yan*), 5 *qian*, quenched 7 times in vinegar, de-oiled Semen Momordicae Cochinensis (*Mu Bie Zi*), 5 *qian*, Lithargyum (*Mi Tuo Seng*), 1 *liang*, and Flos Caryophylli (*Ding Xiang*) and Calomelas (*Ni Fen*), 4 *qian* each. Make the above into pills the size of millet with Massa Medica Fermentata (*Shen Qu*) paste; 15 pills per dose taken with thin gruel.

For glomus lumps with malaria in breast-feeding infants, (use) Rhizoma Ligustici Wallichii (*Chuan Xiong*), 2 *qian*, Radix Rehmanniae (*Sheng Di Huang*) and Rhizoma Atractylodis Macrocephalae (*Bai Zhu*),

---

[1] Diffusing medicinals are those which eliminate congestion and are able to treat non-descension and non-ascension of qi, depression of qi, fire, etc. Thus, even food-dispersing or blood-moving medicinals can be spoken of as diffusing medicinals.

1.5 *qian* each, Pericarpium Citri Reticulatae (*Chen Pi*), Rhizoma Pinelliae Ternatae (*Ban Xia*), Radix Scutellariae Baicalensis (*Huang Qin*), 1 *qian* and stir-fried for each of the above, and Radix Glycyrrhizae (*Gan Cao*, no amount given. Take) all the above as 1 dose boiled with 3 slices of ginger and 5 *fen* of powdered Plastrum Amydae (*Xia Jia*). For food accumulation with stomach heat fuming and steaming[2] in children, use Rhizoma Atractylodis Macrocephalae (*Bai Zhu*), 1 *liang*, Rhizoma Pinelliae Ternatae (*Ban Xia*), and Rhizoma Coptidis Chinensis (*Huang Lian*), 5 *qian* each. Powder the above, mix evenly with *Ping Wei San* (Level the Stomach Powder), and make into pills with gruel; 10-20 pills per dose taken with boiled water.

Chapter Ten

Wind Phlegm Dyspnea & Coughing

Bai Fu Wan (Korean Aconite Pills) suppress cough, transform phlegm, and abate heat. (They) are composed of Rhizoma Pinelliae Ternatae (*Ban Xia*), 2 *qian*, Rhizoma Arisaematis (*Nan Xing*), 1 *liang*, Radix Aconiti Coreani (*Bai Fu Zi*), 5 *qian*, and Alum (*Bai Fan*), 4 *qian*. Powder the above and make into pills the size of Chinese parasol tree seeds with Succus Zingiberis (*Jiang Zhi*); 8-9 pills per dose taken with mint and ginger soup. *Zi Jin Dan* (Purple Gold Elixir) treats phlegm accumulation coughing, dispels wind, and settles fright. (It consists of) Rhizoma Pinelliae Ternatae (*Ban Xia*), 1 *liang*, Rhizoma Arisaematis (*Nan Xing*), iron rust (*Tie Yun Fen, i.e.,* iron rust produced by vinegar), and Radix Aconiti Coreani (*Bai Fu Zi*), 5 *qian* for each of the above, and Alumen (*Ku Fan*). Powder the above and make into pills the size of Chinese parasol tree seeds with Massa Medica Fermentata (*Shen Qu*) paste; 4 pills per dose taken with ginger soup. Another formula to treat wind

---

[2] This is accompanied by signs such as dry mouth, foul breath, strangely stinking stools, and heat in the anus.

phlegm (is made by) grinding one half *liang* of Rhizoma Arisaematis (*Nan Xing*), dip in water 1 finger deep, and dry in the sun. (Then) grind very finely, put in 2 *liang* of Radix Aconiti Coreani (*Bai Fu Zi*), and make into pills the size of Semen Ciceris Arietini (*Ji Dou*) with finely ground wheat flour; 1-2 pills per dose taken with a soup of ginger, honey, and mint.

For wind drool tidal congestion and block[1], use worm-free, mix-fried Semen Gymnocladi Chinensis (*Fei Zao Jiao*), 1 *liang*, crude Alum (*Bai Fan*), 5 *qian*, and Calomelas (*Ni Fen*), one half *qian* [*i.e.*, *Qing Fen* {later editor}]. Mix with water and pour 1-2 *qian* down (the patient's throat). When (the medicinals) have passed the throat, drool will be discharged. Alum is a medicinal able to separate drool below the diaphragm. To treat phlegm dyspnea and exuberant phlegm in children, use Fructus Immaturus Citri Seu Ponciri (*Zhi Shi*), Radix Platycodi Grandiflori (*Jie Geng*), and Pericarpium Arecae (*Da Fu*) with *Er Chen Tang* (Two Aged Decoction. To treat) coughing in children, boil 4 *liang* of fresh Rhizoma Zingiberis (*Sheng Jiang*) and give (the coughing child) a bath (in the decoction. But for) coughing in children whose six pulses are all hidden, (use) Fructus Schizandrae Chinensis (*Wu Wei Zi*), Radix Panacis Ginseng (*Ren Shen*), Sclerotium Poriae Cocoris (*Fu Ling*), Cortex Radicis Mori Albi (*Sang Pi*), Radix Scutellariae Baicalensis (*Huang Qin*), and Radix Glycyrrhizae (*Gan Cao*. While for) dyspnea and coughing in children with fever and disquieted lung qi due to damage by wind evils, (use) Herba Ephedrae (*Ma Huang*), Radix Platycodi Grandiflori (*Jie Geng*), Fructus Perillae Frutescentis (*Zi Su*), Fructus Citri Seu Ponciri (*Zhi Qiao*), Rhizoma Pinelliae Ternatae (*Ban Xia*), Radix Scutellariae Baicalensis (*Huang Qin*), Radix Glycyrrhizae (*Gan Cao*), and Sclerotium Poriae Cocoris (*Fu Ling*). A number of doses effect a cure.

---

[1]　This refers to fulminating dyspnea with rales and phlegm.

Chapter Eleven

Epileptic Mania

(To treat) epileptic mania in children, mix 1 *qian* of powdered Radix Euphorbiae Kansui (*Gan Sui*) with the blood of a pig's heart, roast well, add 1 *qian* of powdered Cinnabar (*Zhu Sha*). Pound and make into pills the size of Semen Cannabis Sativae (*Ma Zi*); some 10 pills taken per dose. (To treat) children with abundant heat and raving bordering on fright (wind), make them drink Succus Bambusae (*Zhu Li*). Adults can be treated in the same way. A child suddenly crying loudly with no reason is bound to death. This is fire breaking out greatly due to extreme qi vacuity.

Chapter Twelve

Night Crying

Infants crying in the night (is impugned to) evil heat overwhelming the heart. (For this, use) Rhizoma Coptidis Chinensis (*Huang Lian*), stir-fried with Succus Zingiberis (*Jiang Zhi*), Radix Glycyrrhizae (*Gan Cao*), and Folium Bambusae (*Zhu Ye*). Boil and take. Or dab carbonized Medulla Junci Effusi (*Deng Xin Hui*) onto the nipples (of the mother) and let the child suckle. (To treat) intestinal cold with constant crying developing into epilepsy, mix powdered Radix Angelicae Sinensis (*Dang Gui*) with breast milk and pour down (the child's throat). Another method (consists of) putting the straw from a chicken coop under the mat without the notice of the mother. (Yet) another method (consists of) putting dry ox droppings the size of the palm under the mat. Another formula to treat child crying ceaselessly like a ghost (is made by) stir-frying 1 character of the powdered lower half of

Periostracum Cicadae (*Chan Tui*) with the upper half cast away. Take with mint soup.

If there are tears, children's fright-crying endlessly is due to abdominal pain. Use *Su He Xiang Wan* (Liquid Styrax Pills) taken with wine. If there are heavenly hung eyes[1], use *Tian Dao Teng Gao* (Ramus Uncariae Cum Uncis Paste).[2] A formula used to treat night crying (consists of) Radix Panacis Ginseng (*Ren Shen*), 1.5 *qian*, Rhizoma Coptidis Chinensis (*Huang Lian*), 1.5 *qian*, stir-fried with Succus Zingiberis (*Jiang Zhi*), mix-fried Radix Glycyrrhizae (*Zhi Gan Cao*), 5 *fen*, Folium Bambusae (*Zhu Ye*), 20 leaves, and Rhizoma Zingiberis (*Jiang*), 1 slice. Boil in water.

---

[1] This refers to upward-looking or upturned eyes. Heaven means up and hung figuratively means the eyes hooked by something intangible. This is a pattern due to evil heat congestion in the chest, accumulated phlegm or drool, or to meat and wine toxins generated in the mother while the child was in utero. Its manifestations are upturned eyes, susceptibility to fright, high temperature, incessant tearing, and, in the extreme, purplish green-blue nails of the hands and feet, spasms, incessant crying like a ghost, and arched back rigidity.

[2] There are two formulas with the same name and same indications. The first is composed Gummum Olibani (*Ru Xiang*), Myrrha (*Mo Yao*), Radix Saussureae Seu Vladimiriae (*Mu Xiang*), Rhizoma Curcumae (*Jiang Huang*), and Semen Momordicae Cochinchinensis (*Mu Bie Zi*). The above are to be made into pills taken with Ramus Uncariae Cum Uncis (*Gou Teng*) soup. The second is composed of Ramus Uncariae Cum Uncis (*Gou Teng*), Rhizoma Corydalis Yanhusuo (*Yan Hu Suo*), Radix Angelicae Sinensis (*Dang Gui*), Radix Glycyrrhizae (*Gan Cao*), Gummum Olibani (*Ru Xiang*), Cortex Cinnamomi (*Rou Gui*), and Secretio Moschi Moschiferi (*She Xiang*).

Chapter Thirteen

Oral Putrescence

One formula (consists of) Radix Sophorae Flavescentis (*Ku Shen*), Minium (*Huang Dan*), Galla Rhi Chinensis (*Wu Bei Zi*), and Pulvis Indigonis (*Qing Dai*), all in equal amounts. Another formula (consists of) Folium Camelliae Sinensis (*Jiang Cha*) and debarked Radix Glycyrrhizae (*Fen Cao*). Powder and apply. For mouth sores in children, apply powdered Alum (*Bai Fan*) dry. (To treat) children with white scales covering all the mouth likened to the mouth of a goose, swab the tongue with well water using a finger wrapped with hair or apply calcined Minium (*Huang Dan*).

Chapter Fourteen

Clenched Jaw

A nasal suppository (for this consists of) Tuber Curcumae (*Yu Jin*), Radix Veratri Nigri (*Li Lu*), and Pediculus Melonis (*Gua Di*), all in equal amounts. Powder, mix with water, and insert into the nose.

Chapter Fifteen

Wind Stroke

(To treat) wind stroke in infants, pour *Su He Xiang Wan* (Liquid Styrax Pills) down (the throat of the sick child) with Succus Zingiberis (*Jiang Zhi*). Then administer *Xing Feng Tang* (Resurrect Wind Decoction)[1] from the *Ju Fang (Collected Formulas)* and *Xiao Xu Ming Tang* (Minor Reinforce Life Decoction) plus Secretio Moschi Moschiferi (*She Xiang*). Boil and take with the stipulated method. Another method (consists of) dissolving *Su He Xiang Wan* in wine and pouring (this) down (the patient's throat) together with a small amount of Succus Zingiberis (*Jiang Zhi*). Then administer *Ba Wei Shun Qi San* (Eight Flavors Normalize the Qi Powder)[2] and finally administer *Xiao Xu Ming Tang*. In severe cases, merely use Radix Saussureae Seu Vladimiriae (*Mu Xiang*) and Rhizoma Arisaematis (*Tian Nan Xing*). Boil with 10 slices of Rhizoma Zingiberis (*Jiang*) and take. If Rhizoma Arisaematis is not available, Radix Saussureae Seu Vladimiriae alone can be taken after being boiled down to a thick decoction.

---

[1] This consists of Radix Ledebouriellae Sesloidis (*Fang Feng*) and Rhizoma Arisaematis (*Nan Xing*), 4 *liang* each, and water-washed and soaked Rhizoma Pinelliae Ternatae (*Sheng Ban Xia*), Radix Scutellariae Baicalensis (*Huang Qin*), and Radix Glycyrrhizae (*Sheng Gan Cao*), 2 *liang* for each of the above. Powder coarsely, 4 *qian* per dose. Boil in water with 10 slices of ginger and take.

[2] This consists of stir-fried Rhizoma Atractylodis Macrocephalae (*Bai Zhu*), Sclerotium Poriae Cocoris (*Fu Ling*), Pericarpium Viridis Citri Reticulatae (*Qing Pi*), Radix Angelicae (*Bai Zhi*), Pericarpium Citri Reticulatae (*Chen Pi*), Radix Linderae Strychnifoliae (*Wu Yao*), and Radix Panacis Ginseng (*Ren Shen*), 1 *liang* for each of the above, and mix-fried Radix Glycyrrhizae (*Zhi Gan Cao*), 5 qian.

(To treat) wind stroke in infants, (boil) *Zhu Fu Tang* (Atractylodes & Aconite Decoction)[3] from the *Ju Fang (Collected Formulas)* with 20 slices of Rhizoma Zingiberis *(Jiang)*, brew with *Su He Xiang Wan*, and administer orally at short intervals. In case of shortness of qi, dizziness of the head, and counterflow frigidity of the hands and feet, administer 50-100 pills of *Yang Zheng Dan* (Nurture the Righteous Elixir)[4] with the previous formula.[5] This never fails to bring an effect. If wind stroke in children under 3 years of age refuses to show improvement (in spite of this medication), administer all at once 1 *jin* of Folium Pini *(Song Ye)* boiled in 1 *dou* of wine down to 3 *sheng*. Recovery follows perspiration immediately.

Chapter Sixteen

Articular Wind

Articular wind is the sudden contraction of the disease of hypertonicity and pain in the hands and feet getting better during the day and worse during the night. First administer *Su He Xiang Wan* (Liquid Styrax Pills) and then *Sheng Wu Yao Shun Qi San* (Raw Lindera

---

[3] This consists of Rhizoma Atractylodis Macrocephalae *(Bai Zhu)*, 2 *liang*, Radix Praeparatus Aconiti Carmichaeli *(Fu Zi)*, 1.5 pieces, and mix-fried Radix Glycyrrhizae *(Zhi Gan Cao)*, 1 *liang*. (Take) 5 coinfuls per dose. Boil with 5 slices of ginger and 1 date.

[4] This consists of Mercurius *(Shui Yin)*, Sulphur *(Liu Huang)*, Cinnabar *(Zhu Sha)*, and Galenitum *(Hei Xi)*, 1 *liang* for each of the above. Heat the above separately, mix together, and make into pills with glutinous rice.

[5] I.e., *Zhu Fu Tang*

Normalize the Qi Powder)[1] and *Wu Ji San* (Five Accumulations Powder). Boil in half a cup each of water and wine and take with 1 character of Secretio Moschi Moschiferi (*She Xiang*).

Low back pain, pain in the legs, deviated mouth and eyes, hemiplegia, and inability to stretch and contract the hands and feet (are due to) qi stroke and wind stroke.[2] Wind will disperse once qi is normalized. Use Rhizoma Atractylodis Macrocephalae (*Bai Zhu*), 4 *liang*, roasted with flour dough, Lignum Aquilariae Agallochae (*Chen Xiang*), 5 *qian*, Rhizoma Gastrodiae Elatae (*Tian Ma*), 1 *liang*, Radix Linderae Strychnifoliae (*Tian Tai Wu Yao*), 3 *liang*, Pericarpium Viridis Citri Reticulatae (*Qing Pi*), Radix Angelicae (*Bai Zhi*), Radix Glycyrrhizae (*Gan Cao*), and Radix Panacis Ginseng (*Ren Shen*), 5 *qian* for each of the above [3 *qian* in a {variant} edition {later editor}]. Boil the above with 3 slices of Rhizoma Zingiberis (*Jiang*) and 5 leaves of Folium Perillae Frutescentis (*Zi Su*) and take on an empty stomach. This is named *Shun Qi San* (Normalize the Qi Powder). It is extremely miraculous.

(To treat) great articular wind[3] with hypertonicity and unbearable pain in the fingers, either the stem, leaves, root, or fruit of Xanthium Sibiricum (*Cang Er*) can be taken in the shape of pills after being powdered.

---

[1] This consists of root-stripped, joint-stripped Herba Ephedrae (*Ma Huang*), pulp-stripped Pericarpium Citri Reticulatae (*Chen Pi*), and Radix Linderae Strychnifoliae (*Wu Yao*), 2 *liang* for each of the above stir-fried Bombyx Batryticatus (*Jiang Can*), Rhizoma Ligustici Wallichii (*Chuan Xiong*), bran-fried Fructus Citri Seu Ponciri (*Zhi Qiao*), stir-fried Radix Glycyrrhizae (*Gan Cao*), Radix Angelicae (*Bai Zhi*), and Radix Platycodi Grandiflori (*Jie Geng*), 1 *liang* for each of the above, and blast-fried Rhizoma Zingiberis (*Pao Jiang*), one half *liang*. Powder the above. (Take) 3 *qian* per dose boiled with 3 slices of ginger and 1 date.

[2] Qi stroke and wind stroke present similar manifestations and undergo similar pathological changes in terms of qi and blood, but they belong to two different patterns. Qi stroke is caused by internal damage by the seven affects, such as like anger and long-lasting stress, and the resultant qi obstruction. In qi stroke there is cold body, absence of phlegm and drool, and a deep pulse. In wind stroke there is warm body, exuberant phlegm and drool and a floating pulse.

[3] The word great here simply means serious or drastic.

Chapter Seventeen

Migratory Red Wind & Cinnabar Toxins[1]

(To treat) migratory red (wind) in the upper with cool diaphragm inside, finely grind Feces Bombycis Mori (*Er Can Sha*) and extract undiluted juice from Radix Typhonii Gigantei (*Jian Dao Cao Gen*) by pounding. Mix these evenly and apply first on the abdomen. Then (apply) on the affected part but with an escape (route) left for (the toxin to move away). When the affected part moves, effect is shown. *Jian Dao Cao Gen* is also called *Ye Ci Gu*. To treat migratory red wind, use Terra Flava Usta (*Fu Long Gan*) mixed with the white of a hen's egg as a dressing. Internally, take Hematitum (*Chi Tu Shui*) brewed with water.

To treat red flood[2] (use) Radix Rehmanniae (*Sheng Di Huang*), Caulis Akebiae Mutong (*Mu Tong*), Herba Seu Flos Schizonepetae Tenuifoliae (*Jing Jie*), Radix Paeoniae Lactiflorae (*Shao Yao*), and Semen Pruni Persicae (*Tao Ren, i.e.,*) bitter medicinals that are also able to exteriorize. (Externally,) apply on the affected part Oleum Musae Basjooris (*Ba Jiao You*). [A {variant} edition instructs to pound and then apply Oleum Musae Basjooris. {later editor}] (This condition) is governed by heat damaging the blood.

---

[1] Migratory wind is a result of dryness and heat in the spleen and lungs with exterior vacuity and consequent invasion of wind evils. It is manifest by migratory swelling with heat, pain, and itching of the skin. It is classified into two kinds, the red and the white, based on the color of the affected skin.

[2] This is a kind of cinnabar toxin characterized by extensive, rouge colored lesions which soon spread over the entire body.

Celestial fire cinnabar toxins[3] in infants arising around the waist is called red flood. Apply smashed Lumbricus (*Qiu Yin Ni*) mixed with oil. To treat cold wind cinnabar toxin[4], extract the juice from Folium Plantaginis (*Che Qian Zi Ye*) by pounding, mix with Terra Flava Usta (*Fu Long Gan*), and apply. This is (also) particularly good if taken orally. To treat cinnabar toxin in infants, apply Pulvis Indigonis (*Lan Dan*, as dressing). Another method is to apply powdered Calcareous Spar (*Han Shui Shi*) and chalk (*Bai Tu*) mixed with rice vinegar. Change (this dressing) whenever it becomes cool.

To treat cinnabar toxins and malign sores when the five colors are constantly changing (*i.e.,* when the color of the sores is constantly changing), apply powdered dry Rhizoma Zingiberis (*Gan Jiang*) mixed with honey. Another formula (consists of) applying Lumbricus (*Di Long*) feces mixed with water. Or apply powdered moss procured from water after it is baked dry. This offers satisfactory effect if it is drunk after boiling water is poured (onto it). (For) various kinds of heat cinnabar toxins, water-ground Catharsius Molossus (*Qiang Lang*) can

---

[3] This is a kind of cinnabar toxin characterized by very red cutaneous lesions as large as the palm of the hand.

[4] This is also known as white cinnabar toxins. It is similar to cinnabar toxins but white in color. It is characterized by itching, pain, and slight swelling at the onset and exacerbation with exposure to wind but relief with warmth.

Cinnabar toxins in newborns is sometimes also called red migratory wind. It is, however, never called this in adults. Cinnabar toxins consist of the sudden breaking out of high fever and aversion to cold with localized heat, pain and moderate swelling in the skin at the initial stage. However, the cutaneous lesions develop and expand very rapidly. Because the affected skin is bright red, it is called cinnabar or cinnabar toxins.

accomplish more than *Zi Xue* (Purple Snow).[5] In addition, for cinnabar toxins, (one) can apply Mirabilitum (*Mang Xiao*) mixed with water.

Migratory red (wind) wandering up and down may cause instant death once it reaches the heart. (To treat this), pound Radix Musae Basjooris (*Ba Jiao Gen*), boil the extracted juice, and apply without any delay.

Chapter Eighteen

Atonic *Bi*[1] of the Body

Ten months after birth, (some) infants' spirit essence may not be well with generalized atonic *bi*. (For this,) burn Vespertilio Superans (*Fu Yi*) to ash, grind finely, and administer one half *qian* with thin gruel 5 ti1mes a day. It is also good if it is fed after being roasted well. (To treat) flaccid head and nape of the neck in infants, mix powdered Radix Acanthopanacis (*Wu Jia Pi*) with wine and apply over the nape bones of the back of the neck.

---

[5] This may refer either to *Zi Xue Dan* (Purple Snow Elixir) or *Zi Xue San* (Purple Snow Powder). It is composed of 1 *jin* of gold (*Jin*), 3 *jin* each of Gypsum (*Shi Gao*), Calcareous Spar (*Han Shui Shi*), and Magnetitum (*Ci Shi*), 5 *liang* each of Cornu Rhinoceroris (*Xi Jiao*) dust, Cornu Antelopis Saigae Tartaricae (*Ling Yang Jiao*) dust, Radix Saussureae Seu Vladimiriae (*Mu Xiang*), and Lignum Aquilariae Agallochae (*Chen Xiang*), 1 *jin* of Radix Scrophulariae Ningpoensis (*Xuan Shen*), 1 *sheng* of Rhizoma Cimicifugae (*Sheng Ma*), 8 *liang* of Radix Glycyrrhizae (*Gan Cao*), 4 *liang* of Flos Caryophylli (*Ding Xiang*), 4 *sheng* each of slaked lime (*Po Xiao*) and Nitre (*Xiao Shi*), one half *liang* of Secretio Moschi Moschiferi (*She Xiang*) powder, and 3 *liang* of Cinnabar (*Zhu Sha*). These ingredients are mixed after a complicated process and used in the form of powder.

[1] This refers to flaccid muscles and joints with or without itching, with or without pain, and with or without numbness.

Chapter Nineteen

Body Heat

(For) body heat in infants, (use) stir-fried Radix Albus Paeoniae Lactiflorae (*Bai Shao Yao*), Rhizoma Cyperi Rotundi (*Xiang Fu*), and Talcum (*Hua Shi*), 1 *liang* for each of the above, Radix Glycyrrhizae (*Gan Cao*), 3 *qian*, and Radix Scutellariae Baicalensis (*Huang Qin*), 1 *qian*. Divide the above into 4 doses, boil each with 3 slices of ginger in 1½ cups of water, and give to the breast-feeding mother.

For thief sweating and tidal fever, (use) Rhizoma Coptidis Chinensis (*Huang Lian*) and Radix Bupleuri (*Chai Hu*) in equal amounts. Make into pills the size of Fructus Ciceris Arietini (*Ji Dou*) with honey; 2 pills (per dose taken) dissolved in wine. (To treat) alternating cold and heat in infants between 1-5 months old, blast-fry Fructus Benincasae Hispidae (*Dong Gua*), extract the juice, and take. This also checks thirst in adults. (To treat) heat in the muscles and skin of infants, (use) Rhizoma Cimicifugae (*Sheng Ma*), Radix Puerariae Lobatae (*Ge Gen*), Radix Paeoniae Lactiflorae (*Shao Yao*), Rhizoma Atractylodis Macrocephalae (*Bai Zhu*), Radix Glycyrrhizae (*Gan Cao*), Radix Scutellariae Baicalensis (*Huang Qin*), Radix Bupleuri (*Chai Hu*), and Sclerotium Poriae Cocoris (*Fu Ling*). Boil and pour the decoction down (the sick child's throat).

For phlegm heat and bone-steaming in infants, (use) Pericarpium Citri Reticulatae (*Chen Pi*), 2 *qian*, Rhizoma Pinelliae Ternatae (*Ban Xia*), 2 *qian*, Radix Glycyrrhizae (Gan Cao), 5 *qian*, Sclerotium Poriae Cocoris (*Fu Ling*), 3 *qian*, Rhizoma Cimicifugae (*Sheng Ma*), 2 *qian*, Radix Puerariae Lobatae (*Ge Gen*), and Radix Albus Paeoniae Lactiflorae (*Bai Shao Yao*), each 1.5 *qian*, Radix Panacis Ginseng (*Ren Shen*), 1 *qian*, and Fructus Schizandrae Chinensis (*Wu Wei Zi*), 30 pieces. All the above as 3 doses. Boil with ginger and dates and take.

Chapter Twenty

Non-closure of the Fontanel

The cause (of this condition) is usually qi vacuity and heat in the mother. Boil and take *Si Wu Tang* (Four Materials Decoction) combined with *Si Jun Zi Tang* (Four Gentlemen Decoction). If there is heat, add wine-processed Rhizoma Coptidis Chinensis (*Huang Lian*) and Radix Glycyrrhizae (*Sheng Gan Cao*). Boil and take. Externally, apply powdered Radix Ampelopsis Japonicae (*Bai Lian*) and bind up (the fontanels) with soft cloth.

Chapter Twenty-one

Miscellaneous Disease in Infants

(To treat) swelling and hardness in the external kidneys[1] and genital sores, apply powdered Lumbricus (*Di Long*) after mixing with saliva. For sloughing scrotum, *i.e.*, swollen scrotum, use Caulis Akebiae Mutong (*Mu Tong*), Radix Glycyrrhizae (*Gan Cao*), Rhizoma Coptidis Chinensis (*Huang Lian*), Radix Angelicae Sinensis (*Dang Gui*), and Radix Scutellariae Baicalensis (*Huang Qin*). Boil and take. Another method (consists of) applying powdered Folium Perillae Frutescentis (*Zi Su Ye*) mixed with water and wrap (the scrotum) with Folium Nelumbinis Nuciferae (*He Ye*). For swelling and pain of the scrotum, mix Succus Radicis Glycyrrhizae (*Sheng Gan Cao Zhi*) with Lumbricus (*Di Long*) feces and dab gently onto (the scrotum). For swelling and pain of the scrotum caused by Lumbricus (*Qiu Yin*) toxins, boil one half *liang* of

---

[1]   *I.e.*, the testicles

Periostracum Cicadae (*Chan Tui*) in 1 bowl of water, wash (with the decoction,) and the pain will be relieved in no time. Administer *Wu Ling San* (Five *Ling* Powder).

For prolapse of the rectum, soak clay from a wall at the northeast corner with boiled water and wash after fuming (with this). For wooden tongue and double tongue, prick to let out blood and a cure will ensue in no time. Dai explains: A wooden tongue is a tongue which is swollen, stiff, and inflexible. He adds that this kind of disorder is ascribed to heat and should be treated by applying Pulvis Fumi Carbonisati (*Bai Cao Shuang*), Talcum (*Hua Shi*), and Mirabilitum (*Mang Xiao*) after powdering and mixing with wine.

Eating soil is (due to) stomach toxic heat. Boil and take soft Gypsum (*Ruan Shi Gao*), Radix Scutellariae Baicalensis (*Huang Qin*), Radix Glycyrrhizae (*Gan Cao*), and Rhizoma Atractylodis Macrocephalae (*Bai Zhu*). Turtle chest (*i.e.,* pigeon chest) requires Rhizoma Atractylodis (*Cang Zhu*), wine-fried Cortex Phellodendri (*Huang Bai*), wine-fried Radix Paeoniae Lactiflorae (*Shao Yao*), Pericarpium Citri Reticulatae (*Chen Pi*), Radix Ledebouriellae Sesloidis (*Fang Feng*), Radix Clematidis Chinensis (*Wei Ling Xian*), Fructus Crataegi (*Shan Zha*), and Radix Angelicae Sinensis (*Dang Gui*). After the bowels are loosened, add Radix Rehmanniae (*Sheng Di Huang*). For turtle back (*i.e.,* hunched back), dab the spinal joints of the back with turtle urine. The method (for obtaining this urine) is to place the turtle on a lotus leaf and, while the turtle is looking around, promptly play a mirror directly on it. Thus it will void urine.

To treat fetal dysentery[2], break a hen's egg, keeping the yolk while the white is removed. Put in 1 *qian* of Minium (*Huang Dan*), seal (the egg) with mud, roast in a fire till (the clay) is dry, and administer (the yolk) with thin gruel. To treat white diarrhea (*i.e.,* diarrhea of white stools), mix evenly 1 *qian* of Realgar (*Xiong Huang*) with 8 *qian* of well fried flour and administer with ginger soup.

---

[2] This refers to dysentery in newborns due to evils in the mother before birth.

To treat white bald sore, stir-fry with wine *Tong Sheng San* (Communicate with the Divinity Powder) with Mirabilitum (*Xiao*) deleted, powder, and take to induce perspiration. For eel-attacking head[3], first boil grass (*Feng Lu Cao*)[4] (growing) on the top of walls and Herba Xanthii Sibirici (*Cang Er Cao*), quench a live charcoal (in this decoction), and wash (the sore). After that, apply a dressing of Resina Pini (*Song Xiang*) as the ruling ingredient. To treat *lai* on the head, apply lard from a horse killed in the last month of the year. Another method to treat *lai* on the head (consists of) heating river water by brewing with reddish white charcoal[5] and washing (the head with it. Yet) another (method consists of) administering wine-processed *Tong Sheng San* in the shape of powder with Radix Et Rhizoma Rhei (*Da Huang*) separately stir-fried with wine. Externally, apply a powdered mixture of Semen Coriandri Sativi (*Hu Sui Zi*), *Xuan Long Wei* [i.e., dust hung on the beams of a roof {later editor}], Terra Flava Usta (*Fu Long Gan*), Rhizoma Coptidis Chinensis (*Huang Lian*), and Alum (*Bai Fan*). Another formula is composed of ash-burnt Cortex Pini (*Song Shu Hou Pi*), 2 *liang*, Resina Liquidambaris Taiwanianae (*Bai Jiao Xiang*), 2 *liang*, heated to a boil, [2 characters missing] Minium (*Huang Dan*), 1 *liang*, ground with water, Alumen (*Ku Fan*), 1 *liang*, finely ground soft Gypsum (*Ruan Shi Gao*), 1 *liang*, Rhizoma Coptidis Chinensis (*Huang Lian*) and Radix Et Rhizoma Rhei (*Da Huang*), 5 *qian* (each), and Calomelas (*Qing Fen*), 4 small cupsful. Powder the above, mix with well heated oil, and apply on the sore. It is necessary to wash off the scabs before applying (this medication).

---

[3]   This refers to sores on the head, usually seen in children. At the beginning, winding, vein-like prominences resembling the work done by earthworms grow. After breaking, they take on the look of mole holes done by mole crickets. Its common name is mole-cricket boils or earthworms' tunnels on the head.

[4]   The translator is not certain of the identity of this herb. He assumes it is not a specific species but just grass growing on the top of walls. Its Chinese, *Feng Lu Cao*, literally translates as Wind Dew Grass.

[5]   This is charcoal which is powdered while it is burning red.

(To treat) head sores in children, burn to ash Folium Phyllostachysis Nigrae (*Ku Zhu Ye*), mix with the white of a hen's egg, and apply. Another formula is composed of Radix Saussureae Seu Vladimiriae (*Mu Xiang*), 3 *qian*, Rhizoma Coptidis Chinensis (*Huang Lian*), 1 *liang*, and Semen Arecae Catechu (*Bing Lang*) and Realgar (*Xiong Huang*), one half *liang* each. Powder the above. Apply dry if (the sore) is wet or after mixing with oil if (the sore) is dry.

(To treat) a new born baby crying frequently with sudden bleeding from the navel, apply a fine powder of Kaolin (*Bai Shi Zhi*, on the navel). Until healed, continue applying after stir-frying the dressing again (each time). It is not permitted to apply a cold dressing after taking off (the old one). To treat a new born whose navel refuses to dry for a long time, bake Radix Angelicae Sinensis (*Dang Gui*), powder, and apply dry. This is also indicated for (a navel) discharging watery pus or with sores due to entrance of urine. Another method (consists of) powdering and applying Alumen (*Bai Ku Fan*) or powdered Terra Flava Usta (*Fu Long Gan*) plus powdered Cortex Phellodendri (*Huang Bai Mo.* Yet) another method (consists of) applying Alum (*Bai Fan*) and calcined Os Albus Draconis (*Bai Long Gu*) in equal amounts, (both) powdered. It is equally good to apply a small amount of carbonized Semen Gossypii Herbacei (*Mian Zi Hui*).

Chapter Twenty-two

Formula for Ceasing Lactation

(This formula consists of) Fructus Gardeniae Jasminoidis (*Sha Zhi Zi*), 3 pieces, ash-burnt with nature preserved, Realgar (*Xiong Huang*), Cinnabar (*Zhu Sha*), and Calomelas (*Qing Fen*), a small amount for each of the above. Powder together, mix evenly with raw sesame oil, and dab on the eyebrows of the child while it is asleep. After waking up, they will no longer eat (*i.e.*, drink) milk.

Chapter Twenty-three

Miscellaneous Formulas

To treat jaundice, obtain 1 cup of sesame oil, heat well in a cauldron, put in 1 *liang* of Ferrous Sulphate (*Lu Fan*), and 1 *jin* of pitted Semen Zizyphi Jujubae (*Hong Zao*). Stir well, collect (the mixture), pound thoroughly, and make into pills the size of Chinese parasol tree seeds; 7 pills per dose taken with any amount of boiled water but not with tea, 7 times a day.

To treat hemorrhoids, obtain 1 Alcedo Athis Bengalensis (*Yu Hu Zi*), wrap with mud, powder after roasting, and then take on an empty stomach with thin gruel. Another method (consists of) obtaining 1 piece of pig's rectum, put inside Semen Coriandri Sativi (*Hu Sui Zi*), bind up (the rectum), and cook well. Keep in the open for a night and then take on an empty stomach.

To treat eel-attacking head, calcine chicken's eggshells with nature preserved, powder, mix with sesame oil, and apply around (the affected part).

To treat *shan*, powder geese eggshells laid the previous year and take on an empty stomach with wine.

To treat visceral toxins[1], burn Folium Indocalami Tessellati (*Hua Ruo*) to ash, boil, and take with wine. Another method (consists of) burning Flos Diospyrosis Kaki (*Shi Hua*) with the pedicle to ash and take with wine.

---

1   This may convey any of three meanings: 1) enduring dysentery due to accumulated toxins in the viscera, 2) internal bleeding due to internal injury manifested by blackened stool or blood in the stool, and 3) purulent piles.

To treat breast node[2], powder Pericarpium Viridis Citri Reticulatae (*Qing Pi*) and Pericarpium Citri Reticulatae (*Chen Pi*) and take brewed with boiled water or wine after a meal.

To treat food reflux retching and vomiting, roast a pig's stomach together with its food (*i.e.*, undigested food) inside in a wood fire, powder, make into pills with dates, and then take.

To treat large and small scrofulas, dip a large handful of Herba Plantaginis (*Che Qian Cao*) in boiling water and take as a salad with ginger and vinegar. Later on, boil and take Radix Lycii Chinensis (*Gou Qi Gen*).

Rice husk stuck in the throat can be gotten out immediately by pouring down (the throat) goose drool.

For any kind of bone penetrating in the flesh and refusing to come back out, boil well Semen Immaturus Pruni Mume (*Bai Mei Rou*), grind thoroughly, and, after it is mixed with powdered elephant's tusk (*Xiang Ya*), apply thickly on the place (where) the bone is stuck. (The bone) will certainly come out.

---

[2] This refers to an oval-shaped, hard lump in the areola of the breast with moderate pain. It is usually due to disharmony of the conception and penetrating vessels and is a product of stagnant qi and phlegm depression.

Appendix

Collection of Missing Case Studies

A person, aged 36, who was addicted to wine in the past, fell in a dead faint after a heavy drink and suffered from paralyzed hands and feet. They were prescribed Radix Astragali Membranacei (*Huang Qi*), 1 *liang*, Rhizoma Gastrodiae Elatae (*Tian Ma*), 5 *qian*, boiled in water mixed with half a cup of sugar cane juice.

A person suffered from wind stroke with both eyes closed, cloudedness, and loss of consciousness. (They were prescribed) *Si Jun Zi Tang* (Four Gentlemen Decoction) plus Succus Bambusae (*Zhu Li*) and Succus Zingiberis (*Jiang Zhi*). Administration was followed by recovery.

A person suffered from wind stroke with numbness and insensitivity of the limbs knowing no pain or itching. This was due to qi vacuity. (They were given) *Si Jun Zi Tang* in large doses plus Rhizoma Gastrodiae Elatae (*Tian Ma*), Tuber Ophiopogonis Japonicae (*Mai Dong*), Radix Astragali Membranacei (*Huang Qi*), and Radix Angelicae Sinensis (*Dang Gui*).

A lustful person living with four concubines suffered from wind stroke with numbness and insensitivity, weakness of the limbs, and hemiplegia. (He was prescribed) *Si Wu Tang* (Four Materials Decoction) plus Radix Panacis Ginseng (*Ren Shen*), Radix Astragali Membranacei (*Huang Qi*), Rhizoma Atractylodis Macrocephalae (*Bai Zhu*), Rhizoma Gastrodiae Elatae (*Tian Ma*), Radix Sophorae Flavescentis (*Ku Shen*), Cortex Phellodendri (*Huang Bai*), Rhizoma Anemarrhenae (*Zhi Mu*), Tuber Ophiopogonis Japonicae (*Mai Dong*), Bombyx Batryticatus (*Jiang Can*), Lumbricus (*Di Long*), and dried Buthus Martensi (*Quan Xie*).

A person suffered from wind stroke with pricking pain all over the body. (They were given) *Si Wu Tang* plus Herba Seu Flos Schizonepetae Tenuifoliae (*Jing Jie*), Radix Ledebouriellae Sesloidis (*Fang Feng*),

Periostracum Cicadae (*Chan Tui*), Semen Viticis (*Man Jing Zi*), and Tuber Ophiopogonis Japonicae (*Mai Men Dong*).

A person, aged 42, suffered from numb and insensitive fingers with a red, numb face. This was a pattern of qi vacuity, (for which) *Bu Zhong Yi Qi Tang* (Supplement the Center & Boost the Qi Decoction) plus one half *qian* each of Radix Saussureae Seu Vladimiriae (*Mu Xiang*) and Radix Praeparatus Aconiti Carmichaeli (*Fu Zi*, were prescribed. Partial) recovery followed administration. Then Tuber Ophiopogonis Japonicae (*Mai Dong*), Radix Et Rhizoma Notopterygii (*Qiang Huo*), Radix Ledebouriellae Sesloidis (*Fang Feng*), and Radix Linderae Strychnifoliae (*Wu Yao*) were added. Complete recovery followed administration (of this).

A person, aged 29, suffered from wind stroke with numb and insensitive limbs and difficulty walking on their feet. (They were prescribed) *Er Chen Tang* (Two Aged Decoction) plus Radix Panacis Ginseng (*Ren Shen*), Rhizoma Atractylodis Macrocephalae (*Bai Zhu*), Radix Angelicae Sinensis (*Dang Gui*), Cortex Phellodendri (*Huang Bai*), Cortex Eucommiae Ulmoidis (*Du Zhong*), Radix Achyranthis Bidentatae (*Niu Xi*), and Tuber Ophiopogonis Japonicae (*Mai Dong*).

A person, aged 56 and addicted to wine, suffered from cold damage with fever and dry mouth as if being burned by fire. (They were given) *Bu Zhong Yi Qi Tang* plus Fructus Seu Semen Hoveniae Dulcis (*Ji Ju Zi*), Radix Angelicae Sinensis (*Dang Gui*), Rhizoma Ligustici Wallichii (*Chuan Xiong*), Radix Paeoniae Lactiflorae (*Shao Yao*), Succus Radicis Rehmanniae (*Di Huang Zhi*), and Succus Sacchari Sinensis (*Gan Zhe Zhi*).

A person, aged 34, suffered from cold damage with fever and generalized nettling pain. (They were prescribed) *Si Wu Tang* plus Radix Panacis Ginseng (*Ren Shen*), Radix Astragali Membranacei (*Huang Qi*), Rhizoma Atractylodis Macrocephalae (*Bai Zhu*), Radix Rehmanniae (*Sheng Di*), and Flos Carthami Tinctorii (*Hong Hua*).

A person suffered from cold damage with lumbago and the left foot cold like ice. (They were prescribed) *Xiao Chai Hu* (Minor Bupleurum

[Decoction]) plus Cortex Phellodendri (*Huang Bai*), Cortex Eucommiae Ulmoidis (*Du Zhong*), and Radix Achyranthis Bidentatae (*Niu Xi*).

A person suffered from cold damage with fire like fever, dry mouth, and massive drinking. (They were given) *Xiao Chai Hu (Tang)* minus Rhizoma Pinelliae Ternatae (*Ban Xia*) but plus Radix Puerariae Lobatae (*Ge Gen*) and Radix Trichosanthis Kirlowii (*Tian Hua Fen*).

A person, aged 29, suffered from cold damage with headache, aching flanks, aching in the limbs, and aching of the diaphragm in the chest. (They also were given) *Xiao Chai Hu Tang* plus Radix Et Rhizoma Notopterygii (*Qiang Huo*), Radix Platycodi Grandiflori (*Jie Geng*), Rhizoma Cyperi Rotundi (*Xiang Fu*), and Fructus Citri Seu Ponciri (*Zhi Qiao*).

A person, aged 36, suffered from cold damage with cough arising in the night and relieved in the day. They were treated as yin vacuity with *Bu Zhong Yi Qi (Tang)* plus Tuber Asparagi Cochinensis (*Tian Dong*), Tuber Ophiopogonis Japonicae (*Mai Dong*), Bulbus Fritillariae (*Bei Mu*), and Fructus Schizandrae Chinensis (*Wu Wei*).

A person suffered from cold damage with cold (up) to the knees. Fructus Schizandrae Chinensis (*Wu Wei Zi*) was added to *Bu Zhong Yi Qi Tang* with Radix Panacis Ginseng (*Ren Shen*) in double amount. Recovery followed administration.

A person, aged 30, suffered from damp qi with aching and pain in the limbs and the feet hardly able to move. (They were prescribed) *Bu Zhong Yi Qi (Tang)* plus Radix Achyranthis Bidentatae (*Niu Xi*), Cortex Eucommiae Ulmoidis (*Du Zhong*), Cortex Phellodendri (*Huang Bai*), Rhizoma Anemarrhenae (*Zhi Mu*), and Fructus Schizandrae Chinensis (*Wu Wei Zi*).

A person, aged 53, suffered from fire like fever. This person had been lustful for wine and sex. Cortex Phellodendri (*Huang Bai*) and Rhizoma Anemarrhenae (*Zhi Mu*) were added to *Bu Zhong Yi Qi Tang* with large amounts of Radix Panacis Ginseng (*Ren Shen*) and Rhizoma Atractylodis Macrocephalae (*Bai Zhu*).

A person suffered from vacuity detriment with coughing and vomiting of blood. (They were given) *Si Wu Tang* plus Radix Panacis Ginseng (*Ren Shen*), Rhizoma Atractylodis Macrocephalae (*Bai Zhu*), Radix Scutellariae Baicalensis (*Huang Qin*), Flos Tussilagi Farfarae (*Kuan Hua*), Fructus Schizandrae Chinensis (*Wu Wei*), Cortex Phellodendri (*Huang Bai*), Rhizoma Anemarrhenae (*Zhi Mu*), Bulbus Fritillariae (*Bei Mu*), Tuber Asparagi Cochinensis (*Tian Dong*), Tuber Ophiopogonis Japonicae (*Mai Dong*), Cortex Radicis Mori Albi (*Sang Pi*), and Semen Pruni Armeniacae (*Xing Ren*).

A person suffered from vacuity detriment with fever, thief sweating, and dream emission. (They were prescribed) *Si Wu Tang* plus Radix Panacis Ginseng (*Ren Shen*), Rhizoma Atractylodis Macrocephalae (*Bai Zhu*), Radix Astragali Membranacei (*Huang Qi*), Cortex Radicis Lycii (*Di Gu Pi*), and Radix Ledebouriellae Sesloidis (*Fang Feng*).

A person suffered from vacuity detriment with tidal fever and weakness of the limbs. (In their case,) *Xiao Chai Hu Tang* was combined with *Si Wu Tang* plus Radix Astragali Membranacei (*Huang Qi*), Rhizoma Atractylodis Macrocephalae (*Bai Zhu*), Tuber Ophiopogonis Japonicae (*Mai Dong*), and Fructus Schizandrae Chinensis (*Wu Wei*).

A person, aged 46 and a heavy drinker, suffered from the pattern of vacuity detriment with continual fever for nights running. (They were prescribed) *Si Wu Tang* plus Succus Sacchari Sinensis (*Gan Zhe Zhi*), Fructus Seu Semen Hoveniae Dulcis (*Ji Ju Zi*), dry Radix Puerariae Lobatae (*Gan Ge*), Fructus Cardamomi (*Bai Dou Kou*), and Pericarpium Viridis Citri Reticulatae (*Qing Pi*).

A person with vacuity detriment spitted out foul smelling phlegm. (They were prescribed) *Si Jun Zi (Tang)* plus Radix Angelicae (*Bai Zhi*), Tuber Asparagi Cochinensis (*Tian Dong*), Tuber Ophiopogonis Japonicae (*Mai Dong*), Fructus Schizandrae Chinensis (*Wu Wei*), Rhizoma Anemarrhenae (*Zhi Mu*), and Bulbus Fritillariae (*Bei Mu*).

A person suffered from vacuity detriment with the four limbs cold like ice. (They were given) *Bu Zhong Yi Qi Tang* plus Cortex Cinnamomi (*Gui Xin*) and dry Rhizoma Zingiberis (*Gan Jiang*), 1 *qian* each.

A person, aged 51, suffered from vacuity detriment with coughing and spitting out threads of blood. (They were prescribed) *Si Wu Tang* with Radix Rehmanniae (*Sheng Di*) instead (of prepared Radix Rehmanniae [*Shu Di*]) plus Cortex Phellodendri (*Huang Bai*), Rhizoma Anemarrhenae (*Zhi Mu*), Radix Scutellariae Baicalensis (*Huang Qin*), Bulbus Fritillariae (*Bei Mu*), Cortex Radicis Mori Albi (*Sang Pi*), Semen Pruni Armeniacae (*Xing Ren*), Flos Tussilagi Farfarae (*Kuan Hua*), Tuber Asparagi Cochinensis (*Tian Dong*), Tuber Ophiopogonis Japonicae (*Mai Dong*), Fructus Schizandrae Chinensis (*Wu Wei*), Flos Asteris Tatarici (*Zi Wan*), 1 *he* of Succus Cephalanoploris Segeti (*Xiao Ji Zhi*), and 7 *fen* of white wax (*Bai La*).

An old person suffered from burning thirst with agitation and fever arising in the afternoon. This was (a case of) yin vacuity. Old people are prohibited from taking Radix Trichosanthis Kirlowii (*Tian Hua Fen*) for fear of damaging their stomach. (Therefore, I prescribed) *Si Wu (Tang)* minus Rhizoma Ligustici Wallichii (*Chuan Xiong*) and plus Rhizoma Anemarrhenae (*Zhi Mu*), Cortex Phellodendri (*Huang Bai*), Fructus Schizandrae Chinensis (*Wu Wei*), Radix Panacis Ginseng (*Ren Shen*), Rhizoma Atractylodis Macrocephalae (*Bai Zhu*), Tuber Ophiopogonis Japonicae (*Mai Dong*), Pericarpium Citri Reticulatae (*Chen Pi*), and Radix Glycyrrhizae (*Gan Cao*).

A person suffered from vacuity detriment with lumps all over their body, (*i.e.,*) phlegm all over the body. (They were prescribed) *Er Chen Tang* plus ground Semen Sinapis Albae (*Bai Jie Zi*) taken after being boiled together with ginger-fried Rhizoma Coptidis Chinensis (*Huang Lian*).

A person suffered from vacuity detriment with massive vomiting of blood. (They were given) *Si Wu Tang* with Radix Rehmanniae (*Sheng Di*) instead (of prepared Radix Rehmanniae [*Shu Di*]) plus Radix Et Rhizoma Rhei (*Da Huang*), Radix Panacis Ginseng (*Ren Shen*), Flos Camelliae Japonicae (*Shan Cha Hua*), and Pulvis Indigonis (*Qing Dai*).

A person suffered from vacuity detriment with intolerable heat in the palms of the hands and soles of the feet. (They were given) *Xiao Chai*

Hu Tang plus Radix Peucedani (*Qian Hu*), Rhizoma Cyperi Rotundi (*Xiang Fu*), and Rhizoma Coptidis Chinensis (*Huang Lian*).

A person, aged 60, suffered from the pattern of vacuity detriment with their whole body near to numbness and insensitivity and fire-like heat in the soles of the feet. (They were) prescribed Radix Panacis Ginseng (*Ren Shen*), Radix Astragali Membranacei (*Huang Qi*), Radix Angelicae Sinensis (*Dang Gui*), Rhizoma Atractylodis Macrocephalae (*Bai Zhu*), Radix Bupleuri (*Chai Hu*), Radix Albus Paeoniae Lactiflorae (*Bai Shao Yao*), Radix Ledebouriellae Sesloidis (*Fang Feng*), Herba Seu Flos Schizonepetae Tenuifoliae (*Jing Jie*), Radix Et Rhizoma Notopterygii (*Qiang Huo*), Rhizoma Cimicifugae (*Sheng Ma*), Radix Achyranthis Bidentatae (*Niu Xi*), and Semen Arctii Lappae (*Niu Bang Zi*).

A female who suffered from uncheckable diarrhea after child-birth was prescribed Radix Panacis Ginseng (*Ren Shen*), 5 *qian*, Rhizoma Atractylodis Macrocephalae (*Bai Zhu*), 7 *qian*, and Radix Praeparatus Aconiti Carmichaeli (*Fu Zi*), 1.5 *qian*. Two doses realized a cure.

A person suffered from diarrhea with rigidity of the limbs, cloudedness and inability to recognize people, and inability to respond to the calls (of other people. They were prescribed) *Si Jun Zi Tang* plus Radix Saussureae Seu Vladimiriae (*Mu Xiang*), Radix Praeparatus Aconiti Carmichaeli (*Fu Zi*), dry Rhizoma Zingiberis (*Gan Jiang*), and Radix Linderae Strychnifoliae (*Wu Yao*). Recovery followed administration.

A person suffered from diarrhea with the hands and feet cold like ice and the body (hot) like fire. (They were prescribed) *Si Jun Zi (Tang)* plus Radix Praeparatus Aconiti Carmichaeli (*Fu Zi*), dry Rhizoma Zingiberis (*Gan Jiang*), Radix Paeoniae Lactiflorae (*Shao Yao*), and Rhizoma Alismatis (*Ze Xie*). Six doses realized a cure.

General Index

L

M

damage xxiii, 35, 398
drool tidal congestion and block 425
fear of exposure to 221
fright xxvii, 399-404, 418
heat tearing complicated by pain 300
hemilateral and ambilateral head 154
intestinal xxv, 240, 241
Lai xxiii, 13
migratory red xxvii, 432
open wound xxvi, 324, 325
pestilential 15
painful xxiv, 162, 191-193, 195, 199, 250, 387
stroke xxiii, xxvii, 3, 5, 7, 8, 10-12, 367, 401, 429-431, 443, 444
stroke in infants 429, 430
summerheat xxiii, 24, 48
water 93
white tiger articular 191
winter, disease caused by a warm 45
Wiseman, Nigel xvii
withdrawal 39, 80, 266
World Health Organization xvii
worm toxins 339
wounds, flogging xxvi, 329
wounds, open incised xxvi, 333
wu yun liu qi xue 41

X

xia wei 23
Xiao Er Bing Yuan Fang Lun 410
Xiao Shu-lin xv, xxii, xxiii, 1
Xu Qian vi
Xu Shu-wei 11
Xu Wen-yi vi, ix

Y

Yi Jing 382
Yi Lei Yuan Rong 312
Yi Xue Fa Ming xv
Yi Yao xv, xvi, xviii, xix, xxi, 3, 13, 14, 18, 116, 147, 150, 153, 154, 158, 170, 180, 199, 210, 233, 293, 319, 320
Yin Tang 404

Yin Zheng Lue Li 42
yong and *ju* 242, 319-321
Yong Quan 30, 284
yong swelling 322
You You Xin Shu 410
Yuan Bing Shi 266, 298

Z

Zhang Chang-sha 19
Zhang Cong-zheng viii, ix, x, xv, 12, 37
Zhang Ji 19
Zhang the Heavenly Scholar 297
Zhang Tian Shi 297
Zhang Zhong-jing 3, 11, 18, 19, 312
Zhang Zi-he viii, xii, 12, 37, 193, 209
Zhen v, viii, x, xiv, xvi, 17, 32, 51, 133, 134, 149, 195, 236, 245, 248, 251, 267, 306, 371, 372, 382, 399
Zheng Hui-qing 411
Zheng Shu-lu 246
Zhong Yao Da Ci Dian xvii
Zhong Yi Nei Ke Lin Chuang Shou Ce xiii
Zhou Ben-dao 222
Zhu Hong 121
Zhu Lin Jing She xxi
Zhu Xi vi, xxi
Zhu Yan-xiu ix
Zhu Zhen-heng v, x, xiv, xvi, 17
Zhu Zi vi, xviii, xxi

Formula Index

J

K, L

M

N, P

Q

R

S

MIGRAINES & TRADITIONAL CHINESE MEDICINE: A Layperson's Guide by Bob Flaws ISBN 0-936185-15-5 $11.95

STICKING TO THE POINT: A Rational Methodology for the Step by Step Formulation & Administration of an Acupuncture Treatment by Bob Flaws ISBN 0-936185-17-1 $14.95

ENDOMETRIOSIS & INFERTILITY AND TRADITIONAL CHINESE MEDICINE: A Laywoman's Guide by Bob Flaws ISBN 0-936185-14-7 $9.95

THE BREAST CONNECTION: A Laywoman's Guide to the Treatment of Breast Disease by Chinese Medicine by Honora Lee Wolfe ISBN 0-936185-13-9 $8.95

NINE OUNCES: A Nine Part Program For The Prevention of AIDS in HIV Positive Persons by Bob Flaws ISBN 0-936185-12-0 $9.95

THE TREATMENT OF CANCER BY INTEGRATED CHINESE-WESTERN MEDICINE by Zhang Dai-zhao, trans. by Zhang Ting-liang & Bob Flaws, ISBN 0-936185-11-2 $16.95

A HANDBOOK OF TRADITIONAL CHINESE DERMATOLOGY by Liang Jian-hui, trans. by Zhang Ting-liang & Bob Flaws, ISBN 0-936185-07-4 $14.95

A HANDBOOK OF TRADITIONAL CHINESE GYNECOLOGY by Zhejiang College of TCM, trans. by Zhang Ting-liang, ISBN 0-936185-06-6 (2nd edit.) $21.95

PRINCE WEN HUI'S COOK: Chinese Dietary Therapy by Bob Flaws & Honora Lee Wolfe, ISBN 0-912111-05-4, $12.95 (Published by Paradigm Press, Brookline, MA)

THE DAO OF INCREASING LONGEVITY AND CONSERVING ONE'S LIFE by Anna Lin & Bob Flaws, ISBN 0-936185-24-4 $16.95

FIRE IN THE VALLEY: The TCM Diagnosis and Treatment of Vaginal Diseases by Bob Flaws ISBN 0-936185-25-2 $16.95

HIGHLIGHTS OF ANCIENT ACUPUNCTURE PRESCRIPTIONS trans. by Honora Lee Wolfe & Rose Crescenz ISBN 0-936185-23-6 $14.95

ARISAL OF THE CLEAR:
A Simple Guide to Healthy
Eating According to
Traditional Chinese
Medicine by Bob Flaws, ISBN
#-936185-27-9 $8.95

**CERVICAL DYSPLASIA &
PROSTATE CANCER:
HPV, A HIDDEN LINK?** by
Bob Flaws, ISBN 0-936185-19-8
$23.95

**PEDIATRIC BRONCHITIS:
ITS CAUSE, DIAGNOSIS
& TREATMENT
ACCORDING TO
TRADITIONAL CHINESE
MEDICINE** trans. by Gao Yu-
li and Bob Flaws, ISBN 0-
936185-26-0 $15.95

**AIDS & ITS TREATMENT
ACCORDING TO
TRADITIONAL CHINESE
MEDICINE** by Huang Bing-
shan, trans. by Fu-Di & Bob
Flaws, ISBN 0-936185-28-7
$24.95

**ACUTE ABDOMINAL
SYNDROMES: Their**
Diagnosis & Treatment by
Combined Chinese-Western
Medicine by Alon Marcus,
ISBN 0-936185-31-7 $16.95

MY SISTER, THE MOON:
The Diagnosis & Treatment
of Menstrual Diseases by
Traditional Chinese
Medicine by Bob Flaws, ISBN
0-936185-34-1, $24.95

**FU QING-ZHU'S
GYNECOLOGY** trans. by
Yang Shou-zhong and Liu Da-
wei, ISBN 0-936185-35-X, $21.95

**FLESHING OUT THE
BONES: The Importance of
Case Histories in Chinese
Medicine** trans. by Charles
Chace. ISBN 0-936185-30-9,
$18.95

**CLASSICAL
MOXIBUSTION SKILLS IN
CONTEMPORARY
CLINICAL PRACTICE** by
Sung Baek, ISBN 0-936185-16-3
$10.95

**THE MEDICAL I CHING:
Oracle of the Healer Within**
by Miki Shima, OMD, ISBN 0-
936185-38-4, $19.95

**MASTER TONG'S
ACUPUNCTURE: An
Ancient Lineage for Modern
Practice**, trans. and
commentary by Miriam Lee,
OMD, ISBN 0-936185-37-6,
$19.95

**A HANDBOOK OF TCM
UROLOGY & MALE
SEXUAL DYSFUNCTION**
by Anna Lin, OMD, ISBN 0-
936185-36-8, $16.95

**PMS: Its Cause, Diagnosis
& Treatment According to
Traditional Chinese
Medicine** by Bob Flaws ISBN
0-936185-22-8 $14.95

**BEFORE COMPLETION:
Essays on the Practice of
TCM** by Bob Flaws, ISBN 0-
936185-32-5, $16.95